Study Guide For

Abrams' Clinical Drug Therapy

RATIONALES FOR NURSING PRACTICE

NINTH EDITION

Study Guide For

Abrams' Clinical Drug Therapy

RATIONALES FOR NURSING PRACTICE

NINTH EDITION

Wolters Kluwer | Lippincott Williams & Wilkins
Health
Philadelphia · Baltimore · New York · London
Buenos Aires · Hong Kong · Sydney · Tokyo

Acquisitions Editor: Hilarie Surrena
Managing Editor: Annette Ferran
Senior Production Editor: Marian A. Bellus
Director of Nursing Production: Helen Ewan
Senior Managing Editor / Production: Erika Kors
Senior Designer: Joan Wendt
Manufacturing Coordinator: Karin Duffield
Compositor: Aptara, Inc.

Ninth Edition

9 8 7 6 5 4 3

ISBN: 978-0-7817-8248-7

Care has been taken to confirm the accuracy of the information presented and to
describe generally accepted practices. However, the authors, editors, and publisher are
not responsible for errors or omissions or for any consequences from application of
the information in this book and make no warranty, expressed or implied, with
respect to the currency, completeness, or accuracy of the contents of the publication.
Application of this information in a particular situation remains the professional
responsibility of the practitioner; the clinical treatments described and recommended
may not be considered absolute and universal recommendations.

The authors, editors, and publisher have exerted every effort to ensure that drug
selection and dosage set forth in this text are in accordance with the current
recommendations and practice at the time of publication. However, in view of
ongoing research, changes in government regulations, and the constant flow of
information relating to drug therapy and drug reactions, the reader is urged to check
the package insert for each drug for any change in indications and dosage and for
added warnings and precautions. This is particularly important when the
recommended agent is a new or infrequently employed drug.

Some drugs and medical devices presented in this publication have Food and Drug
Administration (FDA) clearance for limited use in restricted research settings. It is the
responsibility of the health care provider to ascertain the FDA status of each drug or
device planned for use in his or her clinical practice.

Preface

This Study Guide was written by Denise Pelletier, RN, for the ninth edition of *Clinical Drug Therapy: Rationales for Nursing Practice* by Anne Abrams, Carol Lammon, and Sandy Pennington. The Study Guide is designed to help you practice and retain the knowledge you've gained from the textbook, and it is structured to integrate that knowledge and give you a basis for applying it in your nursing practice. The following types of exercises are provided in each chapter of the Study Guide.

Learning Objectives

The first section of each Study Guide chapter lists the Learning Objectives of the textbook chapter, to remind you of the goals of the chapter as you work your way through the exercises.

Assessing Your Understanding

The second section of each Study Guide chapter concentrates on the basic information of the textbook chapter and helps you to remember key concepts, vocabulary, and principles.

• Fill in the Blanks

Fill in the blank exercises help you to recall important chapter information. They also test key chapter information, encouraging you to recall key points.

• Matching

Matching questions test your knowledge of the definition of key terms.

• Sequencing

Sequencing exercises ask you to remember particular sequences or orders, for instance testing processes and prioritizing nursing actions.

• Short Answers

Short answer questions will cover facts, concepts, procedures, and principles of the chapter. These questions ask you to recall information as well as demonstrate your comprehension of the information.

Applying Your Knowledge

The third section of each Study Guide chapter consists of case study based exercises that ask you to begin to apply the knowledge you've gained from the textbook chapter and reinforced in the first section of the Study Guide chapter. A case study scenario based on the chapter's content is presented, and then you are asked to answer some questions, in writing, related to the case study. In addition to questions related to your knowledge of the drugs themselves, these case scenarios ask you to consider your nursing role, including communication with physicians and patient education.

Practicing for NCLEX

The fourth and final section of the Study Guide chapters helps you practice NCLEX-style questions while further reinforcing the knowledge you have been gaining and testing for yourself through the textbook chapter and the first two sections of the study guide chapter. In keeping with the NCLEX, the questions presented are multiple-choice and scenario-based, asking you to reflect, consider, and apply what you know and to choose the best answer out of those offered. Also included are some questions in the NCLEX alternate format style, such as fill-in-the-blank questions.

Answer Keys

The answers for all of the exercises and questions in the Study Guide are provided at the back of the book, so you can assess your own learning as you complete each chapter.

We hope you will find this Study Guide to be helpful and enjoyable, and we wish you every success in your studies toward becoming a nurse.

The Publishers

Contents

CHAPTER 1

Introduction to Pharmacology

■ Section I: Learning Objectives

1. Differentiate between pharmacology and drug therapy.
2. Distinguish between generic and trade names of drugs.
3. Define a prototypical drug.
4. Select authoritative sources of drug information.
5. Discuss major drug laws and standards.
6. Describe the main categories of controlled substances in relation to therapeutic use and potential for abuse.
7. Identify nursing responsibilities in handling controlled substances correctly.
8. Discuss the role of the Food and Drug Administration (FDA).
9. Analyze the potential impact of drug costs on drug therapy regimens.
10. Develop personal techniques for learning about drugs.

■ Section II: Assessing Your Understanding

ACTIVITY A

Fill in the Blank

1. _____ is the study of drugs (chemicals) that alter functions of living organisms.
2. _____, also called pharmacotherapy, is the use of drugs to prevent, diagnose, or treat signs, symptoms, and disease processes.
3. Drugs given for therapeutic purposes are called _____.
4. Individual drugs that represent groups of drugs are called _____.
5. _____ involves the costs of drug therapy, which include the costs of purchasing, dispensing, storage, and administration; laboratory and other tests used to monitor client responses; and losses due to expiration.

ACTIVITY B

Matching

Match the term in Column A with the definition in Column B.

COLUMN A

1. _____ Generic name
2. _____ Trade or brand name
3. _____ Food, Drug and Cosmetic Act of 1938
4. _____ Durham-Humphrey Amendment
5. _____ Controlled Substances Act

COLUMN B

A. Designates drugs that must be prescribed by a licensed physician or nurse practitioner and dispensed by a pharmacist
B. Regulates the manufacture, distribution, advertising, and labeling of drugs
C. Regulates the manufacture and distribution of narcotics, stimulants, depressants, hallucinogens, and anabolic steroids
D. Often indicates the drug group
E. Name designated and patented by the manufacturer

ACTIVITY C

Sequencing

Since 1962, newly developed drugs have been extensively tested before being marketed for general use. Clinical trials are conducted in four phases, which are given below in random order. Write the correct sequence in which they are performed in the boxes provided.

A. A few doses are given to a certain number of healthy volunteers to determine safe dosages, routes of administration, absorption, metabolism, excretion, and toxicity.

B. Studies help to determine whether the potential benefits of the drug outweigh the risks.

C. A few doses are given to a certain number of subjects who have the disease or symptom for which the drug is being studied, and responses are compared with those of healthy subjects.

D. The FDA evaluates the data from the first three phases for drug safety and effectiveness, allows the drug to be marketed for general use, and requires manufacturers to continue monitoring the drug's effects.

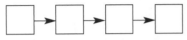

ACTIVITY D

Short Answers

Briefly answer the following questions.

1. Medications may be given for local effects. Give an example of a drug that exhibits its effects locally, and identify the action of the medication.
2. Medications may be given for systemic effects. Explain the mechanism of action for a systemic medication.
3. Identify the advantages of synthetic drugs.
4. Describe why biotechnology is an important source of drugs.
5. Describe the impact of cloning on biotechnology.

■ Section III: Applying Your Knowledge

ACTIVITY E

Case Studies

Consider the scenario and answer the questions.

Sally Smith, a close friend, states that she has a headache that "just won't go away." She asks if she can borrow a prescription medication that you received from your physician last year for persistent migraine headaches.

1. You want to help Sally to relieve the pain that she is experiencing. Discuss the two methods that a consumer may use to procure therapeutic medications.
2. Sally visits her doctor and is instructed to take OTC medications for her pain. Define "OTC" and the regulation of these medications.

3. Sally tells you that she borrowed a friend's prescription drug to control her headache. She states that she felt so good taking the drug that she wants to repeat the experience. Discuss the legal ramifications of self-administration of prescription drugs prescribed to another.

■ Section IV: Practicing for NCLEX

Answer the following questions.

1. The FDA approves many new drugs annually. New drugs are categorized according to their review priority and therapeutic potential. A new drug that is to be reviewed on a priority or accelerated basis would be identified as which of the following?
   a. 1P   c. 1A
   b. 1D   d. 1S

2. The FDA approves drugs for OTC status, including the transfer of drugs from prescription to OTC status. Which of the following are characteristic of prescription drugs that are delegated to OTC status? (Select all that apply.)
   a. They may be administered at a higher dosage than the prescription.
   b. They may be administered at a lower dosage than the prescription.
   c. They may require additional clinical trials to determine the safety and effectiveness of the OTC use.
   d. They may be used for different indications than the original prescription medication.

3. Having drugs available OTC has potential advantages and disadvantages for consumers. Which of the following is one of the advantages?
   a. Reliable self-diagnosis
   b. Increased diagnosis of the identified illness
   c. Faster and more convenient access to effective treatment
   d. Reduction of possible drug interactions

4. When prevention or cure is not a reasonable goal, relief of symptoms can do which of the following? (Select all that apply.)
   a. Improve a client's quality of life
   b. Eliminate pain
   c. Improve ability to function in activities of daily living
   d. Decrease dependence on drugs

5. Drugs are classified according to which of the following features?
   a. Name
   b. Therapeutic uses
   c. Side effects
   d. Actions

6. The names of therapeutic classifications usually reflect which of the following?
   a. Actions of the medication
   b. Conditions for which the medication is used
   c. Possible averse reactions to the medications
   d. Possible generic names for the medication

7. How may drugs be prescribed and dispensed?
   a. By generic name only
   b. By trade name only
   c. By prescription
   d. By generic or trade name

8. Once a drug is patented, which of the following is true?
   a. The drug may be manufactured by other companies.
   b. The drug may be manufactured by other companies under a generic name.
   c. The drug may not be manufactured by other companies until the patent expires.
   d. The drug may be marketed by other companies.

9. The main goal of current drug laws and standards is to ensure which of the following?
   a. That drugs are available to all, regardless of cost.
   b. That drugs marketed for therapeutic purposes are safe and effective.
   c. That drugs are cost effective.
   d. That drugs are patented.

10. Fill in the blank: The _____ regulates vaccines and other biologic products.

11. What does the Comprehensive Drug Abuse Prevention and Control Act regulate?
    a. Classifications of narcotics
    b. Acceptable diagnoses for prescription of narcotics
    c. Manufacture and distribution of narcotics
    d. Abuse of narcotics

12. Which of the following are nurses responsible for? (Select all that apply.)
    a. Storing controlled substances in locked containers
    b. Reporting discrepancies in the narcotic inventory to the physician
    c. Recording prescribed controlled substances on medication administration records
    d. Maintaining an accurate inventory of narcotics

13. Individuals and companies that are legally empowered to handle controlled substances must do which of the following? (Select all that apply.)
    a. Keep accurate records of all transactions.
    b. Be registered with the DEA.
    c. Be registered with the FDA.
    d. Provide for secure storage of controlled substances.

14. The National Institutes of Health Revitalization Act stipulates which of the following?
    a. Men must be included in drug research studies.
    b. Women and minorities must be included in drug research studies.
    c. Animal testing must be completed prior to human drug testing.
    d. Animal testing is not needed prior to human drug testing.

15. Since 1962, newly developed drugs have been extensively tested before being marketed for general use. To test drugs, drug companies *initially* do which of the following?
    a. Test the drugs with animals.
    b. Test the drugs with humans.
    c. Test the drugs in a controlled laboratory experiment.
    d. Test the drugs on volunteers.

16. FDA approval of a drug for OTC availability includes which of the following?

    a. Analysis of the cost of the drug to the consumer

    b. Evaluation of evidence that the consumer can use the drug safely, using information on the product label

    c. Studies involving the safe use of the medication by the consumer

    d. Analysis of the diagnoses for which the medication may be used by the consumer

17. Which of the following should the beginning student of pharmacology use as the primary source of drug data?

    a. The Internet   c. A drug book

    b. The pharmacology text   d. A palm pilot

18. Fill in the blank: A/An _____ is an inactive substance similar in appearance to the actual drug.

19. Which of the following is designated by the Durham-Humphrey Amendment?

    a. Drugs that may be administered by a nurse

    b. Drugs that may be designated as OTC

    c. Drugs that must be prescribed by a licensed physician

    d. Drugs that must be given in conjunction with other drugs to be effective

20. Fill in the blank: The _____ is charged with enforcing the law regarding administration of medications.

CHAPTER 2

Basic Concepts and Processes

■ Section I: Learning Objectives

1. Discuss cellular physiology in relation to drug therapy.
2. Describe the main pathways and mechanisms by which drugs cross biologic membranes and move through the body.
3. Explain each process of pharmacokinetics.
4. Discuss the clinical usefulness of measuring serum drug levels.
5. Describe major characteristics of the receptor theory of drug action.
6. Differentiate between agonist drugs and antagonist drugs.
7. List drug-related and patient-related variables that affect drug actions.
8. Discuss mechanisms and potential effects of drug–drug interactions.
9. Identify signs and symptoms that may occur with adverse drug effects on major body systems.
10. Discuss general management of drug overdose and toxicity.
11. Discuss selected drug antidotes.

■ Section II: Assessing Your Understanding

ACTIVITY A

Fill in the Blank

1. _____ are chemicals that alter basic processes in body cells.
2. Drugs must reach and interact with or cross the _____ to stimulate or inhibit cellular function.
3. _____ involves drug movement through the body (i.e., "what the body does to the drug") to reach sites of action, metabolism, and excretion.
4. _____ is the process that occurs from the time a drug enters the body to the time it enters the bloodstream to be circulated.
5. Liquid medications are absorbed _____ than tablets or capsules because they need not be dissolved.

6. _____ occur when two drugs with similar pharmacologic actions are taken.
7. _____ occurs when two drugs with different sites or mechanisms of action produce greater effects when taken together.
8. _____ by one drug with the metabolism of a second drug may result in intensified effects of the second drug.
9. _____ of one drug from plasma protein-binding sites by a second drug (i.e., a drug with a strong attraction to protein-binding sites may displace a less tightly bound drug) increases the effects of the displaced drug.
10. A/An _____ drug can be given to antagonize the toxic effects of another drug.

ACTIVITY B

Matching

Match the term in Column A with the definition in Column B.

COLUMN A

1. _____ Distribution
2. _____ Protein binding
3. _____ Metabolism
4. _____ Excretion
5. _____ A serum drug level

COLUMN B

A. The method by which drugs are inactivated or biotransformed by the body
B. An important factor in drug distribution
C. A laboratory measurement of the amount of a drug in the blood at a particular time
D. Elimination of a drug from the body
E. Involves the transport of drug molecules within the body after a drug is injected or absorbed into the bloodstream

ACTIVITY C

Sequencing

Given below, in random order, are statements that refer to the movements of a drug in the body. Identify the path that the molecules of most oral drugs must take in order to be effectively absorbed and excreted by writing the correct sequence in the boxes provided.

A. Perform their action, then return to the bloodstream
B. Circulate to their target cells
C. Cross the membranes of cells in the gastrointestinal tract, liver, and capillaries to reach the bloodstream
D. Reenter the bloodstream, circulate to the kidneys, and be excreted in urine
E. Leave the bloodstream and attach to receptors on cells
F. Circulate to the liver, and reach drug-metabolizing enzymes in liver cells

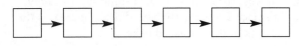

ACTIVITY D

Short Answers

Briefly answer the following questions.

1. Explain how a drug is absorbed systemically.
2. Although cells differ from one tissue to another, their common characteristics include the ability to perform what functions?
3. Identify several factors that may affect the rate and extent of drug absorption.
4. Rapid movement through the stomach and small intestine may increase drug absorption by what mechanisms or factors?
5. Why is drug distribution into the central nervous system (CNS) limited because of the blood–brain barrier?

■ Section III: Applying Your Knowledge

ACTIVITY E

Case Studies

Consider the scenario and answer the questions.

Stanley, age 35, is newly diagnosed with a seizure disorder. His physician arranges for blood levels to be drawn every 2 weeks during the first month that the new drug is administered.

1. Stanley asks you why he needs to have blood drawn every 2 weeks. Define serum drug levels and explain the rationale for obtaining them.
2. Stanley's physician reduces his medication dosage after the first laboratory results because the levels are near toxic. Stanley demonstrates to you that he is taking his medication correctly. He asks why his level might become toxic. Discuss conditions that may foster toxic drug levels in a compliant client.
3. Two months later, the physician notifies Stanley that he has reached a blood therapeutic level and should continue to take the currently prescribed dosage of his medication. Explain the method by which a therapeutic range is determined by the physician.

■ Section IV: Practicing for NCLEX

Answer the following questions.

1. You are explaining to your patient what bioavailability is. Which of the following statements is true of bioavailability?
   a. It is the portion of a dose that reaches the systemic circulation.
   b. It is the portion of a dose that causes toxicity.
   c. It is the portion of a dose that is absorbed by the system to achieve a therapeutic drug level.
   d. It is the portion of a dose that reaches the systemic circulation and is available to act on body cells.

2. A drug is 100% bioavailable when it is administered by which of the following routes?
   a. Oral   c. Intravenous
   b. Parental   d. Rectal

3. Mrs. Anderson is prescribed a medication to control her hypercholesterolemia. Two years later, the physician prescribes a higher dose of her medication due to a process called *enzyme induction*. A student nurse asks you to explain the change in the drug dosage. You explain that with chronic administration some drugs stimulate liver cells to produce which of the following?
   a. smaller amounts of drug-metabolizing enzymes
   b. toxic amounts of drug-metabolizing enzymes
   c. larger amounts of drug-metabolizing enzymes
   d. therapeutic amounts of drug-metabolizing enzymes

VANCOUVER

- WORKS ON GRAM POS ONLY
- SEVERE INFECTIONS ONLY
- PARENTERAL FOR TREATMENT MRSA
  ENDOCARDITIS + OTHER SERIOUS INF x
- ORALLY: C. DIFFICILE COLITIS
  (NOT ABSORBED IN GI)
  ⇒ INHIBITS CELL WALL SYNTHESIS
  ⇒ HI POTENTIAL TOXICITY (OTOTOXICITY
                            NEPHROTOXICITY)
  ⇒ VEIN IRRITATION)
  NARROW THERAPEUTIC RANGE

4. Mr. Elliot is prescribed a combination of medications to treat his disease process. He is exhibiting signs of toxicity related to his new drug regimen. A possible cause of the change in the absorption of his medications may be *enzyme inhibition*. Which of the following is true of enzyme inhibition? (Select all that apply.)

   a. It may occur with concurrent administration of two or more drugs that compete for the same metabolizing enzymes.

   b. It may occur with concurrent administration of two or more drugs that compete for different metabolizing enzymes.

   c. It may necessitate the administration of larger doses of the medication.

   d. It may necessitate the administration of smaller doses of the medication.

5. In the first-pass effect or presystemic metabolism, a drug is extensively metabolized in the liver, with only part of the drug dose reaching the systemic circulation for distribution to sites of action. The first-pass effect occurs when some drugs are given by which of the following routes?

   a. Orally   c. Rectally

   b. Parentally   d. Intravenously

6. Whereas some drugs or metabolites are excreted in bile and then eliminated in feces, others are excreted in bile, reabsorbed from the small intestine, and then returned to the liver. Which of the following is the name of this process?

   a. Enterohepatic recirculation

   b. Interohepatic recirculation

   c. Enterorenal recirculation

   d. Interorenal recirculation

7. For most drugs, serum levels indicate the onset, peak, and duration of drug action. After a single dose of a drug is given, onset of action occurs when the drug level reaches which of the following?

   a. MAX   c. MEC

   b. MIC   d. MAC

8. In clinical practice, measurement of serum drug levels is useful in which of the following circumstances? (Select all that apply.)

   a. When drugs with a narrow margin of safety are given, because their therapeutic doses are close to their toxic doses

   b. When the mediation used is experimental

   c. To document the serum drug levels associated with particular drug dosages, therapeutic effects, or possible adverse effects

   d. To document drug interactions

   e. To monitor unexpected responses to a drug dose, such as decreased therapeutic effects or increased adverse effects

   f. When a drug overdose is suspected

9. Fill in the blank: _____ also called elimination half-life, is the time required for the serum concentration of a drug to decrease by 50%.

10. When a drug is given at a stable dose, how many half-life periods are required to achieve steady-state concentrations and develop equilibrium between tissue and serum concentrations?

    a. 2 to 3   c. 4 to 5

    b. 3 to 4   d. 5 to 6

11. *Pharmacodynamics* involves drug actions on target cells and results in which of the following?

    a. alterations in cellular biochemical reactions and functions

    b. alterations in cellular pharmacologic reactions

    c. alterations in drug absorption

    d. alterations in drug secretion

12. Relatively few drugs act by mechanisms other than combination with receptor sites on cells. Drugs that do not act on receptor sites include which of the following? (Select all that apply.)

    a. Antacids   c. Osmotic diuretics

    b. Salicylates   d. Purines

    e. NSAIDs

13. Mrs. Geonity is prescribed a medication, and the physician modifies the dose on multiple occasions to achieve the maximum therapeutic effect of the drug. She asks you what the rationale is for the dosage changes. How should you respond?
    a. "Dosage determines whether the drug actions may be therapeutic or toxic."
    b. "Dosage varies based on the brand name."
    c. "Your generic drug does not work as efficiently, and the physician increased your dose."
    d. "Your HMO requires that we change the drug dose frequently."

14. Mr. Dow works the evening shift. The physician orders a medication that must be taken three times a day on an empty stomach. He asks you if he can take his evening dose with supper for the sake of convenience. How should you respond?
    a. "If it is only the one meal, the food will not make a difference."
    b. "Food may slow the absorption of the drug."
    c. "Food may increase the effectiveness of the medication."
    d. "It does not matter if the drug is taken on an empty stomach or not."

15. Mr. Ansgow is diagnosed with Parkinson's disease. His physician orders selegiline. As part of his education plan, you instruct the patient to avoid which of the following foods?
    a. Grapefruit   c. Chicken
    b. Cheese   d. Corn

16. Mrs. Adams is diagnosed with atrial fibrillation and prescribed the drug Coumadin. The nurse would instruct her to avoid which of the following foods?
    a. Foods with vitamin B
    b. Foods with vitamin C
    c. Foods with vitamin K
    d. Foods with niacin

17. Mr. Grey is diagnosed with hypercholesterolemia and is prescribed a statin by his physician. As part of his education plan, the nurse should teach Mr. Grey to avoid which of the following foods?
    a. Grapefruit   c. Chicken
    b. Cheese   d. Corn

18. Changes in aging in the geriatric patient that may affect excretion and promote accumulation of drugs in the body include which of the following?
    a. Rigidity of the diaphragm
    b. Increased gastric motility
    c. Decreased mentation
    d. Decreased glomerular filtration rate

19. Mr. Abo, an African American male, asks you why the physician orders a diuretic as part of his treatment plan for hypertension, when the physician ordered an ACE inhibitor for his friend with the same diagnosis. After consulting with the physician, how would you respond?
    a. "Diuretics are more cost-effective."
    b. "Diuretics are shown to be more effective than ACE inhibitors for African American males with hypertension."
    c. "The physician ordered diuretics to reduce the stress on your heart."
    d. "You must take the drug that the doctor orders, because he knows best how to manage your hypertension."

20. Mrs. Smith has a 12-year history of ETOH abuse. She is injured in a motor vehicle accident and requires surgery with general anesthesia. Which of the following would you expect for this client?
    a. A smaller than normal dose of the general anesthetic
    b. A larger than normal dose of the general anesthetic
    c. The same dose of the general anesthetic as another female of her age and medical history
    d. No general anesthesia, because general anesthesia should not be given to a client with her history

CHAPTER 3

Administering Medications

■ Section I: Learning Objectives

1. List the "rights" of drug administration.
2. Discuss knowledge and skills needed to implement the "rights" of drug administration.
3. List requirements of a complete drug order or prescription.
4. Accurately interpret drug orders containing common abbreviations.
5. Differentiate drug dosage forms for various routes and purposes of administration.
6. Discuss advantages and disadvantages of oral, parenteral, and topical routes of drug administration.
7. Identify supplies, techniques, and observations needed for safe and accurate administration of drugs by different routes.

■ Section II: Assessing Your Understanding

ACTIVITY A

Fill in the Blank

1. Drugs given for _____ are called medications.
2. _____ may administer medications in physicians' offices, and _____ often administer medications in long-term care facilities.
3. The _____ system is a method of drug administration in which most drugs are dispensed in single-dose containers for individual clients.
4. _____ are usually kept as a stock supply in a locked drawer or automated cabinet and replaced as needed.
5. _____ is a process designed to avoid medication errors such as omissions, duplications, dosing errors, or drug interactions that occur when a patient is admitted to a healthcare agency, transferred from one department or unit to another within the agency, or discharged home from the agency.

ACTIVITY B

Matching

Match the term in Column A with the definition in Column B.

COLUMN A

1. _____ ad lib
2. _____ PRN
3. _____ mL
4. _____ mcg
5. _____ g

COLUMN B

A. Microgram
B. Gram
C. As desired
D. As needed
E. Milliliter

ACTIVITY C

Sequencing

You are administering a medication using a unit-dose system. Given below, in random order, are the steps used for medication preparation and administration. Place the steps in the correct order, using the boxes provided.

A. The nurse removes the medication and gives it to the client.
B. The nurse identifies the client.
C. The nurse records the drug on the medication administration record.
D. The nurse identifies the medication and compares it with the doctor's order.

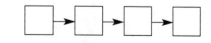

D B C A

ACTIVITY D

Short Answers

Briefly answer the following questions.

1. List the five rights of medication administration.
2. Give three examples of commonly reported medication errors.
3. Describe the components of the Computerized Provider Order Entry (CPOE) medication system.
4. Give three examples of abbreviations that are not acceptable to use in medication administration procedures today according to the JCAHO.
5. Describe the components of a medication order.

■ Section III: Applying Your Knowledge

ACTIVITY E

Case Studies

Consider the scenario and answer the questions.

A physician calls you with a series of verbal orders for Ms. Walden, who is to be discharged today. You are responsible for Ms. Walden's discharge medication education.

1. Describe the parameters for a verbal order.
2. The physician gives Ms. Walden a prescription for a Schedule II controlled drug to be taken after discharge. Describe the parameters for a prescription narcotic; include the method used to refill the prescription.
3. What information would you include in the education plan regarding discharge medications for Ms. Walden?

■ Section IV: Practicing for NCLEX

Answer the following questions.

1. A client refuses a PRN medication; you document the reason for the refusal on the back of the medication administration record and dispose of the medication according to facility policy. By documenting the client's refusal and reason for declining the medication, you are adhering to which of the "rights" for medication administration?

   a. Right dose   c. Right documentation

   b. Right medication   d. Right patient

2. Which of the following is considered essential information to consider about a medication prior to administration?

   a. Cost of the drug   c. Therapeutic effects

   b. The brand name   d. The client's insurance

3. Mrs. Walker requires a PRN pain medication for pain at a level of 5 on a scale of 0 to 10. The physician orders acetaminophen 650 mg, and phone reception is interrupted. What information would you need to clarify the physician's order?

   a. Frequency of administration

   b. Brand name

   c. Cost of the medication

   d. Generic name of the medication

4. Part of your job description is to mentor new nurse graduates during medication administration. The doctor orders acetaminophen 1000 mg by mouth at bedtime for general discomfort for your client. There are several containers of acetaminophen. You instruct the new nurse to do which of the following?

   a. Choose the acetaminophen 325 mg bottle and administer 2 tablets.

   b. Choose the acetaminophen 500 mg bottle and administer 2 tablets.

   c. Choose the acetaminophen 500 g bottle and administer 2 tablets.

   d. Choose the acetaminophen 325 g bottle and administer 2 tablets.

5. The charge nurse on the unit transcribes a physician's order onto the medication administration record. She writes, "Digoxin 0.25 mg PO qod ×3d" on the MAR. How should the order be written to prevent medication error?

   a. Digoxin 0.25 mg PO every other day ×3d

   b. Digoxin 0.25 mg PO qod for three doses

   c. Digoxin 0.25 mg by mouth every other day for three doses

   d. Digoxin 0.25 mg PO qod ×3d

6. The physician orders NPH U100 Insulin 16 units SC every AM for Mrs. Styles. You prepare the insulin dose, and, to ensure safety, you do which of the following?

   a. Give the insulin to the client.

   b. Bring the vial with you.

   c. Ask another nurse to double-check your measurement.

   d. Encourage the client to administer her own insulin.

7. Your physician's order states that a medication must be given IM. You enter the client's room and he states that he will partially remove his pants and asks you to give the injection quickly. You do which of the following?

   a. Agree, because a fast injection is less painful than a slow one.

   b. Refuse, because IM injections may be given only in the deltoid muscle of the arm.

   c. Agree, because you wish to respect the client's wishes.

   d. Refuse, because you are unable to identify anatomic landmarks with the client partially clothed.

8. Mr. Reed has a physician's order to administer Lasix 40 mg by mouth each day at noon. You enter his room and he states, "I was waiting for my Lasix dose; you can give it to me now." You should do which of the following?

   a. Administer the dose.

   b. Clarify the client's identification by checking his name band.

   c. Clarify the client's identification by asking his name.

   d. Call the physician to clarify the order, because the dose is too high.

9. During a medication pass, you notice that the physician ordered a dose of medication that appears to be excessive, based on your knowledge of the medication. You call the physician, and he instructs you to administer the medication anyway. You should do which of the following?

   a. Administer the medication.

   b. Consult with your supervisor, refuse to administer the medication, and notify the physician.

   c. Refuse to administer the medication, and notify the physician.

   d. Ask the physician on-call for a new order.

10. Which of the following specific drugs are often associated with errors and adverse drug events (ADEs)? (Select all that apply.)

    a. Insulin   c. Heparin

    b. Acetaminophen   d. Salicylates

    e. Warfarin

11. Which of the following is a safety feature inherent in using the bar code method to administer drugs?

    a. The bar code on the drug label contains the client's name.

    b. When administering medications, the nurse is only required to scan the bar code on the drug label.

    c. The bar code on the patient's identification band contains the MAR.

    d. A wireless computer network processes the scanned information and gives an error message when the MAR has not been inputted onto the computer.

12. Mrs. Smith has a one-time order of Lasix 60 mg IM. You enter the client's room to administer the medication and she refuses administration of the medication as ordered. She states that Lasix is only given in a pill form and the physician must have made a mistake. As part of your teaching plan, you tell the client which of the following?

    a. "Lasix is available in more than one form. The IM medication will work slower than if given by mouth."

    b. "You are correct; the physician must have made an error."

    c. "The physician orders the medication the way it needs to be administered."

    d. "Lasix is available in more than one form. The IM medication will work faster than if given by mouth."

13. Mrs. Janis' physician orders enteric-coated aspirin 81 mg by mouth once a day. When you attempt to administer the medication, the patient informs you that the aspirin that she takes at home is not coated and works just fine. As part of your education plan, you instruct the client, saying which of the following?

    a. "Enteric-coated tablets and capsules are coated with a substance that is insoluble in stomach acid. This delays dissolution until the medication reaches the intestine, usually to avoid gastric irritation or to keep the drug from being destroyed by gastric acid."

    b. "Enteric-coated tablets and capsules are coated with a substance that is soluble in stomach acid. This delays dissolution until the medication reaches the intestine, usually to avoid gastric irritation or to keep the drug from being destroyed by gastric acid."

    c. "Enteric-coated tablets and capsules are coated with a substance that is insoluble in stomach acid. This delays dissolution until the medication reaches the intestine, usually causing gastric irritation or to keep the drug from being destroyed by gastric acid."

    d. "Enteric-coated tablets and capsules are coated with a substance that is insoluble in stomach acid. This delays dissolution until the medication reaches the liver, usually to avoid gastric irritation or to keep the drug from being destroyed by gastric acid."

14. Mrs. Hone has a new order for Effexor XR. She asks you why she doesn't have to take the medication as frequently as her other antidepressant. As part of your teaching plan, you tell her which of the following?

    a. "XR means that the drug is extended release, which means that there are less consistent serum drug levels and you need to take it less frequently."

    b. "XR means that the drug is delayed release, which means that there are more consistent serum drug levels and you need to take it less frequently."

    c. "XR means that the drug is extended release, which means that there are more consistent serum drug levels and you need to take it less frequently."

    d. "XR means that the drug is extended release, which means that there are more consistent serum drug levels and you need to take it more frequently."

15. Mrs. Hone asks you to open her Effexor XR capsule and mix the contents in applesauce to make it easier to swallow. How should you respond?

    a. "Not a problem; I will mix the medication for you."

    b. "I am sorry, but opening the capsule may cause you to absorb too much medication too quickly."

    c. "The physician gave you this form of your medication because it is easier to take by mouth."

    d. "Effexor XR may only be mixed with food with a physician's order."

16. How many 60-mg tablets of Lasix are needed to give a dose of 120 mg? _____ Show the mathematical formula used to achieve your answer: _____.

17. Which of the following are common parenteral routes? (Select all that apply.)

    a. Subcutaneous   c. Intramuscular

    b. Transdermal   d. Intravenous

18. You are mentoring a new nurse to the unit's medication pass. She asks you why you used two separate needles to prepare a drug for injection using an ampule. Which of the following is a correct response?

   a. "A filter needle is used to withdraw the medication from an ampule or vial because the solution may be too thick to be removed from the drug vial. The filter needle is then replaced with a regular needle before injecting the client."

   b. "A filter needle is used to withdraw the medication from an ampule or vial because broken glass or rubber fragments may need to be removed from the drug solution. A new filter needle may be used before injecting the client."

   c. "A filter needle is used to withdraw the medication from an ampule or vial because broken glass or rubber fragments may need to be removed from the drug solution. The filter needle is then replaced with a regular needle before injecting the client."

   d. "A filter needle is used to withdraw the medication from an ampule or vial because broken glass or rubber fragments may need to be removed from the drug solution. The filter needle need not be replaced with a regular needle before injecting the client."

19. Which of the following is the smallest needle according to its gauge?

   a. 18 gauge   c. 22 gauge
   b. 25 gauge   d. 20 gauge

20. Which of the following are common sites for IM injections? (Select all that apply.)

   a. Deltoid   d. Vastus lateralis
   b. Dorsogluteal   e. Latissimus dorsi
   c. Ventrogluteal

CHAPTER 4

Nursing Process in Drug Therapy

■ Section I: Learning Objectives

1. Assess clients for conditions and factors that are likely to influence drug effects, including age, weight, health status, and lifestyle.
2. Obtain a medication history about the client's use of prescription, over-the-counter (OTC), and social drugs as well as herbal and dietary supplements.
3. Identify nondrug interventions to prevent or decrease the need for drug therapy.
4. Discuss interventions to increase therapeutic effects and decrease adverse effects of drug therapy.
5. Discuss guidelines for rational choices of drugs, dosages, routes, and times of administration.
6. Observe clients for therapeutic and adverse responses to drug therapy.
7. Teach clients and family members how to use prescription and OTC drugs safely and effectively.
8. When indicated, teach clients about the potential effects of herbal and dietary supplements.
9. For clients who use herbal and dietary supplements, provide—or assist them in obtaining—reliable information.
10. Describe major considerations in drug therapy for children, adults, and clients with impaired renal or hepatic function or critical illness.
11. Discuss application of the nursing process in home-care settings.
12. Apply evidence-based data about clients and therapeutic drugs in all steps of the nursing process.

■ Section II: Assessing Your Understanding

ACTIVITY A

Fill in the Blank

1. The _____ _____ is a systematic way of gathering and using information to plan and provide individualized client care and to evaluate the outcomes of care.

2. The nursing process involves both _____ and _____ skills.
3. _____ involves collecting data about client characteristics known to affect drug therapy.
4. _____ _____ describe client problems or needs and are based on assessment data.
5. _____ involve implementing planned activities and include any task performed directly with a client or indirectly on a client's behalf.

ACTIVITY B

Matching

Match the term in Column A with the definition in Column B.

COLUMN A

1. _____ Goal
2. _____ Assessment
3. _____ Intervention
4. _____ Evaluation
5. _____ Nursing Diagnosis

COLUMN B

A. What does the client know about current drugs? Is teaching needed?
B. Deficient Knowledge: Safe and effective self-administration (when appropriate)
C. Experience relief of signs and symptoms
D. Ambulating, positioning, exercising
E. This step involves evaluating the client's status in relation to stated goals and expected outcomes.

ACTIVITY C

Short Answers

Briefly answer the following questions.

1. Describe the assessment phase of the nursing process.
2. Describe and give an example of a nursing diagnosis. Use NANDA for your example.
3. Describe the planning and goals component of the nursing process.
4. Describe the intervention component of the nursing process.
5. When does evaluation occur within the nursing process?

▪ Section III: Applying Your Knowledge

ACTIVITY D

Case Studies

Consider the scenarios and answer the questions.

Case Study 1

You are responsible for the initial assessment for a client returning to the physician's office 10 days after beginning a new medication regimen to control her asthma.

1. You begin your assessment by doing which of the following?
   a. Collecting objective data
   b. Collecting both objective and subjective data
   c. Collecting subjective data only
   d. Taking the client's vital signs

2. You interview the client regarding the effectiveness of the medication as well as any adverse reactions. Your client's statements are considered to be which of the following?
   a. Subjective data
   b. Objective data
   c. An ice-breaker
   d. An important part of the nursing diagnosis

3. Part of your focused assessment includes taking the client's vital signs. Vital signs are an example of which of the following?
   a. Subjective data
   b. Objective data
   c. An ice-breaker
   d. An important part of the nursing diagnosis

Case Study 2

You are responsible for the education plan for a family with a 4-year-old child who is being treated by the physician for rheumatic fever.

1. You verify the age of the child with the mother before calculating the dosage of the medication ordered by the physician. The mother asks you why this information is needed. You state which of the following?
   a. "All aspects of pediatric drug therapy must be guided by the child's age, weight, and disease process."
   b. "All aspects of pediatric drug therapy must be guided by the child's age, height, and weight."
   c. "All aspects of pediatric drug therapy must be guided by the child's age and levels of growth and development."
   d. "All aspects of pediatric drug therapy must be guided by the child's age, weight, and levels of growth and development."

2. The mother asks you why the child is not being given a dosage of the medication closer to what she took when she herself was ill. Wouldn't the higher dosage be more effective against the illness? You reply by saying which of the following?
   a. "When pediatric dosage ranges are listed in drug literature, they should be used."
   b. "Higher dosages may be helpful in this instance; I will call the physician for a change in orders."
   c. "Pediatric dosages are based on height and weight only."
   d. "Pediatric dosages vary from drug to drug and are not based on adult dosages."

3. The child refuses to take the first oral dosage of the medication; the mother tells you just to hold the child's nose and pour the medication into the child's mouth when he opens it. The mother states that this is the method that she uses at home. You do which of the following?

   a. Give the medication to the mother to administer.

   b. Administer the medication intramuscularly and teach the mother to use the same route of administration at home.

   c. State that oral medications should never be forced, because forcing may lead to aspiration.

   d. Administer the medication as suggested by the mother.

■ Section IV: Practicing for NCLEX

Answer the following questions.

1. Mr. Jones is self-administering garlic, St. John's wort, and echinacea. The anesthesiologist asks the client to do which of the following?

   a. Discontinue the herbal medications 1 week prior to surgery.

   b. Maintain his current regimen regardless of the herbal supplements taken.

   c. Discontinue the herbal medications 2 to 3 weeks prior to surgery.

   d. Continue only the garlic and echinacea according to his current medication regimen.

2. Mrs. Abbot recently discovered that she is pregnant. She currently takes herbal medications to control her diabetes and the symptoms related to pregnancy. She asks you if it is safe to take herbal medications while she is pregnant. You state which of the following?

   a. "Most herbal and dietary supplements should be avoided during pregnancy or lactation."

   b. "Most herbal and dietary supplements are safe during pregnancy and are used by many cultures to control the symptoms of nausea."

   c. "Dietary supplements are high in fat and protein; they are safe to take during pregnancy and help to maintain health during lactation."

   d. "Herbal and dietary supplements will cause premature labor."

3. Mr. Gascony, age 76, presents to the physician's office with gastrointestinal pain and diarrhea that is black. When asked about his medication history, he does not include over-the-counter medications. You state that it is important to include them, for which of the following reasons?

   a. Including over-the-counter medications will give you a complete summary of medications.

   b. The client may be taking a combination of medications that cause confusion and place him at risk for falls.

   c. Older clients tend to overdose on over-the-counter medications.

   d. Older people are more likely to have adverse drug reactions.

4. Mr. Rice, who is diagnosed with diabetes mellitus type 2, arrives at the physician's office for a routine checkup. His capillary blood sugar is 312. You question him about his diet and medication compliance. He states that he changed his medications to one that is advertised as "natural" because it should be safer and more effective. You state which of the following?

   a. "Natural medications are more effective; I will consult with the physician regarding a dosage change."

   b. "Natural medications are less effective, and you should not take them."

   c. "Natural does not mean safe or more effective; I will consult the physician about your choice of medications."

   d. "Notify your physician in the future when you change medications."

5. Ms. Rambo presents to the physician's office with a sore throat, fever, and general malaise. She informs you that she has been taking an over-the-counter sore throat medication for 2 weeks without relief. As part of your education plan, you inform the client that she should do which of the following?

   a. Inform the physician before taking any over-the-counter medications.

   b. Read product labels carefully regarding when to stop using the medication or when to consult the physician.

   c. Clarify the use of the over-the-counter medication with the pharmacist at the drug store.

   d. Stop taking any over-the-counter medications when a temperature greater than 101 degrees develops.

6. Mr. Jameson presents in the emergency room with an elevated blood pressure, headache, and dizziness. He states that he has been taking over-the-counter medications for his allergies for 2 weeks. As part of your education plan, you teach the client which of the following?

   a. Over-the-counter medications are contraindicated for clients with a diagnosis of hypertension.

   b. Over-the-counter medications may be contraindicated for clients with a diagnosis of hypertension; read the label carefully.

   c. Over-the-counter medications are safe for clients with a diagnosis of hypertension, and the symptoms are not related to OTC use.

   d. Over-the-counter medications are usually safe for clients with a diagnosis of hypertension, and this episode may be an isolated incident.

7. Mr. Gaines presents to the emergency room with symptoms related to a gastrointestinal bleed. He is currently on warfarin, an anticoagulant, for a diagnosis of recurrent deep vein thrombosis. When questioned about recent OTC drug use, he states that he takes aspirin for recurrent stress-related headaches. As part of your education plan, you state which of the following?

   a. "Consult your physician before taking products containing aspirin if you are taking an anticoagulant."

   b. "Your stress headaches may have contributed to the GI bleed."

   c. "What symptoms do you experience prior to the tension headaches?"

   d. "Aspirin is safe to use in conjunction with your anticoagulants."

8. Mr. Jakes presents to the emergency room with nausea and vomiting as well as right quadrant abdominal pain with rebound tenderness at McBurney's point. He states that he has not had a bowel movement in 3 days and began self-administering laxatives 2 days ago. Upon discharge, you are responsible for the client's education plan. You stress to Mr. Jakes that he should do which of the following?

   a. He should call the physician prior to the administration of laxatives.

   b. He should increase the fiber in his diet to avoid the use of laxatives.

   c. He should take laxatives only if he does not have a bowel movement in 4 days.

   d. He should not take a laxative if he has stomach pain, nausea, or vomiting, to avoid worsening the problem.

9. Mr. Shanks is diagnosed with cardiac disease, and the physician prescribes aspirin 81 mg PO qd. He routinely takes aspirin for headaches related to job stress. As part of your education plan, you instruct the client to do which of the following?

   a. Take only 325 mg of aspirin if he has a headache.

   b. Call his physician's office if he has a headache, because it may be symptomatic of a stroke.

   c. Call his physician's office before taking other products containing aspirin in addition to his current dose.

   d. Take only NSAIDs for his headaches.

10. Sally brings her friend to the emergency department because she is having difficulty waking her. Earlier that evening, they attended a party and drank alcohol. What class of over-the-counter drugs may have contributed to the friend's current state of sedation? (Select all that apply.)

    a. Cold remedies containing dextromethorphan.

    b. Antihistamines.

    c. Laxatives.

    d. NSAIDs.

11. Mr. Case presents to the physician's office and states that his sublingual nitroglycerin no longer relieves his intermittent anginal symptoms. Which of the following might indicate that he requires medication education? (Select all that apply.)

    a. He stores his NTG in a clear bottle that he keeps in the glove compartment in his car.

    b. He keeps the NTG in an antacid bottle by his bedside for convenience.

    c. He administers the NTG at 5-minute intervals when he experiences anginal chest pain.

    d. He keeps his NTG for as long as the bottle has medication in it.

12. If a dose of a medication is missed, most authorities recommend which of the following?

    a. Double the dose the next time that the medication is due.

    b. Take the medication if it is close to the administration time.

    c. Increase the next two doses to maintain the drug's level in the system.

    d. Take the medication as long as there are 2 hours between doses.

13. Which of the following statements would indicate that a mother is administering the *incorrect* dosage of liquid medication to her child?

    a. "I use a calibrated medication cup to administer the medication."

    b. "I use the measuring teaspoon that I cook with."

    c. "I give the medication at the times indicated on the prescription."

    d. "I use a household teaspoon to administer the medication."

14. An antibiotic that is ordered four times a day should be given at which of the following times?

    a. Breakfast, lunch, dinner, and bedtime

    b. Breakfast, lunch, dinner, and with a snack at bedtime

    c. Every 4 hours around the clock

    d. Every 6 hours around the clock

15. Your client states that it is easier to swallow a medication without water than to take it with water. He has always taken his medications in this manner. You state which of the following?

    a. "Water dilutes the medication and reduces its effectiveness."

    b. "Taking oral medications with water helps promote absorption of the drug into the bloodstream."

    c. "Most medications may be taken with or without water."

    d. "Taking medications without water promotes the absorption of the medication in the esophagus."

16. What advice may help a client to prevent an adverse drug interaction secondary to multiple prescription medications?

    a. Get all prescriptions filled at the same pharmacy.

    b. Administer prescription medications on an empty stomach.

    c. Administer prescription medications on a full stomach.

    d. Administer only prescription medications ordered by the primary physician.

17. Mr. Janus is admitted to the hospital with a diagnosis of hypokalemia. He takes the prescription medication furosemide, which is a potassium-wasting diuretic. What action could have been taken to avoid hypokalemia?

    a. Routine prescription blood levels

    b. Patient education regarding polypharmacy

    c. Routine blood work to detect potassium levels

    d. Discontinuance of the medication once symptoms of shortness of breath ceased

18. _____ involves a rigorous process of analyzing, comparing, and summarizing multiple studies.

19. When completing a drug history, the home-care nurse should ask to see all _____ and _____ medications that the client takes and should ask how and when the client takes each one.

20. _____ requirements may vary among clients and within the same client at different times during an illness.

CHAPTER 5

Physiology of the Central Nervous System

■ Section I: Learning Objectives

1. Describe the process of neurotransmission.
2. Describe major neurotransmitters and their roles in central nervous system (CNS) functioning.
3. Discuss signs and symptoms of CNS depression.
4. Discuss general types and characteristics of CNS depressant drugs.

■ Section II: Assessing Your Understanding

ACTIVITY A

Fill in the Blank

1. The central nervous system (CNS), which is composed of the _____ and _____, acts as the control center for regulating physical and mental body processes.
2. _____ carry messages to the CNS, and efferent or motor neurons carry messages away from the CNS.
3. The CNS constantly receives information about blood levels of oxygen and carbon dioxide, body temperature, and sensory stimuli and sends messages to effector organs to adjust the environment toward _____.
4. The CNS carries out its functions by transmitting _____ and _____ signals among components of the CNS and between the CNS and other parts of the body.
5. The CNS is composed of two types of cells: the _____ is the basic functional unit; the _____ protect, support, and nourish the neuron.

ACTIVITY B

Matching

Match the term in Column A with the definition in Column B.

COLUMN A

1. _____ Receptors
2. _____ Synapse
3. _____ Neurotransmitters
4. _____ Hypoxia
5. _____ Cholinergic system

COLUMN B

A. Chemical substances that carry messages from one neuron to another
B. Proteins embedded in the cell membranes of neurons
C. Lack of oxygen
D. Microscopic gap that separates neurons in a chain
E. Uses acetylcholine as its neurotransmitter

ACTIVITY C

Sequencing

Given below, in random order are symptoms of CNS depression. Place them in the correct order, from the mildest to the most severe, using the boxes provided.

A. Loss of reflexes
B. Drowsiness or sleep
C. Respiratory failure
D. Short attention span
E. Death

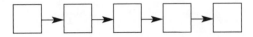

ACTIVITY D
Short Answers

Briefly answer the following questions.

1. Describe the characteristics that allow neurons to communicate with other body cells.
2. Identify three factors that affect the availability and function of neurotransmitters.
3. Identify the areas of the body where norepinephrine may be found.
4. Describe how the CNS functions in health.
5. Describe how the CNS functions in disease.

■ Section III: Applying Your Knowledge

ACTIVITY E
Case Study

Consider the scenario and answer the questions.

Mr. Wentworth presents in the emergency room after feeling chest palpitations. During his drug history, he states that he is taking a new medication for weight loss that his friend gave him. He states that the drug is working well. A sample of the drug is given to the pharmacy and is identified as dexedrine, a CNS stimulant. After his condition is stabilized, you are responsible for his discharge education plan.

1. Mr. Wentworth asks you if he can still continue to take the medication, because his friend has a prescription. Describe the education plan that you would develop to explain the use of prescription medications.

2. Describe the signs and symptoms of CNS stimulant side-effects.

■ Section IV: Practicing for NCLEX

Answer the following questions.

1. Which of the following are conscious processes of the cerebral cortex. (Select all that apply.)
   a. Learning
   b. Memory
   c. Involuntary movement
   d. Verbalization
   e. Voluntary movement

2. The thalamus receives impulses carrying sensations such as heat, cold, pain, and muscle position sense that produce a crude awareness in the thalamus. These sensations are relayed to which of the following?
   a. Cerebral cortex
   b. Hypothalamus
   c. The cholinergic system
   d. Neurotransmitters

3. The _____ helps maintain homeostasis by constantly adjusting water balance, temperature, hormone levels, blood pressure, and other body functions.

4. Which of the following hormones initiates uterine contractions to begin labor and delivery and helps release milk from breast glands during breastfeeding?
   a. Neuroendocrine hormone
   b. ADH
   c. Oxytocin
   d. Myosin

5. When nerve impulses from the hypothalamus excite the vasomotor center, vasomotor tone is increased, and blood pressure does which of the following?
   a. Is stabilized
   b. Is raised
   c. Is lowered
   d. Is in homeostasis

6. The medulla contains groups of neurons that form the vital cardiac, respiratory, and vasomotor centers. If the respiratory center is stimulated, respiratory rate and depth do which of the following?
   a. Become increased
   b. Become decreased
   c. Remain unchanged
   d. Become labored

7. The reticular activating system is a network of neurons that extends from the spinal cord through the medulla and pons to the thalamus and hypothalamus. It receives impulses from all parts of the body, evaluates the significance of the impulses, and decides which impulses to transmit to the cerebral cortex. It also excites or inhibits motor nerves that control both reflex and voluntary movement. Stimulation of these neurons produces which of the following?

    a. Motor depression

    b. Loss of consciousness

    c. Mental alertness

    d. Involuntary movements

8. Many nerve impulses from the limbic system are transmitted through the hypothalamus; this causes physiologic changes in blood pressure, heart rate, respiration, and hormone secretion to occur in response to which of the following?

    a. Emotions   c. Physical stimuli

    b. Thoughts   d. Hormone imbalance

9. The _____, which is connected with motor centers in the cerebral cortex and basal ganglia, coordinates muscle activity.

10. Degenerative changes in the substantia nigra cause dopamine to be released in decreased amounts. This process is a factor in the development of which of the following?

    a. Depression   c. Parkinson's disease

    b. Schizophrenia   d. Obesity

11. Fibers are called _____ because they do not enter the medullary pyramids and cross over.

12. An interruption to the blood supply to the cerebral cortex causes which of the following conditions?

    a. Hypertension   c. Loss of consciousness

    b. Dysrhythmias   d. Apnea

13. Thiamine deficiency can reduce the use of glucose by nerve cells and can cause degeneration of the myelin sheath. Such degeneration in central neurons leads to a form of brain damage known as which of the following?

    a. Wernicke-Korsakoff encephalopathy

    b. Diabetes neuropathy

    c. Vascular insufficiency

    d. CVA

14. Degeneration in _____ leads to polyneuritis and muscle atrophy, weakness, and paralysis.

15. Reflexes (e.g., knee-jerk reflex, pupillary reflexes) are responses to certain nerve impulses received by the spinal cord. They are an example of which of the following?

    a. Voluntary responses

    b. Involuntary responses

    c. Mediated responses

    d. Structured responses

16. When released from the synaptic vesicles, molecules of neurotransmitter cross the synapse, bind to receptors in the cell membrane of the postsynaptic neuron, and excite or inhibit postsynaptic neurons. Free neurotransmitter molecules (i.e., those not bound to receptors) are rapidly removed from the synapse by which of the following sets of mechanisms?

    a. Transportation back into the presynaptic nerve terminal (pre-uptake) for reuse, diffusion into surrounding body fluids, or destruction by enzymes

    b. Transportation back into the synaptic nerve terminal (reuptake) for reuse, diffusion into surrounding body fluids, or destruction by enzymes

    c. Transportation back into the presynaptic nerve terminal (reuptake) for reuse, diffusion into surrounding body fluids, or destruction of enzymes

    d. Transportation back into the presynaptic nerve terminal (reuptake) for reuse, diffusion into surrounding body fluids, or destruction by enzymes

17. A neurotransmitter–receptor complex may have which of the following?

    a. An excitatory or inhibitory effect on the postsynaptic neuron

    b. An inhibitory effect on the postsynaptic neuron

    c. An excitatory effect on the postsynaptic neuron

    d. An excitatory or inhibitory effect on the synaptic neuron

18. The _____ uses *acetylcholine* as its neurotransmitter.

19. _____ is the major inhibitory neurotransmitter in the CNS, with a role in many neuronal circuits (estimated at almost one third of CNS synapses).

20. The rate of serotonin production is controlled by the enzyme tryptophan hydroxylase and the amount of which of the following substances in the diet?

    a. Serotonin   c. Norepinephrine

    b. Tryptophan   d. Epinephrine

CHAPTER 6

Opioid Analgesics and Pain Management

■ Section I: Learning Objectives

1. Discuss the major types and characteristics of pain.
2. Discuss the nurse's role in assessing and managing clients' pain.
3. List characteristics of opioid analgesics in terms of mechanisms of action, indications for use, and major adverse effects.
4. Describe morphine as the prototype of opioid analgesics.
5. Differentiate between ceiling and non-ceiling opioids.
6. Explain why higher doses of opioid analgesics are needed when the drugs are given orally.
7. Contrast the use of opioid analgesics in opioid-naive and opioid-tolerant clients.
8. Assess level of consciousness and respiratory status before and after administering opioids.
9. Teach clients about the safe, effective use of opioid analgesics.
10. Describe the characteristics and treatment of opioid toxicity.
11. Discuss principles of therapy for using opioid analgesics in special populations.
12. Discuss nonopioid drugs used in pain management.

■ Section II: Assessing Your Understanding

ACTIVITY A

Fill in the Blank

1. _____, an unpleasant, uncomfortable sensation, usually indicates tissue damage.
2. _____ analgesics are drugs that relieve moderate to severe pain.
3. _____ are abundant in arterial walls, joint surfaces, muscle fascia, periosteum, skin, and soft tissues; they are scarce in most internal organs.
4. _____ analgesics are used in the management of both acute and chronic pain; other _____ are used mainly for chronic neuropathic pain or bone pain.
5. Because of the potentially fatal adverse effects and risks of drug abuse and dependence, all of the opioid analgesics have _____.

ACTIVITY B

Matching

Match the term in Column A with the definition in Column B.

COLUMN A

1. _____ Hydrocodone
2. _____ Codeine
3. _____ Morphine
4. _____ Fentanyl
5. _____ Methadone

COLUMN B

A. An opium alkaloid that is mainly used to relieve moderate to severe pain
B. A Schedule III drug that is similar to codeine in its analgesic and antitussive effects
C. A potent opioid that is widely used for preanesthetic medication, postoperative analgesia, and chronic pain that requires an opioid analgesic
D. A synthetic drug that is similar to morphine but with a longer duration of action
E. An opium alkaloid and Schedule II drug that is used for analgesic and antitussive effects

ACTIVITY C

Short Answers

Briefly answer the following questions.

1. For a person to feel pain, the signal from the nociceptors in peripheral tissues must be transmitted by a certain route. Describe this route and what happens along the way.
2. Causes of tissue damage may be physical or chemical. Explain how physical or chemical damage activates pain receptors.
3. Explain why most opioid oral drug dosages are larger than those injected.
4. Describe the effects that opioids have on the GI tract.
5. Describe the mechanism by which capsaicin (Zostrix) relieves osteoarthritis pain.
6. Explain why the goal for the postoperative client is pain relief without sedation.

▪ Section III: Applying Your Knowledge

ACTIVITY D

Case Study

Consider the scenario and answer the questions.

Mrs. Leonard is admitted to your unit with severe burns related to a house fire. She is restless, agitated, and complaining of pain: 8 on a scale of 0 to 10. You are responsible for both pain management and the development of an education plan for the client and her family.

1. The family asks you why you are giving the pain medication through an IV rather than by mouth. Explain your rationale.
2. The family states that the pain is not managed by the current treatment because the client is agitated. You develop an education plan for the client's family. Explain the various causes of agitation for this client.

▪ Section IV: Practicing for NCLEX

Answer the following questions.

1. Mrs. Smith is 12 hours status post appendectomy. Her son asks the nurse to reduce the amount of pain medication that his mother is taking. He states, "When I had my appendix out, I needed half the pain medication that she does." You state which of the following?
   a. "I agree she is taking far too much pain medication."
   b. "You should discuss your mother's pain management with the physician."
   c. "Pain is a subjective experience, we all feel pain differently."
   d. "I will call the physician for an order to decrease the dose and the frequency of your mother's pain medication."

2. Mr. James is receiving an opioid analgesic for bone pain related to a fractured femur. On postoperative day 3, he still requests pain medication every 2 to 3 hours. His incision is clean, dry, and intact, and there are no signs or symptoms of an infectious process surrounding the incision. You respond to his request for pain medication by assessing for which of the following?
   a. Drug tolerance
   b. Drug-seeking behavior
   c. Drug addiction
   d. Drug dependence

3. Mrs. Wilson states that her pain is unbearable. You have an order for one or two tablets of an opioid analgesic for pain relief. Which of the following is one method that you may use to assess the intensity of the pain?
   a. Base the pain level by comparing it with other clients with the same diagnosis.
   b. Use a numerical scale of 0 to 10, with 0 being the least amount of pain.
   c. Ask the client to compare her pain with the pain experienced 24 hours ago.
   d. Ask the client to wait for pain medication until she feels that the pain is out of control.

4. Mr. Peters presents in the emergency department and states that he is experiencing pain in his shoulder and chest muscles. The physician orders a cardiac diagnostic assessment. The client asks you why the doctor feels that he has cardiac problems if his shoulder hurts. Which of the following would be an appropriate response?

   a. "At your age, cardiac problems are frequently diagnosed. The assessment is a precaution."

   b. "You may have referred pain. Pain of cardiac origin may radiate to the neck, shoulders, chest muscles, and down the arms, often on the left side."

   c. "Your insurance company requires a cardiac diagnostic assessment whenever you present in the emergency department."

   d. "That is how this physician chooses to assess his clients."

5. You administer an oral opioid analgesic to a client at 6 PM for pain documented as 6 on a scale of 0 to 10. At 6:30 PM, the client states that the pain level is 3 on a scale of 0 to 10, and that level is acceptable to him. The client asks why you returned to reassess the pain. You state that for proper pain management the nurse must do which of the following?

   a. Assess every client in relation to pain, initially to determine if the medication is the correct dose.

   b. Assess every client in relation to pain according to hospital policy.

   c. Assess every client in relation to pain and their activity level.

   d. Assess every client in relation to pain, initially to determine appropriate interventions and later to determine whether the interventions were effective in preventing or relieving pain.

6. Mrs. Zeta is recovering from shingles. She is experiencing sharp pain in the area of the healed pustules on her left rib cage. She does not like how the opioid analgesic that is ordered makes her feel, and she refuses the medication. Which of the following physician's orders would best manage her pain?

   a. Lidoderm in the form of a transdermal gel patch

   b. Heat to the area, 20 minutes on and 2 hours off

   c. Ice to the area, 20 minutes on and 2 hours off

   d. Acetaminophen 500 mg by mouth every 6 to 8 hours

7. Ms. Woods injured her knee in a motor vehicle accident. Her pain is not managed during physical therapy with pain medication alone. After assessing the client for further damage to the joint, the physician orders corticosteroids. Ms. Woods asks you how corticosteroids will improve her mobility and manage her pain. Which of the following is an appropriate explanation?

   a. "Corticosteroids mask inflammation, irritability, and spontaneous discharge in injured nerves and other tissues."

   b. "Corticosteroids can reduce inflammation, irritability, and spontaneous discharge in injured nerves and other tissues."

   c. "Corticosteroids can reduce inflammation, but they may increase irritability and spontaneous discharge in injured nerves and other tissues."

   d. "Corticosteroids can increase inflammation, but they reduce irritability and spontaneous discharge in injured nerves and other tissues."

8. Mr. Smith, a retired Army medic, complains of foot pain related to diabetic neuropathy. He asks you why the physician ordered tricyclic antidepressants (TCAs), stating, "I am not depressed; I just have pain." Which of the following is the appropriate explanation?

   a. TCAs encourage the reuptake of norepinephrine and serotonin in nerve synapses, thereby making these neurotransmitters more available to inhibit pain signals.

   b. TCAs slow down the reuptake of norepinephrine and serotonin in nerve synapses, thereby making these neurotransmitters more available to inhibit pain signals.

   c. TCAs inhibit the reuptake of norepinephrine and serotonin in nerve synapses, thereby making these neurotransmitters more available to inhibit pain signals.

   d. TCAs inhibit the reuptake of norepinephrine and serotonin in nerve synapses, thereby making these neurotransmitters less available to inhibit pain signals.

9. Mrs. Abernathy is experiencing uncontrolled pain related to her peripheral neuropathy. Multiple analgesics have been used to manage her pain without success. The physician orders gabapentin. As part of your teaching plan, you explain to the client that gabapentin works with the nerve cells that carry pain to do which of the following?

   a. Decrease their irritability so that they will be less likely to carry pain signals.

   b. Increase their irritability so that they will be less likely to carry pain signals.

   c. The action of this medication is unknown.

   d. Eliminate their irritability so that they will be less likely to carry pain signals.

10. Mr. Gill presents to the emergency department with a severe headache and pain that is unresolved for 24 hours. While taking his drug history, you note that his pain management involves self-administering 500 mg of acetaminophen, two pills every 4 hours. The physician orders a liver panel. Mr. Gill states, "But it is only acetaminophen, why are you concerned?" As part of the teaching plan, you instruct Mr. Gill that which of the following is the maximum dose of acetaminophen in 24 hours?

    a. 4 grams   c. 3 grams

    b. 2 grams   d. 6 grams

11. The physician orders NSAIDs for your client with a sprained ankle. As part of your education plan, you explain what NSAIDs do. Which explanation is correct?

    a. NSAIDs inhibit inflammatory chemicals that cause, increase, or maintain pain signals.

    b. NSAIDs increase inflammatory chemicals that cause, increase, or maintain pain signals.

    c. NSAIDs reduce inflammatory chemicals that cause, increase, or maintain pain signals.

    d. NSAIDs reduce steroidal chemicals that cause, increase, or maintain pain signals.

12. _____ pain is caused by lesions or physiologic changes that injure peripheral pain receptors, nerves, or the CNS. It is characterized by excessive excitability in the damaged area or surrounding normal tissues, so that nerve cells discharge more easily. As a result, pain may arise spontaneously or from a normally nonpainful stimulus, such as a light touch.

13. Your client describes the pain in his injured ankles as burning and cramping. These symptoms are examples of which type of pain?

    a. Visceral pain   c. Neuropathic pain

    b. Somatic chronic pain   d. Somatic acute pain

14. Which of the following types of pain demands attention less urgently; may not be characterized by visible signs; and is often accompanied by emotional stress, increased irritability, depression, social withdrawal, financial distress, loss of libido, disturbed sleep patterns, diminished appetite, weight loss, and decreased ability to perform usual activities of daily living?

    a. Chronic pain   c. Somatic pain

    b. Acute pain   d. Neuropathic pain

15. Which of the following types of pain may be caused by injury, trauma, spasm, disease processes, and treatment or diagnostic procedures that damage body tissues; is often described as sharp or cutting; is usually proportional in intensity to the amount of tissue damage; and serves as a warning system by demanding the sufferer's attention and compelling behavior to withdraw from or avoid the pain-producing stimulus?

    a. Chronic pain   c. Neuropathic pain

    b. Somatic pain   d. Acute pain

16. A client is admitted to the emergency department for an opioid overdose. What would you expect the physician to order to reverse the action of an opioid?

    a. Naloxone   c. Corticosteroids

    b. Normeperidine   d. Oxycodone

17. Mr. French, age 80, presents to the emergency department with a fractured ankle and multiple abrasions and contusions. He is admitted to the hospital with an order for oxycodone for pain. Oxycodone may be prescribed for a geriatric client because the drug has which of the following characteristics?

    a. It has a long half-life and will manage bone pain more effectively.

    b. It is metabolized by the liver.

    c. It is excreted by the kidney.

    d. It has a short half-life and is less likely to accumulate, causing toxicity or overdosage.

18. A 4-year-old is admitted to the hospital for a fractured tibia. The parents are fearful because their child may not be able to describe his pain in a manner that is necessary for effective pain management. Which of the following is an accurate statement to include as part of your teaching plan for the parents?

    a. "Your child may behave aggressively or complain verbally of discomfort."

    b. "Your child may not experience pain as intensely as an adult."

    c. "Your child may exhibit only nonverbal behavior."

    d. "Your child may become unusually quiet and noncommunicative."

19. A 32-year-old woman in active labor requests opioid analgesics. Your response should be which of the following?

    a. "Opioids administered during labor and delivery may decrease your pain and speed the progress of your labor."

    b. "Opioids administered during labor and delivery may slow the labor process."

    c. "Opioids administered during labor and delivery may depress fetal and neonatal respiration."

    d. "Opioids administered during labor and delivery may improve fetal and neonatal respiration."

20. Which of the following is an antihypertensive drug that may be used to treat opioid withdrawal?

    a. Clonidine

    b. Hydrochlorothiazide

    c. Lisinopril

    d. Prazosin

CHAPTER 7

Analgesic–Antipyretic–Anti-inflammatory and Related Drugs

■ Section I: Learning Objectives

1. Discuss the role of prostaglandins in the etiology of pain, fever, and inflammation.
2. Discuss aspirin and other nonsteroidal anti-inflammatory drugs (NSAIDs) in terms of mechanism of action, indications for use and contraindications to use, nursing process, and principles of therapy.
3. Compare and contrast aspirin, other NSAIDs, and acetaminophen in terms of indications for use and adverse effects.
4. Differentiate among antiplatelet, analgesic, and anti-inflammatory doses of aspirin.
5. Differentiate between nonselective NSAIDs and the cyclooxygenase-2 inhibitor, celecoxib.
6. Teach clients interventions to prevent or decrease adverse effects of aspirin, other NSAIDs, and acetaminophen.
7. Identify factors influencing the use of aspirin, NSAIDs, and acetaminophen in special populations.
8. Discuss the recognition and management of acetaminophen toxicity.
9. Discuss the use of NSAIDs and antigout drugs.
10. Discuss the use of NSAIDs, triptans, and ergot antimigraine drugs.

■ Section II: Assessing Your Understanding

ACTIVITY A

Fill in the Blank

1. Aspirin, NSAIDs, and acetaminophen can also be called _____.
2. _____ sensitize pain receptors and increase the pain associated with other chemical mediators of inflammation and immunity.
3. Body temperature is controlled by a regulating center in the _____.
4. _____ is the normal body response to tissue damage from any source, and it may occur in any tissue or organ. It is an attempt by the body to remove the damaging agent and repair the damaged tissue.
5. Inflammation may be a component of virtually any illness. Inflammatory conditions affecting organs or systems are often named by adding the suffix –_____ to the involved organ or system.

ACTIVITY B

Matching

Match the term in Column A with the definition in Column B.

COLUMN A

1. _____ Acetaminophen
2. _____ Aspirin
3. _____ Ketorolac
4. _____ Bursitis
5. _____ Rheumatoid arthritis

COLUMN B

A. Injectable NSAID often used for pain
B. Inflammation of the bursa
C. Nonprescription drug commonly used as an aspirin substitute because it does not cause nausea, vomiting, or GI bleeding
D. Chronic, painful, inflammatory disorder that affects the synovial tissue of hinge-like joints, tissues around these joints, and eventually other body organs
E. Prototype of the analgesic–antipyretic–anti-inflammatory drugs and the most commonly used salicylate

ACTIVITY C

Sequencing

Because of multiple reports of liver damage from acetaminophen poisoning, the FDA has strengthened the warning on products containing acetaminophen and emphasized that the maximum adult dose of 4 grams daily, from all sources, should not be exceeded. Given below, in random order, are the symptoms of acetaminophen overdosage. Write them in the correct order, from early onset to end-stage, in the boxes provided.

A. Symptoms may subside, but tests of lever function begin to show increased levels.
B. Anorexia, nausea, vomiting, and diaphoresis may occur.
C. Jaundice, vomiting, and CNS stimulation with excitement and delirium occur.
D. Vascular collapse, coma, and death occur.

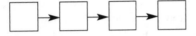

ACTIVITY D

Short Answers

Briefly answer the following questions.

1. Explain how prostaglandins are formed when cellular injury occurs.
2. Describe the role of pyrogens in the febrile process.
3. Identify the systemic manifestations that occur in the inflammatory process.
4. How do aspirin and other NSAIDS reduce inflammation and fever?
5. Aspirin and nonselective NSAIDs are also antiplatelet medications. Describe the antiplatelet process created by ingestion of these drugs.

■ Section III: Applying Your Knowledge

ACTIVITY E

Case Study

Consider the scenario and answer the questions.

Mrs. Anderson presents to her physician's office with long-term joint pain that is interfering with her ability to perform her activities of daily living. She is currently self-administering ibuprofen 400 mg four times a day for pain relief, but the drug is beginning to upset her stomach. The physician diagnoses the client with osteoarthritis and prescribes celecoxib for pain and inflammation. You are responsible for developing an education plan for Mrs. Anderson.

1. Mrs. Anderson asks you to explain why she is in so much pain. Using a model of a joint, explain how DJD causes the pain cycle.
2. Mrs. Anderson is concerned that the new medication will work as well as the ibuprofen. Explain the mechanism of action for COX-2 inhibitors.

■ Section IV: Practicing for NCLEX

Answer the following questions.

1. Mr. Akins presents to the physician's office with inflammation and edema in his left great toe, lasting several days. The physician orders a uric acid level and diagnoses the client with gout. The doctor orders oral colchicine. You are responsible for developing an education plan. Mr. Atkins asks how long it will take for the pain and swelling to subside from his ankle. When colchicine is taken for acute gout, how long does it usually take until pain is relieved?
   a. 7 to 10 days   c. 48 to 72 hours
   b. 24 to 48 hours   d. 3 to 5 days

2. A patient with the diagnosis of chronic gout asks how long he should take his colchicine when he experiences symptoms. Which of the following are the correct instructions for this patient?

   a. Take as directed when pain begins until relief is obtained or nausea, vomiting, and diarrhea occur.

   b. Take for a minimum of 7 to 10 days.

   c. Take for a minimum of 5 to 7 days.

   d. Take as directed when you notice swelling and continue for 7 to 10 days.

3. The patient with chronic gout asks how he can reduce the uric levels in his body when be begins to self-administer colchicine. Which of the following would be your response?

   a. "You should maintain a fluid restriction, drinking no more than 800 to 1000 mL of fluid a day."

   b. "You should increase your caffeine intake; it will help you to eliminate the uric acid crystals."

   c. "Only the medication will reduce the uric acid levels in your body; your fluid intake will not affect the levels."

   d. "Drink 2 to 3 quarts of fluid daily; this will decrease uric acid levels and help prevent formation of uric acid kidney stones."

4. Ms. Ashton complains of a mild headache. The physician orders acetaminophen 325 mg, two tablets by mouth every 4 to 6 hours. Ms. Ashton states that she usually takes ibuprofen for her headaches and asks why the physician ordered acetaminophen. Which of the following explanations would you give?

   a. "Acetaminophen is more effective than ibuprofen for headaches."

   b. "Acetaminophen is less expensive and more efficient for pain relief."

   c. "Acetaminophen is often the initial drug of choice for relieving mild to moderate pain."

   d. "Acetaminophen will reduce the inflammation causing your headache."

5. Mr. Smith's physician orders aspirin 81 mg PO each day as a treatment related to his recent myocardial infarction. The client asks you if he can take acetaminophen instead. Which of the following would be your response?

   a. "Acetaminophen is an effective aspirin substitute for pain or fever but not for prevention of heart attack or stroke."

   b. "Acetaminophen will work just as well; I will call the doctor to notify him of your drug preference."

   c. "Acetaminophen will prevent strokes but not heart attacks."

   d. "You must follow your doctor's order."

6. Celia, age 16, asks you if she can take two Tylenol every 2 hours during exams, because it helps relieve her tension headaches. Which of the following is the most appropriate response?

   a. "Why do you feel so tense regarding exams?"

   b. "Do not exceed recommended doses of acetaminophen due to the risk of life-threatening liver damage."

   c. "Consult your physician."

   d. "Acetaminophen is a benign drug and will relieve your pain."

7. Mr. Adams is taking aspirin 81 mg by mouth each day for prevention of recurrent myocardial infarction. He makes a dentist appointment for a tooth extraction. He calls the physician's office and asks you if he is at risk for bleeding. Which of the following responses is correct?

   a. "Yes, low doses of aspirin may increase your risk of bleeding; I will call you with your new physician's orders."

   b. "No, the dose of aspirin is too low to increase your risk of bleeding."

   c. "Yes, you need to stop the aspirin immediately."

   d. "Your dentist must extract the tooth in a hospital setting to reduce the risk of hemorrhage."

8. Mr. Smith, age 80, presents to the physician's office with complaints of fatigue and a change in the color of his stools. He self-administers ibuprofen 400 mg each night for general discomfort. The physician orders a stool test for guaiac, which yields positive results. The physician discontinues the ibuprofen. You are responsible for a client education plan. Mr. Smith should be educated regarding which of the following as a risk with chronic use of NSAIDs?

   a. GI discomfort   c. GI bleed

   b. GI distress   d. GI upset

9. When an NSAID is given during late pregnancy to prevent premature labor, it may adversely affect the _____ of the fetus.

10. Which of the following is the most effective treatment for a febrile episode in a child aged 6 to 36 months?

   a. Acetaminophen alone

   b. Alternating acetaminophen and ibuprofen every 4 hours over a 3-day period

   c. Ibuprofen alone

   d. Alternating acetaminophen and ibuprofen every 2 hours over a 3-day period

11. Mrs. Sullivan asks why she must consult with her physician when she uses cold products for her children. Your response should be which of the following?

   a. "Your health insurance requires that you notify the physician whenever you administer over-the-counter medications to your children."

   b. "Notification is just a precaution to protect you and your children."

   c. "You really aren't required to do so, it is just a precaution."

   d. "There is a risk of overdose, because acetaminophen is a very common ingredient in OTC cold, flu, fever, and pain remedies."

12. A student nurse asks you why acetaminophen and NSAIDs help to reduce cancer pain. Which of the following is the correct explanation?

   a. Cancer often produces chronic pain from tumor invasion of tissues or complications of treatment. These drugs prevent sensitization of peripheral pain receptors by inhibiting prostaglandin formation.

   b. Cancer rarely produces chronic pain from tumor invasion of tissues or complications of treatment. These drugs eliminate sensitization of peripheral pain receptors by inhibiting prostaglandin formation.

   c. Cancer often produces chronic pain from tumor invasion of tissues or complications of treatment. These drugs potentiate sensitization of peripheral pain receptors by increasing prostaglandin formation.

   d. Cancer rarely produces severe pain from tumor invasion of tissues or complications of treatment. These drugs prevent sensitization of peripheral pain receptors by inhibiting prostaglandin formation.

13. Aspirin increases the risk of bleeding and should generally be avoided for how many weeks before and after surgery?

   a. 3 to 4 weeks   c. 6 to 8 weeks

   b. 1 to 2 weeks   d. 2 to 3 weeks

14. Excessive use of simple analgesics, analgesics containing sedatives or caffeine, triptans, opioids, or ergotamine are believed to play a role in triggering _____.

15. Both categories of migraine abortive drugs (ergot alkaloids and serotonin agonists) exert powerful vasoconstrictive effects and have the potential to do which of the following?

   a. Lower blood pressure

   b. Manage hypertension

   c. Raise blood pressure

   d. Manage hypotension

16. Aspirin is not recommended for children under the age of 15 years due to the risk of _____.

17. Ms. Bean's physician orders an ergot preparation for her migraine headaches. You are responsible for the education plan. Which of the following would be your teaching regarding how the patient is to take her medication?

    a. Take it at the onset of a headache, and lie down in a quiet, darkened room.

    b. Take it when the pain becomes unbearable, so the medication will be more effective.

    c. Take it when sleep alone does not relieve the pain.

    d. Take it whenever you experience a headache.

18. A patient who self-administers the medication butalbital may experience which of the following?

    a. Nausea and vomiting after 6 months of use

    b. Resolution of all headache types

    c. Overuse headaches and withdrawal issues

    d. Weight loss after 6 months of use.

19. Three medications that may be given to reduce serum uric acid levels and prevent joint inflammation and renal calculi are _____, _____, and _____.

20. _____ is a product that helps restore the "shock-absorbing" ability of joint structures.

CHAPTER 8

Antianxiety and Sedative-Hypnotic Drugs

■ Section I: Learning Objectives

1. Discuss the characteristics, sources, and signs and symptoms of anxiety.
2. Discuss the functions of sleep and consequences of sleep deprivation.
3. Describe nondrug interventions to decrease anxiety and insomnia.
4. List characteristics of benzodiazepine antianxiety and hypnotic drugs in terms of mechanism of action, indications for use, nursing process implications, and potential for abuse and dependence.
5. Describe strategies for preventing, recognizing, and treating benzodiazepine withdrawal reactions.
6. Contrast characteristics of selected nonbenzodiazepines and benzodiazepines.
7. Teach clients guidelines for the rational, safe use of antianxiety and sedative-hypnotic drugs.
8. Discuss the use of flumazenil and other treatment measures for overdose of benzodiazepines

■ Section II: Assessing Your Understanding

ACTIVITY A

Fill in the Blank

1. _____ drugs (also known as _____ and _____) promote relaxation, and hypnotics produce sleep.
2. The main drugs used to treat insomnia are the _____ and the _____ hypnotics.
3. _____ is a common disorder that may be referred to as nervousness, tension, worry, or other terms that denote an unpleasant feeling.
4. _____ is a normal response to a stressful situation.
5. _____ is the major inhibitory neurotransmitter in the brain and spinal cord.
6. _____, prolonged difficulty in going to sleep or staying asleep long enough to feel rested, is the most common sleep disorder.

ACTIVITY B

Matching

Match the term in Column A with the definition in Column B.

COLUMN A

1. _____ Hydroxyzine
2. _____ Eszopiclone
3. _____ Chloral hydrate
4. _____ Benzodiazepines
5. _____ Zaleplon

COLUMN B

A. The first oral nonbenzodiazepine hypnotic to be approved for long-term use.

B. Used clinically as antianxiety, hypnotic, and anticonvulsant agents.

C. An antihistamine with sedative and antiemetic properties.

D. Oral nonbenzodiazepine hypnotic approved for the short-term treatment of insomnia.

E. The oldest sedative-hypnotic drug, relatively safe, effective, and inexpensive in usual therapeutic doses.

ACTIVITY C

Short Answers

Briefly answer the following questions.

1. Describe the probable physiological cause for anxiety disorders.
2. Explain the role the serotonin system plays in anxiety.
3. Discuss the impact of sleep on the biologic processes of the body.
4. Define insomnia and discuss the impact of insomnia on the client's health and well-being.
5. Explain the psychological impact that an excessive amount of norepinephrine may have on a client's psychological well-being.

■ Section III: Applying Your Knowledge

ACTIVITY D
Case Studies
Consider the scenarios and answer the questions.

Case Study 1
Mrs. Jones, age 45, suffers from an anxiety disorder. The physician orders buspirone after gradually discontinuing her current benzodiazepine prescription. You develop a teaching plan for Mrs. Jones regarding the administration of the new medication.

1. Mrs. Jones began self-administration of the medication 5 days ago. She calls the physician's office stating that the medication is not working for her. How would you explain the effects of this medication to the patient?
2. Mrs. Jones states that she took her last antianxiety medication to help her sleep; the buspirone is not working as a sleep aid. She asks you why this is so and how the action of buspirone compares with the action of the benzodiazepine prescription that she took in the past. How would you respond?
3. As part of your teaching plan, you explain the possible adverse reactions of buspirone. What are they?

Case Study 2
Mr. Petski, age 35, suffers from long-term insomnia, which is affecting both his work and home life. His profession is high stress, and he complains that he is unable to stop problem-solving when he goes to bed. He had success with short-term hypnotics in the past and asks his physician for a sleep medication. The physician orders eszopiclone. You meet with Mr. Petski to discuss his medication regimen.

1. What information about Mr. Petski's evening habits would indicate an impact on the absorption of the medication as well as its efficacy?
2. Mrs. Petski calls the office stating that her husband appears depressed and anxious. You notify the physician. What is the significance of Mr. Petski's behavior?
3. What change in Mr. Petski's medications or diet may cause adverse reactions?

■ Section IV: Practicing for NCLEX

Answer the following questions.

1. Jane, a college student, is diagnosed with insomnia by her physician. He prescribes eszopiclone for sleep. Jane asks you if she will develop a tolerance to the medication. Which of the following responses is correct?
   a. "If you take the eszopiclone for more than 2 weeks you may develop a tolerance to the hypnotic benefits of the medication and should call your physician."
   b. "During drug testing, tolerance to the hypnotic benefits of eszopiclone was not observed over a 6-month period."
   c. "During drug testing, tolerance to the hypnotic benefits of eszopiclone was observed after administration of the drug for a 6-month period."
   d. "Eszopiclone may be taken indefinitely without tolerance to the hypnotic benefits of the medication."

2. Your patient asks when eszopiclone should be taken to promote sleep. Which of the following is the correct explanation?
   a. Eszopiclone is rapidly absorbed after oral administration, reaching peak plasma levels 30 minutes after administration.
   b. Eszopiclone is rapidly absorbed after oral administration, reaching peak plasma levels 20 minutes after administration.
   c. Eszopiclone is rapidly absorbed after oral administration, reaching peak plasma levels 1 hour after administration.
   d. Eszopiclone is rapidly absorbed after oral administration, reaching peak plasma levels 1 to 2 hours after administration.

3. Mrs. Bright experiences nausea and vomiting whenever she undergoes general anesthesia. Which of the following medications would you expect the physician to order before surgery?
   a. Hydroxyzine   c. Eszopiclone
   b. Ramelton   d. Zaleplon

4. Ms. Dwyers, a 35 year old, is recently divorced and having difficulty coping. She visits her physician, and he diagnoses her with situational anxiety. She is fearful that the anxiety she feels will become chronic. How would you describe situational anxiety to this patient?

   a. A normal response to a stressful situation

   b. An abnormal response to a stressful situation

   c. A method of coping with the divorce

   d. A feeling that will go away on its own

5. Mr. Nickolson's anxiety is interfering with his ability to perform basic activities of daily living and return to work. Which of the following diagnoses will probably be made by his physician?

   a. Intermittent anxiety disorder

   b. Anxiety disorder

   c. Abnormal anxiety disorder

   d. Chronic anxiety disorder

6. Judy S. is prescribed a benzodiazepine for anxiety. She asks you if she can stop the drug when she feels better. Which of the following would be your response?

   a. "Benzodiazepine does not cause physiologic dependence; and withdrawal symptoms will not occur if the drug is stopped abruptly."

   b. "Benzodiazepine may cause physiologic dependence; but withdrawal symptoms will not occur if the drug is stopped abruptly."

   c. "Benzodiazepine may cause physiologic dependence; and withdrawal symptoms will occur if the drug's dosages are tapered."

   d. "Benzodiazepine may cause physiologic dependence; and withdrawal symptoms will occur if the drug is stopped abruptly."

7. Which of the following is the prototype benzodiazepine?

   a. Alprazolam (Xanax)

   b. Diazepam (Valium)

   c. Lorazepam (Ativan)

   d. Clonazepam (Klonopin)

8. The physician orders eszopiclone (Lunesta) for Mr. Jude as a treatment for intermittent insomnia. He states that he feels the prescription works well as a sleep aid, but he is having difficulty with short-term memory loss. Which of the following is this patient experiencing?

   a. An anticipated effect of the drug

   b. An allergic reaction

   c. An adverse reaction

   d. A common side effect

9. Mr. Smith's physician orders ramelton for his long-term insomnia. Mr. Smith is concerned that he will be become dependent on the drug and is hesitant to take it. As part of your teaching plan, you tell Mr. Smith which of the following?

   a. "Ramelton may cause physical dependence."

   b. "Ramelton may cause physical dependence with constant use."

   c. "Ramelton causes physical dependence only if you have a documented sensitivity to the drug."

   d. "Ramelton does not cause physical dependence."

10. Mr. Smith asks, "How long before sleep should I take ramelton?" Which of the following time frames would you give this patient as part of your patient teaching?

    a. 15 minutes   c. 10 minutes

    b. 45 minutes   d. 20 minutes

11. Mr. Peters is prescribed zaleplon for short-term treatment of his insomnia. He states that it only works once in a while. Upon review of his evening habits, you discover which of the following behaviors that may interfere with the absorption of his prescription?

    a. A late, heavy meal before bedtime

    b. Exercise before bedtime

    c. Fasting before bedtime

    d. Doing paperwork before bedtime

12. A combination of zaleplon and alcohol may cause which of the following effects?

    a. Hypertension and respiratory excitement

    b. Respiratory depression and excessive sedation

    c. Cardiac dysrhythmias

    d. A hangover effect

13. Mr. Nobel asks why the over-the-counter drug cimetidine may affect his zaleplon dosage. You state that the physician may need to do which of the following?
    a. Decrease the dose of the zaleplon to 10 mg
    b. Decrease the dose of the zaleplon to 5 mg
    c. Increase the dose of the zaleplon to 15 mg
    d. Increase the dose of the zaleplon to 7 mg

14. Mr. Abernathy is not only having difficulty falling asleep but wakes up frequently during the night. The physician prescribes zolpidem in the CR form. The client asks what makes this form of the drug different. Which of the following explanations would you give the patient?
    a. "Ambien CR contains a slow-releasing layer of medication which aids a person in falling asleep and a second layer which is released rapidly to promote sleep all night."
    b. "Ambien CR contains a rapid-releasing layer of medication which aids a person in falling asleep and a second layer which is also released rapidly to promote sleep all night."
    c. "Ambien CR contains a slow-releasing layer of medication which aids a person in falling asleep and a second layer which is released even more slowly to promote sleep all night."
    d. "Ambien CR contains a rapid-releasing layer of medication which aids a person in falling asleep and a second layer which is released more slowly to promote sleep all night."

15. Mr. Diaz took zolpidem daily for 1 week with good response, then stopped the medication. Two days later, he returns to the physician's office stating that his insomnia is worse than it ever was. You are responsible for the development of a teaching plan for the client, including adverse reactions. After 1 week of regular use, which of the following adverse reactions may occur with zolpidem?
    a. Chronic insomnia
    b. Short-term insomnia
    c. Rebound insomnia
    d. Long-term insomnia

16. Mrs. Rodriguez's physician prescribes alprazolam in addition to the client's antidepressant fluvoxamine. The nurse knows that the physician will modify the benzodiazepine dose by doing which of the following?
    a. Reducing the dose by 50%
    b. Increasing the dose by 25%
    c. Tapering the initial doses of the medication
    d. Increasing the dose by 5%

17. Mr. Anspa, age 70, asks why he is receiving a lower dose of zaleplon than his son. As part of your teaching plan, which of the following explanations would you give?
    a. "Older adults metabolize the drug more quickly, but due to renal dysfunction, the medication must be reduced."
    b. "Older adults metabolize the drug more slowly, and half-lives are longer than in younger adults."
    c. "Older adults metabolize the drug at the same speed as younger adults; I will check the dosage with your physician."
    d. "Older adults do not need as much of the medication for the desired effect as a younger adult does."

18. As a medication nurse, you know that when benzodiazepines are used with opioid analgesics, the analgesic dose should be adjusted in which of the following ways?
    a. It should be increased initially and reduced gradually.
    b. It should be reduced initially and increased gradually.
    c. It should be reduced initially and incrementally thereafter.
    d. It should be increased initially and incrementally thereafter.

19. Mrs. Diaz's physician prescribes a long-acting antianxiety benzodiazepine. She asks why she should take the medication at night when the morning is more convenient. Which of the following teachings would you include in the education plan for Mrs. Diaz?

    a. "If you take the medication in the morning, then you may have difficulty remaining awake at work."

    b. "If you take the medication in the morning, you may have increased anxiety during the day."

    c. "This schedule promotes sleep, and there is usually enough residual sedation to maintain antianxiety effects throughout the next day."

    d. "This schedule is prescribed by the physician and therefore must be followed."

20. _____ is a specific antidote that competes with benzodiazepines for benzodiazepine receptors and reverses toxicity.

CHAPTER 9

Antipsychotic Drugs

■ Section I: Learning Objectives

1. Discuss common manifestations of psychotic disorders, including schizophrenia.
2. Discuss characteristics of phenothiazines and related antipsychotics.
3. Compare characteristics of "atypical" antipsychotic drugs with those of "typical" phenothiazines and related antipsychotic drugs.
4. Describe the main elements of the acute and long-term treatment of psychotic disorders.
5. State interventions to decrease adverse effects of antipsychotic drugs.
6. State interventions to promote compliance with outpatient use of antipsychotic drugs.

■ Section II: Assessing Your Understanding

ACTIVITY A

Fill in the Blank

1. Antipsychotic drugs are used mainly for the treatment of _____.
2. _____ are sensory perceptions of people or objects that are not present in the external environment.
3. _____ are false beliefs that persist in the absence of reason or evidence.
4. Deluded people often believe that other people control their thoughts, feelings, and behaviors or seek to harm them; these beliefs are called _____.
5. Antipsychotic drugs, called _____, are derived from several chemical groups.

ACTIVITY B

Matching

Match the term in Column A with the definition in Column B.

COLUMN A

1. _____ Chlorpromazine
2. _____ Neuroleptic malignant syndrome
3. _____ Extrapyramidal side effects
4. _____ Anticholinergic side effects
5. _____ Antiadrenergic effects

COLUMN B

A. Acute dystonia, parkinsonism, and akathisia
B. The first drug to effectively treat psychotic disorders
C. Blurred vision, constipation, dry mouth, photophobia, tachycardia, and urinary hesitancy
D. Orthostatic hypotension and CNS depression
E. A rare but potentially fatal adverse effect, characterized by rigidity

ACTIVITY C

Short Answers

Briefly answer the following questions.

1. Discuss the signs and symptoms that a patient may experience with the diagnosis of *psychosis* and their impact on the patient's ability to perform activities of daily living and interact within home and work environments?
2. Identify and discuss the factors that may precipitate an acute psychotic episode.
3. Discuss the neurodevelopmental model in relation to the development of schizophrenia.

4. Discuss the role of genetics in the development of schizophrenia.

5. Discuss the impact that the negative symptoms of *schizophrenia* have on a client's ability to cope within home and work environments.

■ Section III: Applying Your Knowledge

ACTIVITY D

Case Studies

Consider the scenarios and answer the questions.

Case Study 1

Mr. Smith is prescribed clozapine by his physician. You are responsible for his education plan.

1. Mr. Smith asks you whether he will have the same extrapyramidal effects with clozapine that he had with his other antipsychotic medication. How would you reply?

2. Explain the rationale for weekly laboratory tests for this client.

3. Mr. Smith returns to the office weekly for his blood work. During an interview 1 month later, he states that he feels able to cope within his environment but gets dizzy often. Discuss the elements of your focused assessment and explain your rationale for this assessment.

Case Study 2

Ms. Case, age 35, is diagnosed with psychosis after an assessment by a psychiatrist in conjunction with her physician. She visits the physician's office with her mother. The physician orders haloperidol. You are responsible for the education plan for this family.

1. Ms. Case's mother states that her daughter is often noncompliant with her medication. After you report this to the physician, how may the medication administration of haloperidol be changed to improve compliance?

2. You discuss signs and symptoms of the extrapyramidal effects of haloperidol. Explain the signs and symptoms in layman's terms.

■ Section IV: Practicing for NCLEX

Answer the following questions.

1. A client who is taking antipsychotic medication presents to the emergency room with symptoms of dyspnea, delirium, tachycardia, and respiratory distress. The physician's initial diagnosis is neuroleptic malignant syndrome. You expect physician's orders for which of the following treatment modalities? (Select all that apply.)

a. Hydration, cooling measures, and benzodiazepines to reduce agitation,

b. Dantrolene to directly relax muscles

c. CNS depressants

d. Bronchodilators

2. Tardive dyskinesia, a late extrapyramidal effect, is generally considered to be irreversible. What is one method used to treat tardive dyskinesia?

a. Increasing the dosage of the medication

b. Discontinuing the medication abruptly

c. Referring the client to a psychiatrist for evaluation

d. Reducing the dosage

3. Mrs. Swett consults her physician because she can't seem to sit still. She is currently taking antipsychotic medications. Her symptoms may be treated with which of the following agents?

a. Cardiotonics   c. Beta-blockers

b. Antihistamines   d. Antiepileptics

4. Mrs. Sage makes an appointment with her physician 2 weeks after beginning her prescription antipsychotic therapy. She states that she is still unable to cope and concentrate at work. Which of the following statements would be appropriate to include in your teaching?

a. "Antipsychotics may take several weeks to achieve maximum therapeutic effect."

b. "The medication should be effective by this time; I will consult the physician."

c. "This medication may need to be changed; I will consult the physician."

d. "Therapeutic effects of antipsychotics should be evaluated every 2 weeks by your physician."

5. The physician prescribed antipsychotic medication for Ms. Janz 2 months ago. She is noncompliant with her medication regimen and is symptomatic. You are responsible for developing a plan of care to facilitate medication compliance. Which of the following would your plan include?

   a. A written contract to ensure compliance

   b. Coordination of the efforts of several health and social service agencies or providers

   c. Immediate hospitalization for medication noncompliance lasting 1 week

   d. Administration of daily oral medications by the community health nurse

6. Mr. Dowe is admitted to your mental health unit with symptoms of acute psychosis. The physician orders haloperidol IV by bolus injection. The dose depends on the severity of the agitation. What initial dose would you expect the physician to order?

   a. 7 to 10 mg   c. 2 to 4 mg

   b. 3 to 5 mg   d. 0.5 to 10 mg

7. Mr. Bagman is admitted to your emergency department via ambulance. He is attempting to pull out his IV line and is exhibiting symptoms of agitation and thrashing about. The physician orders a benzodiazepine-type sedative. What information is needed prior to administration of the drug?

   a. Whether the client has a history of agitation

   b. Whether the client is currently taking antibiotics

   c. Whether the client is experiencing drug intoxication or withdrawal

   d. Whether the client is currently taking a diuretic

8. Mr. Bath's physician orders antipsychotic medications for him. He experiences little or no side effects from the medications and is able to function successfully in both his home and work environments. Six weeks later he is diagnosed with hepatitis B. He begins to experience adverse reactions to his medications. A possible reason for the adverse reactions might be that, in the presence of liver disease, which of the following may happen?

   a. Metabolism may be accelerated and drug elimination half-lives shortened, causing an increased risk of adverse effects.

   b. Metabolism may be slowed and drug elimination half-lives shortened, with resultant accumulation and increased risk of adverse effects.

   c. Metabolism may be slowed and drug elimination half-lives prolonged, with resultant accumulation and increased risk of adverse effects.

   d. Metabolism may be accelerated and drug elimination half-lives prolonged, with resultant accumulation and increased risk of adverse effects.

9. Ms. Anspar is diagnosed with renal insufficiency. You develop a teaching plan based on her diagnosis and antipsychotic drug usage. She asks you why it is so important to have renal function tests routinely. You reply that, if renal function test results become abnormal, which of the following may be a consequence?

   a. The drug may need to be lowered in dosage or discontinued.

   b. The drug will be discontinued immediately.

   c. The drug will be continued with caution.

   d. The drug dosages will be increased to increase absorption.

10. Mr. Rhodes presents at the physician's office with yellow sclera. He is concerned that he has hepatitis. Mr. Rhodes began a new medication regimen about 1 month ago that includes phenothiazines. He states that the medications work well for him. Jaundice associated with phenothiazine administration is considered to be which of the following?

    a. An adverse reaction

    b. A hypersensitivity reaction

    c. A rare occurrence

    d. A life-threatening occurrence

11. Mr. Adams, an African American man, routinely takes haloperidol to manage his psychosis. Recently, he presented to the physician's office with signs of tardive dyskinesia, and his physician modified the drug regimen over time. Mr. Adams will now take the drug olanzapine and discontinue the haloperidol. To reduce his fears, you could tell this patient which of the following?

    a. "The signs of tardive dyskinesia will diminish over time."

    b. "African Americans always experience tardive dyskinesia with antipsychotics."

    c. "When compared with haloperidol, olanzapine has been associated with fewer extrapyramidal reactions in African Americans."

    d. "The olanzapine does not produce side effects in African American males."

12. Mrs. Keys is diagnosed with Alzheimer-type dementia. She resides in a long-term care facility. Mrs. Keys' daughter asks the physician to prescribe an antipsychotic to control her mother's outbursts of anger and depression. The physician orders a psychiatric consultation for the client. Mrs. Keys' daughter asks, "Why doesn't the doctor just order an antipsychotic?" You explain the decision by saying which of the following?

    a. "Clients with dementia routinely become agitated due to their disease process."

    b. "Clients with dementia respond poorly to antipsychotic medications."

    c. "Clients with dementia respond well to antipsychotic medications."

    d. "Use of antipsychotic drugs exposes clients to adverse drug effects and does not resolve underlying problems."

13. Mrs. Keys' physician orders a low-dose antipsychotic to manage her acute agitation. Her daughter states that her mother is improved but her cognitive functions are the same, if not worse, than last month. Which of the following is the explanation for this development?

    a. Antipsychotics cause a gradual return of cognitive ability.

    b. Antipsychotics reduce memory loss.

    c. Antipsychotics increase the risk of long-term memory loss.

    d. Antipsychotics do not improve memory loss and may further impair cognitive functioning.

14. Jane Nils is 9 years old and receives antipsychotics to manage her disease. Jane's mother asks why her daughter receives such a high dose of the medication compared with an adult. Which of the following explanations is correct?

    a. Children usually have a slower metabolic rate than adults and may therefore require relatively high doses for their size and weight.

    b. Children usually have a faster metabolic rate than adults and may therefore require relatively low doses for their size and weight.

    c. Children usually have a faster metabolic rate than adults and may therefore require relatively high doses for their height and weight.

    d. Children usually have a faster metabolic rate than adults and may therefore require relatively high doses for their size and weight.

15. Mr. Ghee is scheduled for major abdominal surgery in the morning. He is concerned that he is receiving a lower than normal dose of his antipsychotic. You explain that antipsychotics may do which of the following?

    a. Potentiate the effects of general anesthetics

    b. Diminish the effects of general anesthetics

    c. Cause increased tardive dyskinesia when used with anesthetics

    d. Cause a hypertensive crisis when combined with anesthetics

16. Acute dystonia is manifested by which of the following? (Select all that apply.)

    a. Severe spasms of muscles of the face, neck, tongue, or back

    b. Oculogyric crisis

    c. Opisthotonus

    d. Anuria

    e. Hypoxia

17. Acute dystonia is treated with intramuscular or intravenous administration of which of the following agents?

    a. Cardiotonics

    b. Diphenhydramine

    c. Cholinergic medications

    d. Narcan

18. _____ is approved for the treatment of schizophrenia and acute mania associated with bipolar disorder. It is the first in a new category of drugs called partial dopamine agonists.

19. A/An _____ is a drug that has the ability to block a receptor if it is overstimulated and to stimulate a receptor if it is understimulated.

20. Mr. Sikes takes quetiapine for his bipolar disease. His physician orders cimetidine for his GI distress. When used in conjunction with quetiapine, the cimetidine dose will be adjusted in which of the following ways?

a. Increased

b. Decreased

c. Remain the same

d. Titrated based on the client's WBC count

CHAPTER 10

Antidepressants and Mood Stabilizers

■ Section I: Learning Objectives

1. Describe the major features of depression and bipolar disorder.
2. Discuss the characteristics of antidepressants in terms of mechanism of action, indications for use, adverse effects, principles of therapy, and nursing process implications.
3. Compare and contrast the various categories of antidepressants: selective serotonin reuptake inhibitors (SSRIs), tricyclic antidepressants (TCAs), mixed serotonin-norepinephrine reuptake inhibitors (SNRIs), monoamine oxidase inhibitors (MAOIs), and other atypical antidepressants.
4. Discuss selected characteristics of atypical antidepressants.
5. Describe the use of lithium in bipolar disorder.
6. Describe the use of atypical antipsychotics in the manic phase of bipolar disorder.
7. Discuss interventions to increase the safety of lithium therapy.
8. Describe the nursing role in preventing, recognizing, and treating overdoses of antidepressant drugs and lithium.
9. Analyze important factors in using antidepressant drugs and lithium in special populations.

■ Section II: Assessing Your Understanding

ACTIVITY A

Fill in the Blank

1. _____ _____ is a major depressive episode occurring after the birth of a child.
2. _____ _____ is associated with impaired ability to function in usual activities and relationships.

3. _____ _____ _____ ____ is characterized by episodes of major depression plus mania and occurs equally in men and women.
4. _____ _____ _____ ____ is characterized by episodes of major depression plus hypomanic episodes and occurs more frequently in women.
5. The average depressive episode lasts about _____ _____.

ACTIVITY B

Matching

Match the term in Column A with the definition in Column B.

COLUMN A

1. _____ SSRIs
2. _____ TCAs
3. _____ MAOIs
4. _____ SNRIs
5. _____ Antidepressants

COLUMN B

A. Considered to be third-line medications in the treatment of depression because of a high incidence of food and drug interactions that can potentially lead to hypertensive crisis
B. Second-line medications in the treatment of depression, producing a high incidence of adverse effects
C. Similar to SSRIs in terms of therapeutic effects but produce more anticholinergic, CNS sedation, and cardiac conduction abnormalities
D. Must be taken for 2 to 4 weeks before depressive symptoms improve
E. Considered to be first-line medications in the treatment of depression because they have a more favorable side effect profile

ACTIVITY C

Short Answers

Briefly answer the following questions.

1. Discuss the methods used to prevent antidepressant toxicity and the interventions used to treat toxicity.
2. For clients with certain concurrent medical conditions, antidepressants may have adverse effects. Discuss disease-specific adverse reactions related to antidepressants.
3. Why is lithium considered the drug of choice for bipolar disorder?
4. Dosages of antidepressant drugs should be individualized according to clinical response. Discuss the method of dosage adjustment used with SSRIs and venlafaxine.
5. Discuss both the causes and the signs and symptoms of serotonin syndrome.

■ Section III: Applying Your Knowledge

ACTIVITY D

Case Studies

Consider the scenarios and answer the questions.

Case Study 1

Ms. Roth cares for her 70-year-old mother, Millie, in her home. Until recently, Millie was an active member of the household, often helped with the grandchildren's homework, and served as a member of the local senior center. However, since Millie underwent abdominal surgery for a small-bowel obstruction and experienced a routine recovery 1 month ago, she has been refusing to eat and shows little interest in her environment or her grandchildren. The physician prescribes an antidepressant for Millie and orders follow-up care with the community health nurse.

1. One week later, you visit the home. Ms. Roth reports that her mother is the same and states that a larger dose of the antidepressant may be needed. How would you respond?
2. One month later, the physician increases the dose of the antidepressant. What behaviors should the family recognize and report to the physician?

Case Study 2

Mr. Jones' physician ordered fluoxetine 2 months ago for a diagnosis of situational depression. Mr. Jones arrives at the physician's office in an agitated state and complains of chronic insomnia. The physician orders discontinuance of the antidepressant, as recommended by the PDR.

1. What other signs and symptoms might Mr. Jones describe when you take a detailed history before his appointment with the physician?
2. You meet with Mr. Jones 1 week later. He states that he still is experiencing insomnia and agitation. How would you explain this?

■ Section IV: Practicing for NCLEX

Answer the following questions.

1. Mrs. Nate is prescribed fluoxetine during the third trimester of her pregnancy for depression. After birth, her child exhibits symptoms of neonatal withdrawal syndrome. When would you expect the symptoms to abate?
   a. In a few days
   b. After 6 weeks
   c. In a few hours
   d. With administration of fluoxetine

2. Mr. Finch takes an SSRI for his depression. He discontinues the SSRI and asks why he cannot begin his prescription for an MAOI immediately. You respond that combination therapy may cause _____.

3. Children, adolescents, and young adults ages 18 to 24 may have an increased risk of which of the following effects when taking antidepressant medications?
   a. Manic episodes   c. Somnolence
   b. Suicidal episodes   d. Postural hypotension

4. Bipolar disorder type II is characterized by episodes of major depression plus hypomanic episodes and occurs more frequently in which of the following categories of patients?
   a. Men   c. Women
   b. Children   d. The elderly

5. Mr. Gatz, age 35, is slowly recovering from an abdominal aortic aneurysm repair and cerebral vascular accident 6 weeks ago. His physical condition is unstable at this time. His physician prescribes a low-dose antidepressant for him based on a diagnosis of situational depression. Mr. Gatz's wife asks if a higher dose might be more beneficial. Which of the following would you teach the family regarding this patient's dosage?

   a. Dosage is based on the client's diagnosis.

   b. Dosage must be titrated based on the client's weight.

   c. A higher dose may cause postural hypertension.

   d. Dosage must be cautious and slow and the client's responses carefully monitored.

6. Mr. Alexander has a history of hepatic dysfunction secondary to alcoholism. Based on Mr. Alexander's diagnostic history, which of the following would you expect his physician to order?

   a. A higher dose of the antidepressant

   b. A lower dose of the antidepressant

   c. More frequent doses of the antidepressant

   d. No antidepressants, because they would be contraindicated for this client

7. Which of the following are the antidepressant drugs of choice for older adults?

   a. SSRIs

   b. TCAs

   c. MAOIs

   d. Older adults should not receive antidepressant medications

8. Which of the following antidepressant medications would *not* be a drug of choice for an adolescent?

   a. SSRIs   c. MAOIs

   b. TCAs   d. ACE inhibitors

9. If a TCA is prescribed for a child older than 12 years of age, which of the following tests would routinely be ordered by the physician?

   a. CBC and chemistry panel and plasma drug levels

   b. Hemoglobin and hematocrit and plasma drug levels

   c. Chest x-ray and plasma drug levels

   d. Blood pressure, ECG, and plasma drug levels

10. Mr. Haven asks the physician for antidepressant therapy for his son James, age 14. The physician orders a psychiatric consultation before prescribing medication, for which of the following reasons?

    a. It is unsafe to administer antidepressants to an adolescent without a psychiatric consultation.

    b. It is probably best to reserve drug therapy for those who do not respond to nonpharmacologic treatments such as cognitive behavioral therapy.

    c. A definitive diagnosis has not been established.

    d. Adolescents require higher doses of antidepressants than adults do.

11. Mr. Murphy, an African American, is prescribed a TCA for his depression. He asks you why the dose he receives is lower than that of his Caucasian friend. Which of the following responses is correct?

    a. African Americans tend to metabolize TCAs more slowly than Caucasian do.

    b. African Americans tend to metabolize TCAs more quickly than Caucasian do.

    c. African Americans experience side effects with higher doses.

    d. African Americans experience suicidal ideation with higher doses.

12. Mrs. Ball's bipolar disorder symptoms have been successfully managed with lithium for many years. She is scheduled for a CABG and is instructed to stop her lithium 1 to 2 days before surgery and resume when full oral intake of food and fluids is allowed. She asks why she must stop the medication. Which of the following explanations would you give?
    a. "You will not have bipolar symptoms during surgery or immediately afterward because of the anesthetics."
    b. "Lithium will cause hypertension during surgery."
    c. "Lithium may prolong the effects of anesthetics and neuromuscular blocking drugs."
    d. "Lithium may cause cardiac complications during surgery."

13. Ms. Meese discontinues her SSRI abruptly. Which of the following signs and symptoms of withdrawal would you expect to see when she arrives at the physician's office 1 week later? (Select all that apply.)
    a. Dizziness
    b. Lethargy or anxiety/hyperarousal
    c. Chest pain
    d. Headache
    e. Gastrointestinal upset

14. Mr. Janis presents to your emergency department with tactile hallucinations, choreiform movements, and convulsions. His wife states that he may have overdosed on lithium. Treatment may include which of the following? (Select all that apply.)
    a. Correction of fluid and electrolyte imbalances
    b. Hemodialysis
    c. Administration of Narcan
    d. Medication-induced coma

15. How frequently should the serum concentration of lithium be monitored when therapy is initiated?
    a. Monthly in the morning, 12 hours after the last dose of lithium
    b. Four times weekly in the morning, 12 hours after the last dose of lithium
    c. Weekly in the morning, 12 hours after the last dose of lithium
    d. Two or three times weekly in the morning, 12 hours after the last dose of lithium

16. Dosages of antidepressant drugs should be individualized according to _____ _____.

17. Mr. Smith wishes to discontinue his antidepressant secondary to sexual dysfunction. Which of the following antidepressant medications may be ordered by his physician because it does not interfere with sexual function?
    a. Mirtazapine   c. Duloxetine
    b. Bupropion   d. Venlafaxine

18. Because the available drugs have similar efficacy in treating depression, the choice of an antidepressant depends on which of the following factors? (Select all that apply.)
    a. Cost
    b. Age
    c. Gender
    d. Medical conditions
    e. The specific drug's adverse effects

19. Mr. Jones is taking warfarin and presents to the physician's office with calf pain and a positive Homan's sign. He tells the physician that he has been depressed lately and is taking an herbal remedy. Which of the following herbal antidepressants may reduce the effectiveness of his warfarin?
    a. St. John's wort   c. Watercress
    b. Feverfew   d. Wallwort

20. _____ is a naturally occurring metallic salt that is used in clients with bipolar disorder, mainly to treat and prevent manic episodes.

CHAPTER 11

Antiseizure Drugs

■ Section I: Learning Objectives

1. Identify types and potential causes of seizures.
2. Discuss major factors that influence the choice of an antiseizure drug for a client with a seizure disorder.
3. Recognize characteristics and effects of commonly used antiseizure drugs.
4. Differentiate between older and more recent antiseizure drugs.
5. Compare advantages and disadvantages of monotherapy and combination drug therapy for seizure disorders.
6. Apply the nursing process with clients receiving antiseizure drugs.
7. Describe strategies for prevention and treatment of status epilepticus.
8. Discuss the use of antiseizure drugs in special populations.

■ Section II: Assessing Your Understanding

ACTIVITY A

Fill in the Blank

1. A _____ involves a brief episode of abnormal electrical activity in nerve cells of the brain that may or may not be accompanied by visible changes in appearance or behavior.
2. A _____ is a tonic-clonic type of seizure characterized by spasmodic contractions of involuntary muscles.
3. A/An _____ is also called an antiepileptic drug (AED) or an anticonvulsant.
4. When seizures occur in a chronic, recurrent pattern, they characterize a disorder known as _____.
5. _____ _____ begin in a specific area of the brain and often indicate a localized brain lesion such as birth injury, trauma, stroke, or tumor.

ACTIVITY B

Matching

Match the term in Column A with the definition in Column B.

COLUMN A

1. _____ Ethosuximide
2. _____ Diazepam
3. _____ Phenytoin
4. _____ Fosphenytoin
5. _____ Carbamazepine

COLUMN B

A. The prototype and one of the oldest and most widely used AEDs.
B. The AED of choice for absence seizures; may be used with other AEDs for treatment of mixed types of seizures
C. A water-soluble prodrug formulation that is rapidly hydrolyzed to phenytoin after IV or IM injection
D. A benzodiazepine used in seizure disorders
E. Used to treat trigeminal neuralgia and bipolar disorder

ACTIVITY C

Short Answers

Briefly answer the following questions.

1. Discuss the probable causes for seizure activity in a client.
2. Describe the characteristics of epilepsy.
3. Describe the causes of epilepsy for a child and an adult.
4. Describe the difference between the tonic and clonic phases of a seizure.
5. What is the difference between a tonic-clonic seizure and an absence seizure?

■ Section III: Applying Your Knowledge

ACTIVITY D
Case Studies
Consider the scenarios and answer the questions.

Case Study 1
Mr. Alphonse is on a business trip to your state. He is brought to the emergency department unconscious with tonic-clonic seizures lasting for several minutes. You find an empty bottle of anticonvulsants in his brief case. The physician diagnoses Mr. Alphonse with status epilepticus.

1. Identify what other life-threatening signs and symptoms of status epilepticus you must recognize and report to the physician for prompt treatment.
2. What is the probable cause of Mr. Alphonse's seizure activity?

Case Study 2
Ms. Jones is recovering from an operable brain tumor. Her seizures were managed in the hospital with phenytoin. You are responsible for her predischarge education plan.

1. Ms. Jones asks if she can modify the dosage times from every 12 hours to every 8 to 12 hours, because she does not want to interrupt her sleep habits. How would you respond?
2. You teach Ms. Jones to report adverse effects to her physician. What are the adverse effects of phenytoin?
3. Ms. Jones asks you if she can switch to the brand name for the phenytoin when she returns home. How would you answer?

■ Section IV: Practicing for NCLEX

Answer the following questions.

1. Which of the following are causes of seizures classified as secondary? (Select all that apply.)
   a. Tumors
   b. Metabolic disorders
   c. Anginal episode
   d. Withdrawal of alcohol or sedative-hypnotic drugs

2. As a community health nurse, you begin education with the client and family by requesting that they keep a diary of the occurrence of seizures. This is important because the diary may assist the physician to do which of the following?
   a. Titrate the AEDs
   b. Estimate client compliance with medication
   c. Include the client in the decision-making process
   d. Keep the client and the family focused on the symptoms of the disease process

3. The community health nurse also assists the physician in the decision-making process for AED drug titration by performing which of the following functions?
   a. Counting the number of pills in the AED drug bottle to ensure compliance
   b. Administering the AED medication to the client
   c. Ensuring that the client makes the appointments for serum drug levels
   d. Monitoring the client for signs and symptoms of seizure activity during the monthly visit

4. Which of the following is a possible effect of phenytoin administered along with continuous nasogastric enteral feedings?
   a. Increasing absorption of the AED
   b. Decreasing the absorption of the AED
   c. Not affecting absorption of the AED
   d. Precipitating signs of overdosage

5. Which of the following is a sign of phenytoin toxicity?
   a. Seizure activity   c. Memory loss
   b. Loss of concentration   d. Nystagmus

6. A patient with hepatitis develops a seizure disorder. The physician would most likely modify the dosage in which of the following ways? (Select all that apply.)
   a. Reducing the dose
   b. Increasing the dose
   c. Giving the medication more frequently
   d. Giving the medication less frequently

7. What is the drug of choice for a newborn with seizure activity?

   a. IM phenobarbital   c. IM phenytoin

   b. IV phenobarbital   d. PO phenytoin

8. Which of the following signs and symptoms must a parent be alert for in a young school-age child with a seizure disorder taking AEDs?

   a. Poor study habits related to lack of concentration

   b. Hyperactivity and inability to concentrate

   c. Excessive sedation and interference with learning and social development

   d. Anger and agitation in the classroom setting

9. Older adults are at high risk for adverse drug effects and adverse drug–drug interactions with AEDs due to which of the following factors? (Select all that apply.)

   a. Multiple medical conditions

   b. Multiple drugs

   c. Decreased protein binding and liver and kidney function

   d. Rapid absorption of AEDs

10. The older adult taking AEDs has an increased risk for which of the following conditions?

    a. Falls   c. Cardiac dysfunction

    b. Seizure activity   d. Renal dysfunction

11. Older adults taking carbamazepine may develop _____, especially if they also take sodium-losing diuretics (e.g., furosemide, hydrochlorothiazide).

12. Mr. Rich presents in the emergency department with tonic-clonic seizure activity. What is the IV drug of choice for treatment to obtain rapid control of the seizure?

    a. Topiramate   c. Zonegran

    b. Valproic acid   d. Benzodiazepine

13. The physician prescribes oxcarbazepine for Mrs. Smith. What information should be included in the education plan for this patient if she relies on oral contraceptives?

    a. It increases the effectiveness of the oral contraceptive, and the dosage should be reduced.

    b. It is contraindicated with oral contraceptives, and the contraceptive should be discontinued.

    c. It does not affect the absorption of the oral contraceptive.

    d. It decreases effectiveness oral contraceptives, and a barrier type of contraception is recommended.

14. The effectiveness of drug therapy is evaluated primarily by which of the following methods?

    a. Client response in terms of therapeutic or adverse effects

    b. Serum drug levels

    c. Physician evaluation every 3 months

    d. Routine EEGs

15. Mrs. Lopez's seizure disorder has been successfully controlled by AEDs for years. She and her husband decide that it is time to start a family. She asks you if it is safe for the fetus for her to continue her AEDs as prescribed. What should you tell her about AEDs?

    a. They are safe during pregnancy.

    b. They are considered teratogenic.

    c. They may interfere with conception.

    d. They are contraindicated during the third trimester.

16. _____ (_____) is chemically a sulfonamide and is contraindicated for use in clients who are allergic to sulfonamides.

17. Which of the following medications may be used for both bipolar and seizure disorders?

    a. Topiramate   c. Zonegran

    b. Valproic acid   d. Benzodiazepine

18. Mr. Hickey, a licensed practical nurse, is prescribed topiramate for a seizure disorder. He asks you how long he needs to take the medication to achieve a steady-state concentration. He is concerned that his seizure activity will not be controlled when he returns home from the hospital. Which of the following is an appropriate response?

    a. "The average elimination half-life is about 21 hours, and steady-state concentrations are reached in about 4 days with normal renal function."

    b. "The average elimination half-life is about 8 hours, and steady-state concentrations are reached in about 2 days with normal renal function."

    c. "The average elimination half-life is about 48 hours, and steady-state concentrations are reached in about 8 days with normal renal function."

    d. "The average elimination half-life is about 15 hours, and steady-state concentrations are reached in about 3 days with normal renal function."

19. Ms. Raman suffers from severe and frequent seizure activity. Her physician prescribes levetiracetam. She asks why this drug will be more effective than the other drugs that she has taken in the past. Which of the following would be your response?

    a. Levetiracetam reaches steady-state plasma concentrations after 1 day of twice-daily administration.

    b. Levetiracetam reaches steady-state plasma concentrations after 2 days of twice-daily administration.

    c. Levetiracetam reaches steady-state plasma concentrations after 3 days of twice-daily administration.

    d. Levetiracetam reaches steady-state plasma concentrations after 5 days of twice-daily administration.

20. _____ (_____) is commonly used to treat chronic pain syndromes, including neuropathies (i.e., diabetic and others).

CHAPTER 12

Antiparkinson Drugs

■ Section I: Learning Objectives

1. Describe major characteristics of Parkinson's disease.
2. Differentiate between the types of commonly used antiparkinson drugs.
3. Discuss therapeutic and adverse effects of dopaminergic and anticholinergic drugs.
4. Discuss the use of antiparkinson drugs in selected populations.
5. Apply the nursing process in clients experiencing parkinsonism.

■ Section II: Assessing Your Understanding

ACTIVITY A

Fill in the Blank

1. _____ _____ is a chronic, progressive, degenerative disorder of the central nervous system (CNS) characterized by resting tremor, bradykinesia, rigidity, and postural instability.
2. Idiopathic parkinsonism results from progressive destruction of or degenerative changes in dopamine-producing nerve cells in the _____ _____ of the _____ _____; the area in the midbrain that controls smooth voluntary movement.
3. The first symptom of Parkinson's disease is often a _____ _____ that begins in the fingers and thumb of one hand (pill-rolling movements).
4. Drugs used in Parkinson's disease help correct the neurotransmitter imbalance by _____ levels of dopamine.
5. Dopaminergic drugs _____ the amount of dopamine in the brain by various mechanisms.

ACTIVITY B

Matching

Match the term in Column A with the definition in Column B.

COLUMN A

1. _____ Selegiline
2. _____ Bromocriptine
3. _____ Levodopa
4. _____ Carbidopa
5. _____ Amantadine

COLUMN B

A. Ergot derivative that directly stimulates dopamine receptors in the brain
B. Inhibits the enzyme AADC
C. Inhibits metabolism of dopamine by monoamine oxidase
D. Synthetic antiviral agent initially used to prevent influenza A virus
E. Most effective drug available for the treatment of Parkinson's disease

ACTIVITY C

Short Answers

Briefly answer the following questions.

1. Explain the roles of dopamine and acetylcholine in Parkinson's disease.
2. Describe the symptoms of Parkinson's disease.
3. Discuss the rationale for the administration of antiparkinson drugs to alleviate the symptoms of Parkinson's disease.
4. Why has the FDA issued a black box warning regarding selegiline-transdermal?
5. For what reason is levodopa contraindicated in narrow-angle glaucoma?

■ Section III: Applying Your Knowledge

ACTIVITY D
Case Studies

Consider the scenarios and answer the questions.

Case Study 1

Mrs. Genus is diagnosed with idiopathic parkinsonism, and her physician prescribes both levodopa and, as an adjunct therapy, rasagiline. You develop an education plan regarding her drug regimen.

1. Mrs. Genus asks why she must take both drugs, when levodopa works well for her with periodic off times. What answer would you give her?
2. Mrs. Genus asks if she needs to modify her diet. How would you respond?
3. Mrs. Genus' physician tapers her fluoxetine and will discontinue it before beginning the rasagiline. Explain the rationale behind the discontinuance of the medication.

Case Study 2

Mrs. Piney presents to her physician's office with insomnia. The physician diagnoses the client with Ekbom's syndrome and orders ropinirole. You are responsible for the development of an education plan regarding her new diagnosis and drug regimen.

1. Mrs. Piney asks you, "What are the symptoms of Ekbom's syndrome?" What do you tell her?
2. She asks, "Why do I have to take another drug? Will it really help?" What explanation would you give the patient?

■ Section IV: Practicing for NCLEX

Answer the following questions.

1. Classic symptoms of Parkinson's disease include which of the following? (Select all that apply.)
   a. Resting tremor
   b. Activity-generated tremor
   c. Bradykinesia
   d. Rigidity
   e. Postural instability

2. _____ increases dopamine activity by increasing dopamine release and reducing neuronal reuptake.

3. Apomorphine increases dopamine activity by directly stimulating _____ _____.

4. Parkinsonism is a progressive neurodegenerative disorder characterized by a deficit of _____ and a relative excess of _____.

5. Mr. Plume is diagnosed with Parkinson's disease. You visit him 1 week after hospitalization to assess his progress and medication regimen compliance. He states that there is no significant improvement in his symptoms. You tell him which of the following?
   a. "Noticeable improvement may not occur for several weeks after the initial drug dose."
   b. "Noticeable improvement usually occurs 7 to 10 days after the initial drug dose."
   c. "You should have noticed improvement by now; I will notify your physician."
   d. "Are you sure that you are taking the medication as ordered?"

6. Mr. Plume's symptoms begin to abate with a multidisciplinary approach to his care. Which of the following specialists would participate in his plan of care to improve his independence in activities of daily living? (Select all that apply.)
   a. Physical therapist
   b. Pharmacist
   c. Occupational therapist
   d. Dietitian

7. Mrs. Clinton begins tolcapone therapy, and her physician arranges for laboratory testing to be completed on a routine basis. Which of the following laboratory studies would be ordered by the physician?
   a. CBC
   b. Liver transaminase enzymes
   c. Hemoglobin and hematocrit
   d. BUN and creatinine

8. Mr. Burt is diagnosed with chronic renal failure. He routinely takes amantadine for his Parkinson's disease with success. Why would his physician consider discontinuing the amantadine?

   a. With amantadine, 50% of the drug is excreted via the kidneys.

   b. With amantadine, metabolism occurs in the kidneys.

   c. With amantadine, catabolism occurs in the kidneys.

   d. With amantadine, excretion is primarily via the kidneys.

9. In the older adult, the dosage of levodopa/carbidopa may need to be reduced because of which of the following age-related conditions?

   a. Increase in peripheral AADC, the enzyme that carbidopa inhibits

   b. Decrease in peripheral AADC, the enzyme that carbidopa inhibits

   c. Cardiac incompetency and resultant congestive heart failure

   d. Pulmonary incompetency and resultant chronic obstructive pulmonary disease

10. Mrs. Bunting is prescribed centrally active anticholinergics for her Parkinson's disease. Six weeks later, her daughter asks the physician to hospitalize Mrs. Bunting for a psychiatric evaluation. The physician does which of the following?

    a. Evaluates the client for adverse reactions from the centrally active anticholinergics

    b. Increases the centrally active anticholinergics to decrease the client's symptoms

    c. Admits the client to the hospital for a psychological evaluation

    d. Immediately discontinues the centrally active anticholinergic medication

11. Mr. Dorsey is prescribed levodopa for his Parkinson's disease. The dosage has been modified on multiple occasions. Mr. Dorsey asks you how the doctor decides what will be the optimal dose. Which of the following is your reply?

    a. "The optimal dose is the highest one that allows the client to function adequately."

    b. "The optimal dose is the one that allows the client to function adequately."

    c. "The optimal dose is the lowest one that allows the client to function adequately."

    d. "The optimal dose is the one that maximizes client function."

12. Mr. Swett, diagnosed with Parkinson's disease 8 years ago, presents to the physician's office with signs of prominent bradykinesia and rigidity. The physician orders levodopa/carbidopa. As part of your education plan, you explain which of the following about the combination of levodopa/carbidopa?

    a. It may be effective with end-stage bradykinesia and rigidity.

    b. It is probably the most effective drug when bradykinesia and rigidity become prominent.

    c. It will provide palliation therapy.

    d. It is the treatment of last resort.

13. Mrs. Pointer is diagnosed with advanced idiopathic parkinsonism, and her physician prescribes combination therapy. She asks you what is the advantage of combination therapy over monotherapy. How do you reply? (Select all that apply.)

    a. It provides better control of symptoms.

    b. It provides increased dosage of individual drugs.

    c. It provides reduced dosage of individual drugs.

    d. It provides for maintenance of symptoms.

14. Mrs. Ramsey is diagnosed with Parkinson's disease and is having difficulty performing her activities of daily living. Her physician orders pramipexole. Pramipexole may be used alone for which of the following purposes?

    a. To maintain ability to perform activities of daily living

    b. To delay physical impairment related to Parkinson's disease

    c. To delay mental impairment related to Parkinson's disease

    d. To improve motor performance and improve ability to participate in usual activities of daily living

15. Mr. Boyle is recently diagnosed with Parkinson's disease. His symptoms are well managed by his current medication regimen. He wishes to receive levodopa therapy, because his friends tell him it is the best treatment for his disease. As part of your education plan, you state which of the following?

    a. "Only the physician can determine the correct medication for your disease process."

    b. "Levodopa is usually reserved for clients with significant symptoms and functional disabilities."

    c. "Levodopa is the drug of last resort and your symptoms are not that bad yet."

    d. "I will ask the physician if he can change your drug regimen."

16. Levodopa acts to replace _____ in the basal ganglia of the brain.

17. Mr. Boyle's physician orders levodopa for the treatment of his Parkinson's disease. The client asks you whether the levodopa will cure his condition. Which of the following is a correct statement about the effects of levodopa?

    a. It does not alter the underlying disease process, but it may improve a client's quality of life.

    b. It will cure the Parkinson's disease.

    c. It will control the symptoms for 10 to 12 years.

    d. It is the treatment of last resort and may control his symptoms.

18. Anticholinergic drugs are contraindicated to treat Parkinson's symptoms for clients with the diagnosis of _____.

19. Acetylcholine should be used with caution in the elderly because it may impair _____ _____.

20. Anticholinergic drugs are used in idiopathic parkinsonism to decrease which of the following? (Select all that apply.)

    a. Salivation

    b. Contractures

    c. Spasticity

    d. Tremors

    e. Slurred speech

CHAPTER 13

Skeletal Muscle Relaxants

■ Section I: Learning Objectives

1. Discuss common symptoms and disorders for which skeletal muscle relaxants are used.
2. Differentiate between the uses and effects of selected skeletal muscle relaxants.
3. Describe nonpharmacologic interventions to relieve muscle spasm and spasticity.
4. Apply the nursing process with clients experiencing muscle spasm or spasticity.

■ Section II: Assessing Your Understanding

ACTIVITY A

Fill in the Blank

1. _____ _____ _____ are used to decrease muscle spasm or *spasticity* that occurs in certain neurologic and musculoskeletal disorders.
2. _____ _____ or cramp is a sudden, involuntary, painful muscle contraction that occurs with musculoskeletal trauma.
3. Spasms may be _____ (alternating contraction and relaxation).
4. Spasms may be _____ (sustained contraction).
5. _____ involves increased muscle tone or contraction and stiff, awkward movements.

ACTIVITY B

Matching

Match the term in Column A with the definition in Column B.

COLUMN A

1. _____ Tizanidine
2. _____ Metaxalone
3. _____ Dantrolene
4. _____ Methocarbamol
5. _____ Baclofen

COLUMN B

A. Used to relieve discomfort from acute, painful musculoskeletal disorders
B. An alpha$_2$-adrenergic agonist, similar to clonidine, that is used to treat spasticity in clients with MS, spinal cord injury, or brain trauma
C. Used mainly to treat spasticity in MS and spinal cord injuries.
D. Acts directly on skeletal muscle to inhibit muscle contraction.
E. Used to relieve discomfort from acute, painful musculoskeletal disorders; also may be used to treat tetanus.

ACTIVITY C

Short Answers

Briefly answer the following questions.

1. Discuss the pathophysiology related to multiple sclerosis.
2. What personal and environmental factors may influence the symptoms of multiple sclerosis?
3. Identify two drugs used to treat different stages of multiple sclerosis and their actions.
4. Describe the general characteristics of skeletal muscle relaxants.
5. Identify two indications for the use of skeletal muscle relaxants.

■ Section III: Applying Your Knowledge

ACTIVITY D

Case Studies

Consider the scenarios and answer the questions.

Case Study 1

Mrs. Robb is diagnosed with multiple sclerosis. She is a career woman, active in her community, and a member of the PTA at her children's school. The physician orders muscle relaxants to help her cope with the symptoms that she is experiencing. You are the community health nurse assigned to her case and responsible for the care plan for this client

1. Mrs. Robb asks what she might do to improve her mobility and maintain her ability to be self-sufficient. What disciplines would be included in a plan of care involving the client's safety and functionality?
2. The oral baclofen that the physician orders causes drowsiness and confusion, which interferes with Mrs. Robb's ability to help her children with their homework at night. What information about the absorption of baclofen would assist her to modify her dosage times (with physician approval) to meet her psychosocial goals?
3. Mrs. Robb's symptoms are in remission. She asks you if she can discontinue the baclofen right away. You suggest that she confer with her physician. What explanation would you give her for your suggestion?

Case Study 2

Mr. Jean has a history of malignant hyperthermia. He is scheduled for an inguinal hernia repair in 3 days. His surgeon consults with the anesthesiologist. When Mr. Jean visits the surgeon, they discuss the prophylactic use of dantrolene. You are responsible for the preoperative education plan for Mr. Jean.

1. How would you describe malignant hyperthermia to this patient?
2. The surgeon orders dantrolene to be taken 2 days before surgery. Mr. Jean asks why they just can't give him the medication during surgery if he has symptoms again. How would you respond?

3. Mr. Jean experiences symptoms of malignant hyperthermia during the surgery and is treated with IV dantrolene. Would you expect the dantrolene to be continued postoperatively? What adverse reactions related to dantrolene would be taught to both Mr. Jean and his family?

■ Section IV: Practicing for NCLEX

Answer the following questions.

1. Drugs used to relieve spasticity with MS are _____ and _____.

2. To treat muscle spasm and spasticity, the physician may order which of the following therapies? (Select all that apply.)
   a. Physical therapy   c. Occupational therapy
   b. Speech therapy   d. Radiation therapy

3. Both muscle spasms and spasticity can cause which of the following? (Select all that apply.)
   a. Pain   c. Disability
   b. Hypoxia   d. Dysphasia

4. _____ results from damage to nerves in the brain and spinal cord.

5. Muscle spasms usually result from which of the following?
   a. Self-administration of NSAIDs
   b. Self-administration of antipyretics
   c. Trauma to the affected skeletal muscle
   d. Alternating use of heat and cold to the sprained muscle tissue

6. Mrs. Bette's physician orders baclofen for her spasticity. You are her home care nurse. Which of the following blood tests would you schedule routinely for your client?
   a. CBC and electrolytes
   b. Liver function tests
   c. Cardiac function tests
   d. Hemoglobin and hematocrit

7. Your education plan for Mrs. Bette related to her safe functioning at home would include which of the following factors? (Select all that apply.)

   a. Assessment of drug effects

   b. Monitoring of functional abilities

   c. Nonpharmacologic interventions to help prevent or relieve spasticity

   d. Discontinuance of medication regimen when the client is in remission

8. Mr. Zee routinely takes baclofen as a skeletal muscle relaxant for a neuromuscular disorder. His last lab results indicate that he is experiencing renal insufficiency. Based on these data, what would you expect the physician to do?

   a. Increase the dose

   b. Titer the dose

   c. Maintain the current dose

   d. Reduce the dose

9. Mr. Sicts, age 80, is placed on a CNS depressant to manage the symptoms of a neuromuscular disease. Which of the following would be one of your nursing diagnoses?

   a. Risk for infection

   b. Risk for falls

   c. Risk for immobility

   d. Risk for cardiac disease

10. The physician orders short-term skeletal muscle relaxants for Tim Gatz, age 11. You are responsible for the family education plan. You teach the parents that the medications should be used only under which of the following conditions?

    a. When close supervision is available for monitoring drug effects

    b. When the spasms cause uncontrolled pain

    c. When the client needs to be alert during pain management

    d. During school hours to increase alertness and management of spasms

11. Baclofen and tizanidine may be given for spasticity to clients with a diagnosis of MS. Which drug may cause fewer adverse effects?

    a. Baclofen (Lioresal)

    b. Tizanidine (Zanaflex)

12. Mr. Pirelli's physician ordered tizanidine for symptoms related to his spinal cord injury and gave him latitude with dosing. He asks you how soon before activities that cause pain should he administer his medication. You state that oral tizanidine begins to act within 30 to 60 minutes and peaks in how long?

    a. 2 to 4 hours   c. 1 to 2 hours

    b. 1 to 3 hours   d. 2 to 3 hours

13. Mrs. Aziz presents to the emergency department with severe pain and receives methocarbamol by injection. As part of your safety care plan, you should instruct the client that she may experience which of the following common adverse reactions?

    a. Pain at the injection site

    b. Shortness of breath and dizziness

    c. Palpitations and chest pain

    d. Fainting, incoordination, and hypotension

14. Mr. Fresco suffers from severe muscle spasms; his current drug regimen does not adequately manage his pain. He drinks a six-pack of beer each night and has for 30 years. He asks his physician to change his medication to metaxalone because his friend tells him it will make the pain manageable. The physician *does not* order metaxalone, for which of the following reasons?

    a. There is a risk of oversedation due to his alcohol use.

    b. It is not the drug of choice for severe muscle spasms.

    c. There are addictive effects of the medication when used in combination with alcohol.

    d. It is contraindicated in patients with hepatic impairment.

15. Cyclobenzaprine (Flexeril) is contraindicated in clients with _____ disorders.

16. Mr. Shatz injured his back at work and asks how long he may take the cyclobenzaprine for the spasms that he is experiencing. Which of the following is the correct response?

    a. 1 week   c. 3 weeks.

    b. 10 days   d. 2 weeks

17. Mr. DeParte suffers from acute musculoskeletal pain. The physician orders carisoprodol, and his pain is adequately managed. He asks if he might take the drug for long-term pain management. Which of the following statements is the correct response?

    a. "Long-term use can cause physical dependence."

    b. "Long-term use is indicated for your disease process."

    c. "Long-term use may facilitate your return to work."

    d. "Long-term use can cause adverse reactions when used with your antiepileptic drug."

18. Mr. Smyth works in an auto assembly line. His physician orders a skeletal muscle relaxant for short-term back spasms. Which instruction would be part of your education plan for this patient?

    a. "Do not take the medication when working with machinery."

    b. "The medication is safe, and you may return to work when your pain is managed."

    c. "You need to take the medication on a full stomach before physical therapy."

    d. "The side effects of skeletal muscle relaxants will not interfere with most activities of daily living, including work."

19. _____ is the only skeletal muscle relaxant that acts peripherally on the muscle itself; it inhibits the release of calcium in skeletal muscle cells, thereby decreasing the strength of muscle contraction.

20. _____ and _____ increase the effects of gamma-aminobutyric acid, an inhibitory neurotransmitter.

CHAPTER 14

Substance Abuse Disorders

■ Section I: Learning Objectives

1. Identify risk factors for development of drug dependence.
2. Describe the effects of alcohol, cocaine, marijuana, and nicotine on selected body organs.
3. Compare and contrast characteristics of dependence associated with alcohol, benzodiazepines, cocaine, and opiates.
4. Describe specific antidotes for overdoses of central nervous system (CNS) depressant drugs and the circumstances indicating their use.
5. Outline major elements of treatment for overdoses of commonly abused drugs that do not have antidotes.
6. Describe interventions to prevent or manage withdrawal reactions associated with alcohol, benzodiazepines, cocaine and other CNS stimulants, and opiates.

■ Section II: Assessing Your Understanding

ACTIVITY A

Fill in the Blanks

1. _____ _____ is a significant health, social, economic, and legal problem. It is often associated with substantial damage to the abuser and society.
2. Most drugs of abuse are those that affect the _____ and alter the state of consciousness.
3. Most drugs of abuse are also associated with _____ if used repeatedly.
4. Many drugs of abuse activate the _____ system in the brain by altering neurotransmission systems.
5. Characteristics of drug _____ include craving a drug, often with unsuccessful attempts to decrease its use and compulsive drug-seeking behavior.

ACTIVITY B

Matching

Match the term in Column A with the definition in Column B.

COLUMN A

1. _____ Methadone
2. _____ Clonidine
3. _____ Midazolam or propofol
4. _____ Naltrexone
5. _____ Flumazenil

COLUMN B

A. Useful for treating delirium tremens because doses can be easily titrated to manage symptoms
B. Blocks euphoria produced by heroin, acts longer, and reduces preoccupation with drug use
C. Opiate antagonist that reduces craving for alcohol and increases abstinence rates
D. Given to reduce symptoms associated with excessive stimulation of the sympathetic nervous system
E. Specific antidote that can reverse benzodiazepine-induced sedation, coma, and respiratory depression

ACTIVITY C

Short Answers

Briefly answer the following questions.

1. Define substance abuse.
2. List commonly abused drugs.
3. What physical or emotional effects are sought by those who use drugs of abuse?
4. Discuss methods used to obtain drugs of abuse by the general population.
5. What are the characteristics of drug dependence?

■ Section III: Applying Your Knowledge

ACTIVITY D

Case Studies

Consider the scenarios and answer the questions.

Case Study 1

Mr. Rather was involved in a motor vehicle accident 6 months ago in which a friend died. He received opioid analgesics for his skeletal pain during his recovery period. He comes to the physician's office today for anther prescription for his pain but refuses any analgesics but opioids. Based on the care plan for his surgery, he should not require pain medication, his injuries are healed, and rehabilitation is complete. His wife states that he is taking pain medications routinely. The physician suspects drug dependence.

1. What symptoms might the wife and the patient describe that would lead the physician to suspect physical dependence?
2. Mr. Rather's wife also states that when her husband discusses his friend's death he takes more medication. Why would the interdisciplinary team also suspect psychological dependence?
3. Mr. Rather's wife states that she suspects that her husband bought the drugs that he is using on the streets. She states also that he seems to take more and more as time passes to relieve the pain. How would you describe tolerance to Mr. Rather and his wife?

Case Study 2

Mr. Rather discusses his options regarding safe withdrawal from his medications with the physician. The drugs of abuse that he has routinely self-administered are cocaine, alcohol, and opiates.

1. Mrs. Rather, who is herself a medical assistant, asks you what the physiologic basis is for the drug dependence. How would you reply?
2. Mr. Rather states that he has attempted to stop taking the drugs but finds that he just can't bring himself to; they make him forget. Explain the action of the drugs on the brain's reward system.
3. Mrs. Rather is concerned because her husband sometimes buys drugs on the street. What are some of the risks associated with this behavior?

■ Section IV: Practicing for NCLEX

Answer the following questions.

1. As an adjunct to Mr. Wilson's alcohol withdrawal management program, the physician orders disulfiram. You are responsible for his education program. When he arrives home after discharge, he pours himself a beer. Which of the following symptoms would he expect to experience? (Select all that apply.)
   a. Flushing, tachycardia, bronchospasm
   b. Hypotension, anemia, and confusion
   c. Sweating, nausea and vomiting
   d. Paranoia, mania, and depression

2. Mr. Weiss returns home after a coronary artery bypass graft and celebrates his survival by overindulging in alcohol. He does not have a history of alcohol abuse. His drug regimen includes warfarin. Which of the following adverse reactions related to the combination of the drugs would you expect?
   a. Decreased anticoagulant effects and increased risk of clot formation
   b. No significant drug reaction related to only one incident
   c. Increased anticoagulant effects and decreased risk of bleeding
   d. Increased anticoagulant effects and risk of bleeding

3. Mrs. Song has a history of chronic alcohol usage and subsequent liver damage. She develops a deep vein thrombosis and is sent home from the hospital on warfarin. Which of the following adverse reactions related to the combination of the drugs would you expect?
   a. Decreased anticoagulant effects and increased risk of clot formation
   b. No significant drug reaction related to only one incident
   c. Increased anticoagulant effects and decreased risk of bleeding
   d. Increased anticoagulant effects and risk of bleeding

4. With oral antidiabetic drugs that decrease blood sugar, alcohol has which of the following effects?

   a. It diminishes hypoglycemic effects.

   b. It exacerbates hyperglycemic effects.

   c. It potentiates hypoglycemic effects.

   d. It causes polyuria, polydipsia, and subsequent dehydration.

5. With antihypertensive agents, alcohol has which of the following effects?

   a. It diminishes vasodilation and hypotensive effects.

   b. It potentiates vasodilation and hypotensive effects.

   c. It potentiates vasoconstriction and hypotensive effects.

   d. It causes euphoria, mania, and confusion.

6. Mrs. Small's physician prescribes antianxiety medication. You are responsible for her education plan. She asks if she can take the antianxiety medication when she drinks socially with her friends. Which of the following should be your response?

   a. "If you limit alcohol consumption to two drinks, you should be safe."

   b. "Combining alcohol with antianxiety medication may be lethal and should be avoided."

   c. "The drug and alcohol may be co-administered safely."

   d. "The antianxiety medication will increase your blood alcohol level rapidly; you should use a designated driver."

7. Because they are rapidly absorbed from the large surface area of the lungs, smoking or inhaling the vapors is a preferred route of administration for which of the following drugs? (Select all that apply.)

   a. Cocaine   c. Ativan

   b. Marijuana   d. Heroin

8. When questioned about her alcohol usage, Ms. Askew states that she drinks three martinis a night. Which of the following assumptions can you make?

   a. This is the correct amount consumed.

   b. She normally consumes four to six martinis a night.

   c. She is giving you information you expect to hear.

   d. She may have understated the amount of alcohol consumed.

9. You work at a hospital-based methadone clinic. When interviewing heroin users, which of the following assumptions can you make?

   a. Heroin addicts may overstate the amount used in attempts to obtain higher doses of methadone.

   b. Heroin addicts may understate the amount used due to the adverse effects of the methadone.

   c. Heroin addicts will understate the amount used so that they will experience increased euphoria from an increased dosage of methadone.

   d. Heroin addicts will identify the correct amount of drug abused to maintain the sense of euphoria similar to their current drug.

10. _____, _____, _____, and _____ are often used to combat the anxiety and nervousness induced by cocaine, methamphetamine, and other CNS stimulants.

11. Healthcare professionals are considered to be at high risk for development of substance abuse disorders, at least partly because of which of the following factors?

   a. Easy access

   b. Low cost

   c. Lax regulations related to use

   d. None of the above; healthcare professionals are considered low-risk

12. Which of the following statements is true about psychological rehabilitation efforts?

    a. They do not make an impact on addiction treatment because it is a physical dependence.

    b. They should be part of any treatment program for a drug-dependent person.

    c. They are rarely covered by health insurance.

    d. They are successful when used in facility-based rehabilitation programs.

13. Mrs. Johnson presents to the physician's office with her son James, age 12. She found him in the garage this morning sniffing gasoline to get high. You are assigned the education plan for the family. Which of the following would you include as areas of the body where damage might occur?

    a. Heart and lungs

    b. Pancreas and gallbladder

    c. Vascular system

    d. Liver, kidneys, and bone marrow

14. Ms. Keizer presents to the emergency department confused and disheveled and states that she was raped. She attended a party earlier in the evening. Which of the following substances, often called a date-rape drug, might have been added to her drink?

    a. THC   c. Ketamine

    b. Cocaine   d. GHB

15. Mr. Angus, age 19, arrives at the emergency department with his friend. His friend states that they were smoking marijuana and Mr. Angus suddenly began having hallucinations, began exhibiting bizarre behavior, then became unconscious. You find that Mr. Angus is hypertensive and suspect that the marijuana was laced with which of the following substances?

    a. Ketamine   c. THC

    b. GHB   d. PCP

16. Mr. Jones, age 54, recently suffered from myocardial infarction. His medical history indicates that he has been smoking 2 packs of cigarettes per day since the age of 16. He asks the physician for the nicotine patch. Which of the following would you expect the physician to do?

    a. Order the patch

    b. Suggest other methods of nicotine withdrawal

    c. Order a reduced dosage of the patch

    d. State that nicotine cessation at this time may cause further cardiac damage

17. Ms. Ellis began using cocaine for the energy rush and uses on a daily basis. She presents to her physician with symptoms of anxiety and psychosis and is referred to a cocaine withdrawal program. Which of the following treatment methods does such a program include? (Select all that apply.)

    a. Psychotherapy   c. Behavioral therapy

    b. Cessation therapy   d. 12-Step program

18. Which of the following is an accurate statement about heroin addicts?

    a. They inject upon waking and cycle throughout the day until sleep.

    b. They inject approximately every 4 to 6 hours to maintain the high.

    c. They inject several times daily, cycling between desired effects and symptoms of withdrawal.

    d. They experience withdrawal symptoms based on the route of administration.

19. The physician orders hospitalization for the patient who withdraws from benzodiazepines. Which of the following is the rationale behind this order?

    a. Withdrawal can cause cardiac arrhythmias and subsequent cardiac arrest.

    b. Withdrawal can precipitate renal failure.

    c. Convulsions are more likely to occur during the first 48 hours of withdrawal and delirium after 48 to 72 hours.

    d. Liver failure is a risk for such patients.

20. _____ is metabolized at the same rate regardless of the amount present in body tissues.

CHAPTER 15

Central Nervous System Stimulants

■ Section I: Learning Objectives

1. Describe general characteristics of central nervous system (CNS) stimulants.
2. Discuss reasons for decreased use of amphetamines for therapeutic purposes.
3. Discuss the rationale for treating attention deficit/ hyperactivity disorder with CNS stimulants.
4. Identify effects and sources of caffeine.
5. Identify nursing interventions to prevent, recognize, and treat stimulant overdose.

■ Section II: Assessing Your Understanding

ACTIVITY A

Fill in the Blanks

1. _____ is characterized by persistent hyperactivity, a short attention span, difficulty completing assigned tasks or schoolwork, restlessness, and impulsiveness.
2. _____ is a sleep disorder characterized by daytime "sleep attacks" in which the person goes to sleep at any place or at any time.
3. Two disorders treated with CNS stimulants are _____ and _____.
4. _____ is the most common psychiatric or neurobehavioral disorder in children
5. Studies indicate that children with ADHD are more likely to have _____ _____, mood disorders, and substance-abuse disorders as adolescents and adults.

ACTIVITY B

Matching

Match the terms in Column A with the definition in Column B.

COLUMN A

1. _____ Amphetamines and methylphenidate
2. _____ Xanthines
3. _____ Caffeine
4. _____ Atomoxetine (Strattera)
5. _____ Amphetamine, dextroamphetamine (Dexedrine), and methamphetamine (Desoxyn)

COLUMN B

A. Stimulate the cerebral cortex, increasing mental alertness and decreasing drowsiness and fatigue
B. Used in the treatment of narcolepsy and ADHD
C. Closely related drugs that share characteristics of the amphetamines as a group
D. Frequently consumed CNS stimulant worldwide, mostly obtained from dietary sources (e.g., coffee, tea, soft drinks)
E. Second-line drug for the treatment of ADHD in children and adults, with a low risk of abuse and dependence compared with the other drugs used for ADHD

ACTIVITY C

Short Answers

Briefly answer the following questions.

1. Discuss the psychosocial characteristics of ADHD.
2. Describe the signs and symptoms of narcolepsy.
3. In addition to drug treatments, what might be done to treat narcolepsy?
4. Describe the characteristics of CNS stimulants.
5. How do amphetamines affect brain function?

■ Section III: Applying Your Knowledge

ACTIVITY D
Case Studies
Consider the scenarios and answer the questions.

Case Study 1

Mrs. Stratos, age 35, works in a high-stress job that requires long hours and high levels of concentration. She presents to the physician's office with complaints of palpitations and chronic insomnia. Upon assessment, you note that she is alert and oriented to person, place, and time. Both her blood pressure and pulse are elevated compared with her last office visit. She paces back and forth during the assessment and states that she is unable to sit still. You note that she has pallor and dark circles under her eyes. She states that she drinks two cups of coffee in the morning and one before she leaves work in order to remain awake while driving home at night.

1. What is the appropriate nursing diagnosis for Mrs. Stratos?
2. What should you explore as part of the patient history?
3. During the history taking, you discover that Mrs. Stratos drinks four energy drinks per day, which results in excessive caffeine intake. What is your plan for this patient?

Case Study 2

Jane, age 7, is placed on medication for ADHD. As her nurse, you are responsible for the education plan for the parents.

1. Jane's mother says to you, "The dose of the medication may be increased by half a tablet in the morning if Jane has difficulty concentrating." What do you think of this statement? How would you respond to the mother?
2. What signs and symptoms should Jane's mother be instructed to report to the physician?
3. In a child taking stimulants, what should you be monitoring for?

■ Section IV: Practicing for NCLEX

Answer the following questions.

1. Joseph Bean, a college student, presents to the emergency room with palpitations and signs and symptoms of CNS stimulation. He states that he has been awake for 72 hours studying and keeps awake using power drinks and caffeine. Which of the following statements indicate that his education plan has been effective?
   a. "Caffeine can cause life-threatening health problems with excessive intake."
   b. "Energy drinks do not contain caffeine; if they are not combined with excessive caffeine intake they will not cause adverse side effects."
   c. "Caffeine did not cause my symptoms. I have the flu."
   d. "Caffeine is not an ingredient of energy drinks."

2. Which of the following are the characteristic symptoms of narcolepsy? (Select all that apply.)
   a. Difficult to rouse in the morning
   b. Unpredictable sleep during daytime hours
   c. Transient insomnia
   d. Daytime drowsiness

3. Which of the following effects do CNS stimulants have on behavior and attention in patients with ADHD?
   a. Restoring   c. Improving
   b. Deteriorating   d. Contravening

4. When does ADHD usually start and resolve?
   a. Starts in childhood and resolves by adolescence
   b. Starts in childhood and resolves by adulthood
   c. Starts in childhood and resolves before adolescence
   d. Starts in childhood and may persist through adulthood

5. ADHD is characterized by which of the following? (Select all that apply.)
   a. Hyperactivity
   b. Improved retention
   c. Impulsivity
   d. Short attention span

6. Mr. Adams, age 75, is given an order for a CNS stimulant secondary to a new diagnosis of narcolepsy. He begins to experience signs and symptoms of excessive CNS stimulation. He is likely to also experience an exacerbation of which preexisting condition?
   a. Diabetes
   b. Cardiac dysrhythmias
   c. Gout
   d. Hyperparathyroidism

7. Which of the following may affect medication dosage adjustment for the child with ADHD as he or she matures?
   a. Onset of puberty
   b. Change in hepatic metabolism
   c. Brain growth
   d. Musculoskeletal growth

8. Methylphenidate is commonly prescribed and usually given daily for the first 3 to 4 weeks for which of the following purposes?
   a. To determine parent and child compliance with the medication regimen
   b. To determine medication blood levels in order to modify the dose
   c. To assess the education plan and modify the plan to meet the client's needs
   d. To assess beneficial and adverse effects

9. Drug therapy is indicated in which of the following circumstances? (Select all that apply.)
   a. Symptoms are mild to moderate.
   b. Symptoms are moderate to severe.
   c. Symptoms are identified by the parents and teacher.
   d. Symptoms are present for several months.
   e. Symptoms interfere in social, academic, or behavioral functioning.

10. Mr. Gaines arrives at the emergency department with signs and symptoms of CNS stimulant toxicity. Treatment includes which of the following? (Select all that apply.)
    a. Monitor for musculoskeletal changes
    b. Monitor cardiac function
    c. Increase sensory stimulation
    d. Minimize external stimulation

11. After caffeine is ingested orally, it achieves peak blood level within what period of time?
    a. 30 to 45 minutes   c. 10 to 15 minutes
    b. 45 to 60 minutes   d. 15 to 20 minutes

12. As an added ingredient, which of the following effects may caffeine have?
    a. Decreasing analgesia
    b. Decreasing anxiety
    c. Reducing dysrhythmias
    d. Increasing analgesia

13. Theophylline preparations are xanthines used in the treatment of respiratory disorders, such as asthma and bronchitis, with the desired effect being bronchodilation and improvement of breathing. In this setting, which of the following roles does CNS stimulation hold?
    a. It is an integral component of the medication preparation.
    b. It is an adverse effect.
    c. It does not interfere with the action of the medication.
    d. It is often used as an adjunct medication.

14. Mr. McNally is diagnosed with narcolepsy by his physician. He asks the physician to prescribe modafinil, because it works so well for his friend. The physician will not prescribe the medication. Which of the following aspects of the patient's history would lead to this decision?
    a. Gout and a history of tophi
    b. Ischemic changes on his electrocardiograms
    c. Pancreatitis
    d. Cirrhosis of the liver

15. Mr. Goya asks whether a guarana product will keep him awake longer than caffeine. As part of your education plan, which of the following statements could you accurately make?
    a. "The caffeine content of a guarana product is unknown."
    b. "Guarana is caffeine free."
    c. "The caffeine content of guarana is essentially the same as coffee."
    d. "The amount of caffeine in guarana is higher than in coffee."

16. The main goal of therapy with CNS stimulants is to relieve symptoms of the disorders for which they are given. Which of the following is a secondary goal?
    a. To prevent adverse reactions
    b. To serve as a study aid
    c. To have clients use the drugs appropriately
    d. To prevent side effects

17. CNS stimulants are dangerous when used by which of the following people? (Select all that apply.)
    a. Drivers to maintain an alert state
    b. Athletes
    c. Clients diagnosed with cardiac dysrhythmias
    d. Clients diagnosed with gout

18. A limited number of tablets of CNS stimulants are routinely prescribed. Which of the following is the reason for this limitation?
    a. The cost is prohibitive when prescribed in a large number.
    b. It reduces the likelihood of drug dependence or diversion.
    c. Changes in dosages are common.
    d. HMOs will not reimburse the cost for larger numbers.

19. CNS stimulants are not recommended for ADHD in children younger than what age?
    a. 6 years   c. 4 years
    b. 5 years   d. 3 years

20. In general, authorities recommend no more than _____ mg of caffeine per day for healthy adults and little to none for people with heart disease.

CHAPTER 16

Physiology of the Autonomic Nervous System

■ Section I: Learning Objectives

1. Identify physiologic effects of the sympathetic nervous system.
2. Differentiate subtypes and functions of sympathetic nervous system receptors.
3. Identify physiologic effects of the parasympathetic nervous system.
4. Differentiate subtypes and functions of parasympathetic nervous system receptors.
5. Describe signal transduction and the intracellular events that occur when receptors of the autonomic nervous system are stimulated.
6. State names and general characteristics of drugs affecting the autonomic nervous system.

■ Section II: Assessing Your Understanding

ACTIVITY A

Fill in the Blanks

1. The _____ _____ is composed of two main divisions, the central nervous system (CNS) and the peripheral nervous system (PNS).
2. The _____ includes the brain and spinal cord.
3. The _____ includes all the neurons and ganglia found outside the CNS.
4. _____ neurons carry sensory input from the periphery to the CNS and modify motor output through the action of reflex arcs.
5. The _____ portion of the PNS is further subdivided into the somatic nervous system and the autonomic nervous system.

ACTIVITY B

Matching

Match the term in Column A with the definition in Column B.

COLUMN A

1. _____ Acetylcholine
2. _____ Ligands
3. _____ Acetylcholine and norepinephrine
4. _____ The sympathetic nervous system
5. _____ Ganglia

COLUMN B

A. Bundles of nerve tissue composed of the terminal end of the presynaptic neuron and clusters of postsynaptic neuron cell bodies
B. The main neurotransmitters of the ANS
C. Synthesized from acetylcoenzyme A and choline
D. Collectively, neurotransmitters, such as acetylcholine and norepinephrine, as well as medications and hormones that can bind to receptors in the ANS
E. Stimulated by physical or emotional stress, such as strenuous exercise or work, pain, hemorrhage, intense emotions, and temperature extremes

ACTIVITY C

Short Answers

Briefly answer the following questions.

1. Discuss the synthesis and action of norepinephrine within the body.
2. Discuss the function of norepinephrine.
3. What are the functions stimulated by the parasympathetic nervous system?
4. What is the role of nicotinic and muscarinic receptors within the body?
5. What is the role of dopamine as it relates to the functioning of the body?

■ Section III: Applying Your Knowledge

ACTIVITY D

Case Studies

Consider the scenarios and answer the questions.

Case Study 1

You are participating in a study group to discuss the autonomic drugs and their effect on body systems. During a question and answer period you address the following topics.

1. Describe the effects of the sympathomimetic, adrenergic, and alpha- and beta-adrenergic agonists.
2. What are the drugs that have the same effects on the body as stimulation of the parasympathetic?
3. What do sympatholytic, antiadrenergic, and alpha- and beta-adrenergic blocking drugs do?
4. What do parasympatholytic, anticholinergic, and cholinergic blocking drugs do?

Case Study 2

You are participating in a study group. Your topic is the sympathetic nervous system and its effect on body systems. During a question and answer period you address the following topics.

1. What is the "fight-or-flight" reaction? What does it entail?
2. What are some specific body responses related to a perceived threat?

■ Section IV: Practicing for NCLEX

Answer the following questions.

1. Which of the following statements is true about the number of receptors in the ANS
   a. It is fixed from birth.
   b. It is fixed but may be regulated when the body experiences stress.
   c. It is dynamic and can be upregulated or downregulated as needed.
   d. It is dynamic only when the body experiences stress or threat.

2. Cholinergic receptors include _____ and _____ receptors; there are several subtypes.

3. Adrenergic receptors include alpha and beta receptors as well as which of the following types of receptors?
   a. Anticholinergic   c. Dopamine
   b. Cholinergic   d. Anhydrous

4. Drugs that block activity of ANS receptors prevent the actions of both endogenous neurotransmitters and ANS _____.

5. Drugs that activate ANS receptors function like which of the following neurotransmitters to stimulate the ANS?
   a. Exogenous   c. Anticholinergic
   b. Cholinergic   d. Endogenous

6. Stimulation of receptors in the parasympathetic nervous system produces what kind of effects?
   a. Cholinergic   c. Synergistic
   b. Anticholinergic   d. Adrenergic

7. Stimulation of receptors in the sympathetic nervous system produces what kind of effect?
   a. Antiadrenergic   c. Cholinergic
   b. Adrenergic   d. Anticholinergic

8. Release of neurotransmitters allows nerve impulses in the ANS to bridge synapses and travel from presynaptic to postsynaptic nerves, eventually stimulating receptors located on _____ organs.

9. Drugs that act on the ANS usually affect which of the following body parts?

    a. Specific organs   c. The entire body

    b. Specific tissues   d. Specific glands

10. Muscarinic$_1$ receptors are expressed primarily in which branch of the nervous system?

    a. ANS

    b. Parasympathetic nervous system

    c. CNS

    d. Sympathetic nervous system

11. _____ _____ is one of the products of phospholipid metabolism and acts as a second messenger to increase the intracellular concentration of calcium.

12. Which of the following are some of the specific body responses to parasympathetic stimulation? (Select all that apply.)

    a. Dilation of blood vessels in the skin

    b. Decreased heart rate, possibly bradycardia

    c. Increased secretion of digestive enzymes and motility of the gastrointestinal tract

    d. Dilation of the smooth muscle of bronchi

13. Approximately 75% of all parasympathetic nerve fibers are in the _____ nerves.

14. Activation of alpha$_1$ receptors in smooth muscle cells is thought to open ion channels and cause which of the following effects?

    a. Vasodilation

    b. Gastrointestinal dilation

    c. Bladder incontinence

    d. Vasoconstriction

15. In the brain, some of the norepinephrine released into the synaptic cleft between neurons returns to the nerve endings from which it was released and stimulates presynaptic alpha$_2$ receptors. This negative feedback prevents which of the following effects?

    a. Calcium-mediated release of norepinephrine from storage vesicles into the synapse

    b. Calcium-mediated release of epinephrine from storage vesicles into the synapse

    c. Increased sympathetic outflow and an antiadrenergic effect

    d. Decreased sympathetic outflow and an adrenergic effect

16. When norepinephrine and epinephrine act on body cells that respond to sympathetic nerve or catecholamine stimulation, they interact with two distinct adrenergic receptors, _____ and _____.

17. Dopamine receptors are located in the brain, in blood vessels of the kidneys and other viscera, and probably in presynaptic sympathetic nerve terminals. Activation (agonism) of these receptors may result in which of the following effects?

    a. Stimulation or inhibition of insulin production

    b. Stimulation or inhibition of the CNS

    c. Stimulation or inhibition of cellular function

    d. Stimulation or inhibition of the ANS

18. The two divisions of the ANS are usually _____ in their actions on a particular organ.

19. Norepinephrine is synthesized from the amino acid _____ by a series of enzymatic conversions that also produce dopamine and epinephrine.

20. The functions of the ANS can be broadly described as activities designed to do which of the following? (Select all that apply.)

    a. Maintain a constant internal environment (homeostasis)

    b. Respond to stress or emergencies

    c. Repair body tissues

    d. Stimulate or inhibit insulin production

CHAPTER 17

Adrenergic Drugs

■ Section I: Learning Objectives

1. Identify effects produced by stimulation of alpha- and beta-adrenergic receptors.
2. List characteristics of adrenergic drugs in terms of effects on body tissues, indications for use, adverse effects, nursing process implications, principles of therapy, and observation of client responses.
3. Discuss the use of epinephrine to treat anaphylactic shock, acute bronchospasm, and cardiac arrest.
4. Identify clients at risk for the adverse effects associated with adrenergic drugs.
5. List commonly used over-the-counter preparations and herbal preparations that contain adrenergic drugs.
6. Discuss principles of therapy and nursing process for using adrenergic drugs in special populations.
7. Describe signs and symptoms of toxicity due to noncatecholamine adrenergic drugs.
8. Discuss treatment of overdose with noncatecholamine adrenergic drugs.
9. Teach the client about safe, effective use of adrenergic drugs.

■ Section II: Assessing Your Understanding

ACTIVITY A

Fill in the Blanks

1. _____ drugs produce effects similar to those produced by stimulation of the sympathetic nervous system and therefore have widespread effects on body tissues.
2. Adrenergic medications, such as phenylephrine, pseudoephedrine, and _____, are synthetic chemical relatives of naturally occurring neurotransmitters and hormones.
3. Specific effects of adrenergic medications depend mainly on the type of adrenergic _____ activated by the drug.

4. Some adrenergic drugs are _____ formulations of naturally occurring neurotransmitters and hormones, such as norepinephrine, epinephrine, and dopamine.
5. Major therapeutic uses and adverse effects of adrenergic medications derive from drug action on the _____, blood vessels, and lungs.

ACTIVITY B

Matching

Match the term in Column A with the definition in Column B.

COLUMN A

1. _____ Epinephrine (Adrenalin)
2. _____ Ephedrine
3. _____ Pseudoephedrine (Sudafed)
4. _____ Isoproterenol (Isuprel)
5. _____ Phenylephrine (e.g., Neo-Synephrine)

COLUMN B

A. Mixed-acting adrenergic drug that acts by stimulating alpha$_1$ and beta receptors and causing release of norepinephrine from presynaptic terminals.
B. Drug stimulating alpha$_1$ and beta receptors, used as a bronchodilator and nasal decongestant
C. Synthetic catecholamine that acts on beta$_1$- and beta$_2$-adrenergic receptors
D. Synthetic drug that acts on alpha-adrenergic receptors to produce vasoconstriction.
E. Prototype of the adrenergic drugs

ACTIVITY C

Short Answers

Briefly answer the following questions.

1. Identify three clinical indications for the use of adrenergic drugs.
2. What is the role of adrenergic drugs during cardiac arrest?
3. What is the role of adrenergic drugs in the treatment of asthma?
4. What is the role of adrenergic drugs in the treatment of allergic reactions?
5. Identify two miscellaneous uses of adrenergic drugs and explain why they are used.

■ Section III: Applying Your Knowledge

ACTIVITY D

Case Study

Consider the scenario and answer the questions.

Mrs. Wilson, age 35, is diagnosed with bronchial asthma. She is noncomplaint with her medication regimen secondary to the cost of her prescriptions. She presents to the emergency department today with symptoms associated with respiratory distress. You note auditory expiratory wheezing, perioral cyanosis, and a pulse oximetry of 83% in room air.

1. What would you expect to be the physician's treatment of choice to reduce bronchospasm?
2. When you interview Mrs. Wilson, you learn that she uses Primatene Mist as an over-the-counter asthma treatment at home. Why might you be concerned regarding over-the-counter asthma treatments? What are possible advantages of this approach?
3. What are the established treatment guidelines for patients with asthma?
4. What is another concern about products such as Primatene Mist?
5. What is a common ingredient in OTC anti-asthma tablets (e.g., Bronkaid, Primatene)?
6. What patient populations should not take over-the-counter asthma treatments on a regular basis?

■ Section IV: Practicing for NCLEX

Answer the following questions.

1. Dietary supplements containing _____ are prohibited in the United States.

2. Which of the following receptors does phenylephrine stimulate?
   a. Alpha$_2$ c. Beta$_2$
   b. Beta$_1$ d. Alpha$_1$

3. Contraindications to adrenergic drugs include which of the following conditions? (Select all that apply.)
   a. Cardiac dysrhythmias
   b. Hyperthyroidism
   c. Hypersensitivity to sulfites
   d. Hypersensitivity to penicillins

4. Local anesthetics containing adrenergics should not be used on which part of the body?
   a. The abdomen   c. The back
   b. The chest   d. The fingers

5. A benefit of epinephrine in cardiac arrest situations due to asystole or pulseless electrical activity is the added ability to do which of the following?
   a. Increase oxygenation to the brain
   b. Stimulate electrical and mechanical activity
   c. Reduce seizure activity
   d. Increase oxygenation to the myocardium

6. Epinephrine is recommended as a vasopressor in cardiac arrest situations; however, current ACLS guidelines state that _____ may replace either the first or second dose of epinephrine in all cardiac arrest algorithms.

7. Use of beta-adrenergic blocking drugs (e.g., propranolol) may have which of the following effects?
   a. Increasing the effectiveness of epinephrine in cases of anaphylaxis
   b. No change in the effectiveness of epinephrine
   c. Decreasing the effectiveness of epinephrine in cases of anaphylaxis
   d. None of the above; epinephrine is contraindicated when the patient is taking beta-adrenergic drugs

8. Mrs. Bates is taking propranolol for migraine prophylaxis. She presents to the emergency department in cardiac distress. Part of the treatment modality includes the use of epinephrine. You understand that, because of the propranolol, the physician may order which of the following?

   a. Higher than usual doses of epinephrine

   b. Lower than usual doses of epinephrine

   c. The same dose of epinephrine as stated in the emergency department protocol

   d. Discontinuation of epinephrine

9. Individuals who are susceptible to severe allergic reactions should carry epinephrine in the form of a/an _____.

10. _____ is the drug of choice to treat anaphylaxis.

11. Mr. Nyman presents to the physician's office with allergic rhinitis. What would you expect the physician to order?

    a. An adrenergic drug

    b. A bronchodilator

    c. An antihistamine

    d. An anticholinergic drug

12. Mr. Jacques, age 75, is diagnosed with chronic obstructive lung disease; he also has a history of cardiac dysrhythmias, hyperlipidemia, and hypertension. His physician orders a metered-dose inhaler, and you are responsible for the client's education plan. You teach Mr. Jacques to report which of the following?

    a. Gastrointestinal upset   c. Persistent edema

    b. Skin lesions   d. Palpitations

13. Mr. Wilson is diagnosed with hepatitis C. He regularly takes an adrenergic medication. Secondary to the diagnosis of hepatitis C, which of the following would you expect the physician to do?

    a. Increase the dosage of the adrenergic medication

    b. Make no change in the dosage of the adrenergic medication

    c. Discontinue the adrenergic medication

    d. Decrease the dose of the adrenergic medication

14. Mr. Bates is diagnosed with diabetes type 2, asthmatic bronchitis, benign prostatic hyperplasia, and hyperlipidemia. He takes an adrenergic medication as part of his daily drug regimen. As part of his education plan, which of the following signs and symptoms would you teach Mr. Bates to observe for?

    a. Muscle cramping   c. Painful urination

    b. Indigestion   d. Constipation

15. Mr. Simpson is prescribed an adrenergic ophthalmic medication. Which of the following should be included in the teaching plan?

    a. The drug is only absorbed locally.

    b. Side effects are limited to inflammation of the conjunctiva.

    c. Allergic and adverse reactions are rare.

    d. Hypertension may be a side effect of the medication.

16. _____ is most often used to relieve congestion of the upper respiratory tract and may be given topically, as nose drops.

17. Angel Rodriguez, age 6, is given parenteral epinephrine for the treatment of bronchospasm. You understand that children may experience which of the following conditions secondary to parenteral epinephrine?

    a. Hypotension

    b. Rebound shortness of breath

    c. Syncope

    d. Rhinitis

18. Ephedrine and ephedra-containing herbal preparations are often abused as an alternative to amphetamines. Which of the following are identified as herbal preparations? (Select all that apply.)

    a. Ma huang   c. Crack

    b. Herbal ecstasy   d. Smack

19. Mr. Janis takes a nasal adrenergic medication for his allergic rhinitis. Part of your education plan should include the fact that overuse of adrenergic drugs may cause which of the following effects?

    a. Tolerance   c. Increased effectiveness

    b. Addiction   d. Decreased congestion

20. The usual goal of vasopressor drug therapy is to maintain tissue perfusion and a mean arterial pressure of at least what level?

    a. 40 to 60 mm Hg   c. 60 to 89 mm Hg

    b. 20 to 40 mm Hg   d. 80 to 100 mm Hg

CHAPTER 18

Antiadrenergic Drugs

■ Section I: Learning Objectives

1. List characteristics of antiadrenergic drugs in terms of effects on body tissues, indications for use, nursing process implications, principles of therapy, and observation of patient response.
2. Discuss alpha$_1$-adrenergic blocking drugs and alpha$_2$-adrenergic agonists in terms of indications for use, adverse effects, and other selected characteristics.
3. Compare and contrast beta-adrenergic blocking drugs in terms of cardioselectivity, indications for use, adverse effects, and other selected characteristics.
4. Teach patients about the safe, effective use of antiadrenergic drugs.
5. Discuss principles of therapy and nursing process for using antiadrenergic drugs in special populations.

■ Section II: Assessing Your Understanding

ACTIVITY A

Fill in the Blanks

1. _____ drugs decrease or block the effects of sympathetic nerve stimulation, endogenous catecholamines, and adrenergic drugs.
2. A basal level of sympathetic tone is necessary to maintain normal body functioning, including regulation of _____ _____, blood glucose levels, and stress response.
3. The goal of antiadrenergic drug therapy is to suppress _____ stimulation—not the normal physiologic responses to activity, stress, and other stimuli.
4. Antiadrenergic effects can occur when either alpha$_1$ or beta receptors are blocked by adrenergic _____ or when presynaptic alpha$_2$ receptors are stimulated by agonist drugs.

5. Most antiadrenergic drugs have _____ or blocking effects when they bind with alpha$_1$, beta$_1$, beta$_2$, or a combination of receptors in peripheral tissues.

ACTIVITY B

Matching

Match the term in Column A with the definition in Column B.

COLUMN A

1. _____ Clonidine (Catapres)

2. _____ Methyldopa (Aldomet)

3. _____ Prazosin (Minipress)

4. _____ Tamsulosin (Flomax)

5. _____ Phentolamine (Regitine)

COLUMN B

A. Oral agent that reduces blood pressure within 1 hour, reaches peak plasma levels in 3 to 5 hours, and has a plasma half-life of approximately 12 to 16 hours (longer with renal impairment)

B. The first alpha$_1$ antagonist designed specifically to treat BPH

C. Similar to phenoxybenzamine but more useful clinically

D. Prototype drug, well absorbed after oral administration, reaches peak plasma concentrations in 1 to 3 hours; action lasts approximately 4 to 6 hours

E. Older drug with low to moderate absorption; peak plasma levels reached in 2 to 4 hours, and peak antihypertensive effects occur in approximately 2 days

ACTIVITY C

Short Answers

Briefly answer the following questions.

1. Describe the mechanism of action of alpha$_2$-adrenergic agonists such as clonidine (Catapres).
2. Describe the mechanism of action of alpha$_1$-adrenergic blocking drugs such as tamsulosin.
3. Describe the mechanism of action of beta-adrenergic blocking agents.
4. Describe the mechanism of action for nonselective alpha-adrenergic blocking drugs such as phentolamine.
5. What effect does a beta$_1$-receptor blockade have on the human body?

■ Section III: Applying Your Knowledge

ACTIVITY D

Case Study

Consider the scenario and answer the questions.

Mr. Jenks presents to the physician's office with complaints about difficulty voiding, frequency, and urgency. The physician diagnoses him with benign prostatic hypertrophy and prescribes alfuzosin (Uroxatral). You are responsible for Mr. Jenks' education plan regarding his new medication regimen.

1. What kind of drug is alfuzosin?
2. Mr. Jenks is concerned that the medication will not be effective enough to prevent the need to get up to void several times a night; after all, the medication is given only once a day. What can you teach Mr. Jenks concerning the half-life and duration of his medication? To promote absorption of alfuzosin, what should you teach Mr. Jenks concerning taking the medication?
3. Mr. Jenks is visiting a dermatologist for a chronic athlete's foot infection that is not responding to traditional over-the-counter treatments. The dermatologist orders ketoconazole. One week later Mr. Jenks presents to the physician's office with dizziness and headache. Based on Mr. Jenks' recent drug history, what do you suspect? If Mr. Jenks were exposed to and developed hepatitis C with subsequent liver damage, why would the physician discontinue alfuzosin?
4. What are the common adverse effects related to alfuzosin therapy?

■ Section IV: Practicing for NCLEX

Answer the following questions.

1. Mrs. Benton is diagnosed with supraventricular tachycardia. What would you expect the physician to order?
   a. Alpha-blocker   c. Ace inhibitor
   b. Beta-blocker   d. Antihypertensive

2. Mrs. Anspar is diagnosed with a vasospastic disorder. What would you expect the physician to order?
   a. Alpha$_1$-adrenergic blocking drug
   b. Alpha$_2$-adrenergic stimulating drug
   c. Beta$_1$-adrenergic blocking drug
   d. Beta$_2$-adrenergic blocking drug

3. Mr. Gonzalez is diagnosed with essential hypertension. What would you expect the physician to order?
   a. Beta$_2$ antagonist   c. Beta$_1$ agonist
   b. Alpha$_1$ agonist   d. Alpha$_2$ agonist

4. The mechanism of action for clonidine (Catapres) is reflected in the drug's ability to do which of the following?
   a. Stimulate the release of norepinephrine in the brain
   b. Inhibit the release of norepinephrine in the brain
   c. Stimulate the release of epinephrine in the brain
   d. Inhibit the release of epinephrine in the brain

5. Antiadrenergic drugs decrease or block the effects of which of the following? (Select all that apply.)
   a. Sympathetic nerve stimulation
   b. Endogenous catecholamines (e.g., epinephrine)
   c. Adrenergic drugs
   d. Antiarrhythmic drugs

6. Mrs. Bates presents to the emergency room with dizziness, a headache scaled as a 10 on a scale of 0 to 10, and blood pressure of 260/140 mm Hg. The physician diagnoses the patient with urgent hypertension and orders clonidine. What would you expect the loading dose to be?

   a. 2 mg

   b. 0.5 mg

   c. 0.2 mg

   d. 0.6 mg

7. A dose of _____ mg should not be exceeded when using clonidine to treat malignant hypertension.

8. Mr. Gallia presents to the emergency department with complaints of chest pain, nausea, vomiting, and diaphoresis. Based on ECG and laboratory data, he is diagnosed with an acute MI. Part of the treatment regimen includes administration of which of the following agents?

   a. Beta-blocker

   b. Ace inhibitor

   c. Antihypertensive

   d. Antihistamine

9. Mrs. Banff had a CVA and MI and is now receiving a beta-blocker. She must be closely monitored for which of the following effects?

   a. Malignant hypertension

   b. Hypotension

   c. Hypokalemia

   d. Hyperkalemia

10. Mr. Gonzalez is receiving $alpha_1$-adrenergic blocking drugs. As a home care nurse, you understand that he is at increased risk for falls due to which of the following conditions?

    a. Angina

    b. Hypertension

    c. Hypotension

    d. Orthostatic hypotension

11. Mr. Gates is taking beta adrenergic medication. Which of the following should you teach him to do before taking each dose?

    a. Monitor his blood pressure

    b. Monitor his radial pulse

    c. Withhold food

    d. Compare the label on the medication with the physician's order

12. Mr. Gaines is diagnosed with cirrhosis of the liver. He is currently receiving metoprolol for hypertension. What would you expect the physician to do?

    a. Increase the dose of the medication

    b. Discontinue the medication

    c. Decrease the dose of the medication

    d. Maintain the current dose of the medication

13. Atenolol and nadolol are both eliminated primarily in the _____.

14. Mrs. Gonzalez, age 65, presents to the physician's office for her primary care visit. She is diagnosed with chronic renal failure, diabetes type 2, hypertension, and congestive heart failure. Her medication regimen includes the use of atenolol. Based on her diagnoses, what would you expect the physician to do?

    a. Increase the dose of her beta-blockers

    b. Decrease the dose of her beta-blockers

    c. Maintain the current dose of her beta-blockers

    d. Discontinue the beta-blockers

15. In a client with renal impairment, the dosage of acebutolol and nadolol should be reduced if creatinine clearance is less than _____ milliliters per minute.

16. Mr. Chantal, age 85, is receiving an $alpha_2$-adrenergic agonist to treat his hypertension. The physician chooses to discontinue the medication and use an alternative treatment modality. What would you expect the physician to do?

    a. Stop the medication immediately and begin the alternative treatment

    b. Taper the dosage of the medication over 2 days

    c. Taper the dosage of the medication over 1 to 2 weeks

    d. Taper the medication over 5 to 7 days

17. Older adults undergoing cataract surgery are at risk of a surgical complication, intraoperative _____ _____ syndrome, if they are taking selective $alpha_1$-blockers for BPH or hypertension.

18. When beta-blockers are given to children, general guidelines indicate that the dosage should be adjusted according to which of the following factors?

    a. Age
    b. Symptomology
    c. Sex
    d. Body weight

19. Beta-adrenergic blocking drugs are used in children for disorders similar to those in adults. They are contraindicated in children with which of the following conditions?

    a. A resting blood pressure greater than 140/80 mm Hg

    b. A resting heart rate greater than 150 beats per minute

    c. Congestive heart failure

    d. A resting heart rate of less than 60 beats per minute

20. Mr. Garnett presents to the emergency department with symptoms of anaphylaxis. His current medication regimen includes beta-blockers. Bronchodilation does not occur when epinephrine is administered secondary to which of the following drug-induced conditions?

    a. $Alpha_1$ blockade
    b. $Alpha_2$ blockade
    c. $Beta_1$ blockade
    d. $Beta_2$ blockade

CHAPTER 19

Cholinergic Drugs

■ Section I: Learning Objectives

1. Describe effects and indications for use of selected cholinergic drugs.
2. Discuss drug therapy for myasthenia gravis.
3. Discuss the use of cholinergic drug therapy for paralytic ileus and urinary retention.
4. Discuss drug therapy for Alzheimer's disease.
5. Describe major nursing care needs of patients receiving cholinergic drugs.
6. Describe signs, symptoms, and treatment of overdose with cholinergic drugs.
7. Discuss atropine and pralidoxime as antidotes for cholinergic drugs.
8. Discuss principles of therapy for using cholinergic drugs in special populations.
9. Teach patients about safe, effective use of cholinergic drugs.

■ Section II: Assessing Your Understanding

ACTIVITY A

Fill in the Blanks

1. _____ drugs stimulate the parasympathetic nervous system in the same manner as acetylcholine.
2. In normal neuromuscular function, _____ is released from nerve endings and binds to nicotinic receptors on cell membranes of muscle cells to cause muscle contraction.
3. _____ _____ is an autoimmune disorder in which autoantibodies are thought to destroy nicotinic receptors for acetylcholine on skeletal muscle.
4. Alzheimer's disease, the most common type of dementia in adults, is characterized by abnormalities in the cholinergic, serotonergic, noradrenergic, and _____ neurotransmission systems.
5. Acetylcholine stimulates _____ receptors in the gut to promote normal secretory and motor activity.

ACTIVITY B

Matching

Match the term in Column A with the definition in Column B.

COLUMN A

1. _____ Bethanechol (Urecholine)
2. _____ Neostigmine (Prostigmin)
3. _____ Edrophonium (Tensilon)
4. _____ Physostigmine salicylate (Antilirium)
5. _____ Donepezil (Aricept)

COLUMN B

A. Used to treat mild to moderate Alzheimer's disease
B. Synthetic derivative of choline
C. Short-acting cholinergic drug used to diagnose myasthenia gravis
D. The only anticholinesterase capable of crossing the blood–brain barrier
E. The prototype anticholinesterase agent

ACTIVITY C

Short Answers

Briefly answer the following questions.

1. What is the function of cholinergic drugs on body systems?
2. What is the role of acetylcholine as it relates to normal brain function?
3. What is the role of acetylcholine as it relates to the gastrointestinal system?
4. What is the role of acetylcholine as it relates to the urinary system?
5. What is the mechanism of action for direct-acting cholinergic drugs?

■ Section III: Applying Your Knowledge

ACTIVITY D

Case Study

Consider the scenario and answer the questions.

Mr. Davis, age 35, presents to the physician's office with complaints of generalized weakness. The physician orders tests to evaluate his condition and diagnoses Mr. Davis with myasthenia gravis. You are responsible for the education plan for both the disease process and the medications prescribed for the condition.

1. Mr. Davis is relieved to understand that the symptoms that he is experiencing are related to a disease process and he can begin treatment. He asks you to explain his diagnosis. How would you respond?
2. How is myasthenia gravis diagnosed? The physician orders neostigmine. How does this fit in?
3. Mr. Davis does not want to self-administer the neostigmine by injection, so the physician prescribes the medication so that it may be administered orally. What can you tell the patient about oral doses of neostigmine? What can you tell him about long-term use of the medication?

■ Section IV: Practicing for NCLEX

Answer the following questions.

1. Mr. Bates is treated in the critical care unit for overdose of indirect cholinergic drugs. What is the treatment of choice in this situation?
   a. An anticholinesterase reactivator
   b. Atropine
   c. Pralidoxime
   d. A cholinesterase reactivator

2. Mr. Chin is experiencing paralysis due to overdose of indirect cholinergic drugs. You understand that atropine will reverse muscarinic effects due to overdose of cholinergic drugs, but which of the following will it not reverse?
   a. Cholinergic effects of skeletal-muscle weakness or paralysis
   b. Nicotinic effects of skeletal-muscle weakness or paralysis
   c. Ketoacidosis in the skeletal muscle
   d. Lactic acid accumulated in the skeletal muscle

3. _____ is used to differentiate between myasthenic crisis (too little cholinergic medication) and cholinergic crisis (too much cholinergic medication).

4. Indirect-acting cholinergic or anticholinesterase drugs are indicated to treat myasthenia gravis as well as which of the following conditions?
   a. Muscular dystrophy
   b. Musculoskeletal cancer
   c. Alzheimer's disease
   d. Cerebrovascular dementia

5. Mrs. Belts had surgery 24 hours ago to repair a hernia. You find that she has not had a bowel movement since the day before the surgery. She is experiencing abdominal distention, and during auscultation you note an absence of bowel sounds. Further examination and testing reveal a paralytic ileus. The physician orders bethanechol. What type of drug is bethanechol?
   a. Anticholinergic medication
   b. Direct-acting cholinergic drug
   c. Indirect-acting cholinergic drug
   d. Indirect-acting anticholinergic medication

6. Indirect-acting cholinergic drugs also stimulate nicotinic receptors in skeletal muscles, resulting in which of the following?
   a. Increased smooth muscle tone
   b. Decreased musculoskeletal pain
   c. Improved skeletal muscle tone and strength
   d. Decreased muscle spasticity

7. Both direct-acting cholinergic drugs and indirect-acting cholinergic drugs (or anticholinesterase drugs) have widespread _____ effects when they activate muscarinic receptors in cardiac muscle, smooth muscle, exocrine glands and the eye.

8. Mr. Baton, age 75, is diagnosed with myasthenia gravis. As his home care nurse, how can you assist him with medication compliance?
   a. Pre-pouring his medications one week at a time
   b. Ensuring that all medications have safety caps
   c. Persuading his son to call once a week to encourage him to take his medications
   d. Asking the housekeeper to administer the medications

9. Mr. Gates is diagnosed with hepatitis C and myasthenia gravis. His prescriptions include neostigmine. You are concerned because Mr. Gates may experience which of the following?
   a. Increased absorption of the medication
   b. Increased adverse effects
   c. Increased resistance to the medication
   d. Decreased absorption of the medication

10. Mr. Gibbons, age 65, takes cholinergic medication. He presents to the emergency room with symptoms associated with GI distress. He is diagnosed with a small-bowel obstruction. Which of the following actions would you expect the physician to take?
    a. Increase the dose of the cholinergic medication to facilitate peristalsis
    b. Decrease the dose of the cholinergic medication to slow peristalsis
    c. Maintain the same dosage of the cholinergic medication because it will not affect the diagnosis
    d. Discontinue the cholinergic medication to prevent injury to the areas proximal to the obstruction

11. Individuals with peptic ulcer disease should not use cholinergic drugs because they increase _____ _____ secretion.

12. Mrs. Baton is taking cholinergic medication to control bladder retention. She presents to the emergency department with confusion, shortness of breath, and an apical pulse of 42 beats per minute and irregular. Which of the following actions would you expect the physician to take?
    a. Increase the cholinergic medication to increase cardiac contractility
    b. Increase the cholinergic medication to increase oxygenation to the heart through vasodilation
    c. Decrease the cholinergic medication to alleviate the symptom of confusion
    d. Discontinue the cholinergic medication secondary to the diagnosis of bradycardia

13. Patients with hyperthyroidism should avoid cholinergic drugs. Which of the following is a symptom associated with the administration of cholinergic medication to an individual with the diagnosis of hyperthyroidism?
    a. Hyperglycemia   c. Increased TSH
    b. Decreases TSH   d. Reflex tachycardia

14. You understand that cholinergic medications are contraindicated in clients with asthmatic bronchitis because they may have which of the following effects?
    a. Cause bronchodilation
    b. Decrease secretions
    c. Cause secretions to thicken
    d. Cause bronchoconstriction

15. A direct-acting drug, _____, is used to treat urinary retention due to urinary bladder atony and postoperative abdominal distention due to paralytic ileus.

16. Direct-acting cholinergic drugs affect the bladder by causing which of the following? (Select all that apply.)
    a. Increased tone and contractility
    b. Relaxation of the sphincter
    c. Increased bladder capacity
    d. Reduction in UTIs

17. Direct-acting cholinergic drugs cause
_____ respiratory secretions.

18. Indirect-acting cholinergic or anticholinesterase drugs decrease the inactivation of _____ in the synapse by the enzyme acetylcholinesterase.

19. When indirect-acting cholinergic drugs are used to treat Alzheimer's disease, they improve symptoms by doing which of the following?
    a. Improving cholinergic neurotransmission to the brain
    b. Improving anticholinergic neurotransmission to the brain
    c. Improving medication absorption through the blood–brain barrier
    d. Causing vasodilation of the cerebral arteries

20. Anticholinesterase drugs are classified as either reversible or irreversible inhibitors of _____.

CHAPTER 20

Anticholinergic Drugs

■ Section I: Learning Objectives

1. List characteristics of anticholinergic drugs in terms of effects on body tissues, indications for use, nursing process implications, observation of patient response, and teaching patients.
2. Discuss atropine as the prototype of anticholinergic drugs.
3. Discuss clinical disorders or symptoms for which anticholinergic drugs are used.
4. Describe the mechanism by which atropine relieves bradycardia.
5. Review anticholinergic effects of antipsychotics, tricyclic antidepressants, and antihistamines.
6. Discuss principles of therapy and nursing process for using anticholinergic drugs in special populations.
7. Describe the signs and symptoms of atropine or anticholinergic drug overdose and its treatment.
8. Teach patients about the safe, effective use of anticholinergic drugs.

■ Section II: Assessing Your Understanding

ACTIVITY A

Fill in the Blanks

1. _____ drugs block the action of acetylcholine on the parasympathetic nervous system.
2. _____ amines are uncharged, lipid-soluble molecules.
3. Some belladonna derivatives and synthetic anticholinergics are _____ amines.
4. When given at high doses, a few anticholinergic drugs are also able to block _____ receptors in autonomic ganglia and skeletal muscles.
5. Because cholinergic _____ receptors are widely distributed in the body, anticholinergic drugs produce effects in a variety of locations, including the central nervous system (CNS), heart, smooth muscle, glands, and the eye.

ACTIVITY B

Matching

Match the term in Column A with the definition in Column B.

COLUMN A

1. _____ Ipratropium or tiotropium
2. _____ Atropine
3. _____ Homatropine hydrobromide
4. _____ Hyoscyamine
5. _____ Scopolamine

COLUMN B

A. Prototype of anticholinergic drugs, a naturally occurring belladonna alkaloid that can be extracted from the belladonna plant or prepared synthetically

B. A belladonna alkaloid used in gastrointestinal and genitourinary disorders characterized by spasm, increased secretion, and increased motility

C. May be given by inhalation for bronchodilating effects

D. When given parenterally, depresses the CNS and causes amnesia, drowsiness, euphoria, relaxation, and sleep

E. A semisynthetic derivative of atropine used as eye drops to produce mydriasis and cycloplegia

ACTIVITY C

Short Answers

Briefly answer the following questions.

1. Describe the characteristics of tertiary amines and give examples of two medications in this category.
2. Describe the characteristics of quaternary amines.
3. Describe the general characteristics of anticholinergic drugs.
4. How do anticholinergic drugs affect the cardiovascular system?
5. How do anticholinergic drugs affect the respiratory system?

■ Section III: Applying Your Knowledge

ACTIVITY D

Case Study

Consider the scenario and answer the questions.

Mrs. Benz, age 78, is diagnosed with COPD by her physician. The physician orders tiotropium bromide. You are responsible for her education plan.

1. Mrs. Benz asks you how the medication will help her to breathe easier. How would you respond?
2. Mrs. Benz asks you if it might just be easier to take the capsule by mouth than in the inhalation device. She asks, "Wouldn't it work just as well?" How would you respond? What other patient education concerning this medication is in order?
3. Mrs. Benz then asks if she can take the medication twice on days she goes golfing, so that she will breathe easier. How would you respond to this?
4. Mrs. Benz is later diagnosed with mild to moderate renal insufficiency. What would you expect the physician to do? Would the patient's age be a factor in the physician's decision?

■ Section IV: Practicing for NCLEX

Answer the following questions.

1. _____ is the antidote for muscarinic agonist poisoning.

2. Anticholinergic overdose is characterized by which of the following signs and symptoms? (Select all that apply.)
   a. Hyperthermia
   b. Moist mucus membranes
   c. Mydriasis
   d. Urinary retention

3. _____ is the specific antidote for anticholinergic overdose.

4. Mrs. Briggs, age 57, has a history of two myocardial infarctions in the past 3 years. She presents to the physician's office with symptoms of an overactive bladder. She requests an anticholinergic medication that she saw advertised on television. You would expect the physician to do which of the following?
   a. Order the anticholinergic medication
   b. Order blood work to rule out a urinary tract infection and order the medication
   c. Order a urinalysis to rule out a urinary tract infection and order the medication
   d. Explain to the client that the medication is contraindicated because of her medical history

5. You are caring for Mr. Banks. He asks why he needs the preoperative anticholinergic medication ordered by the anesthesiologist. You explain that anticholinergic drugs are given preoperatively to prevent anesthesia-associated complications such as which of the following?
   a. Tachycardia   c. Hypertension
   b. Bradycardia   d. Dehydration

6. Mr. Brady, age 75, is experiencing extrapyramidal symptoms secondary to an antipsychotic drug. Which of the following drugs would you expect the physician to order to relieve these symptoms?
   a. Beta-blockers   c. ACE inhibitors
   b. Anticholinergics   d. Physostigmine salicylate

7. _____ is the drug of choice to treat bradycardia.

8. Which of the following medications may be given to children because of its bronchodilation effects in the treatment of asthma and chronic bronchitis?

   a. Ipratropium   c. Hyoscyamine
   b. Atropine   d. Scopolamine

9. Opthalmic anticholinergic preparations are indicated for _____ and _____ effects to aid in eye examination and surgery.

10. Mr. Bates is diagnosed with IBS and the physician orders an antispasmodic. Which of the following drugs would you expect the physician to order?

    a. Atropine   c. Glycopyrrolate
    b. Hyoscyamine   d. Ipratropium

11. You are asked to create a presentation for your anatomy and physiology class on cholinergic receptors. You explain that cholinergic (muscarinic) receptors are widespread throughout the body and are located in which of the following body parts? (Select all that apply.)

    a. Mitochondria   c. Eyes
    b. Heart   d. Glands

12. Most anticholinergic drugs interact with muscarinic cholinergic receptors in the brain, secretory glands, heart, and smooth muscle and are sometimes called _____ drugs.

13. Anticholinergic drugs block the action of acetylcholine on which of the following systems?

    a. Sympathetic nervous system
    b. Parasympathetic nervous system
    c. Musculoskeletal system
    d. Genitourinary system

14. Mr. Belcher is prescribed an anticholinergic drug by his physician. He likes to hike with his grandchildren. As his home care nurse, you realize that part of Mr. Belcher's education plan should include heat stroke prevention, because anticholinergic medications have which of the following effects?

    a. Increasing sweating and the risk for heat stroke and dehydration
    b. Causing postural hypotension and increased risk for falls and from exposure to the elements
    c. Causing bradycardia in older adults, which increases the risk for falls and from exposure to the elements
    d. Preventing sweating and heat loss and increasing the risk of heat stroke

15. A client presents to your emergency department with evidence of bradydysrhythmias. Which of the following is the treatment of choice for bradydysrhythmias?

    a. Atropine 0.5 mg administered IV every 3-5 minutes
    b. Atropine 1 mg administered IV every 3-5 minutes
    c. Atropine 0.25 mg administered IV every 3-5 minutes
    d. Atropine 4 mg administered IV every 3-5 minutes

16. Mr. Giancarlo, age 80, who lives in a long-term care facility, is prescribed anticholinergic medications by his physician. Recently he has complained of blurred vision. You call the physician regarding these symptoms. You would expect to modify Mr. Giancarlo's care plan to include which of the following?

    a. Falls prevention
    b. Dietary modifications
    c. Use of restraints
    d. Occupational therapy

17. Mrs. Beach, age 45, is diagnosed with overactive bladder, asthmatic bronchitis, and narrow-angle glaucoma. She asks the physician to prescribe the same anticholinergic medication that her friend uses for her overactive bladder. Which of the following would you expect the physician to do?

    a. Order the medication

    b. Order the medication with scheduled routine blood work

    c. Decline the prescription preference because of the diagnosis of asthmatic bronchitis

    d. Decline the prescription because of the diagnosis of narrow-angle glaucoma

18. Mr. Wright is diagnosed with irritable bowel syndrome. The physician orders anticholinergic medication. What is the reason for this decision?

    a. To reduce the inflammation to the intestines

    b. To increase the frequency of the bowel movements

    c. To reduce the frequency of bowel movements

    d. To prevent a gastrointestinal bleed

19. Mr. Devlin has been a paraplegic for 5 years. He complains of increased incontinence, and the physician orders anticholinergic medication. What is the reason for this decision?

    a. To increase bladder capacity

    b. To strengthen the detrusor muscles

    c. To decrease bladder capacity

    d. To decrease irritation to the wall of the bladder

20. Mr. Levitz is diagnosed with Parkinson's disease. The physician orders anticholinergic drugs. What is the reason for this decision?

    a. To improve his gait

    b. To decrease spasticity

    c. To prevent fractures

    d. To improve swallowing

CHAPTER 21

Physiology of the Endocrine System

■ Section I: Learning Objectives

1. Examine the relationship between the endocrine system and the central nervous system.
2. Describe general characteristics and functions of hormones.
3. Compare steroid and protein hormones in relation to site of action and pharmacokinetics.
4. Examine hormonal action at the cellular level.
5. Describe the second messenger roles of cyclic adenosine monophosphate and calcium within body cells.
6. Differentiate between physiologic and pharmacologic doses of hormonal drugs.

■ Section II: Assessing Your Understanding

ACTIVITY A

Fill in the Blanks

1. The main connecting link between the nervous system and the endocrine system is the _____, which responds to nervous system stimulation by producing hormones.
2. A/An _____ _____ _____ occurs when hormone secretion is stimulated as they are needed and inhibited when they are not needed.
3. _____ are extremely important in regulating body activities.
4. _____-derived hormones usually circulate in an unbound, active form.
5. _____ modify rather than initiate cellular reactions and functions.

ACTIVITY B

Matching

Match the term in Column A with the definition in Column B.

COLUMN A

1. _____ Hypothalamus
2. _____ ACTH, cortisol, and growth hormone
3. _____ Endocrine tissues
4. _____ Lipid-soluble steroid and thyroid hormones
5. _____ Estrogen and progestin secretion

COLUMN B

A. Function through hormones, which act as chemical messengers to transmit information between body cells and organs
B. Have a longer duration of action because they are bound to plasma proteins
C. Controls secretion of almost all hormones from the pituitary gland
D. Secreted in 24-hour (circadian) cycles
E. Related to the 28-day menstrual cycle

ACTIVITY C

Short Answers

Briefly answer the following questions.

1. Identify the components of the endocrine system.
2. What role does the endocrine system play in the regulation of body systems?
3. Define the term *hormones* and state their function.
4. Explain the function of erythropoietin.
5. White blood cells produce cytokines. What is the role of cytokines in the body?

■ Section III: Applying Your Knowledge

ACTIVITY D

Case Study

Consider the scenario and answer the questions.

You are working on a medical unit and caring for clients with glandular hypofunction and others with glandular hyperfunction.

1. What kinds of structural and functional factors are associated with hypofunction of a gland?
2. Sometimes an endocrine gland may produce adequate hormone but the hormone does not function normally. What might explain this situation?
3. An endocrine gland may atrophy and become less able to produce its hormone. What causes it to atrophy?
4. What are some causes of excessive stimulation and enlargement of an endocrine gland? What does glandular hyperfunction usually result in?

■ Section IV: Practicing for NCLEX

1. Chronic exposure to abnormal levels of hormones may cause which of the following situations?
   a. Receptors capable of potentiating hormonal levels within the gland
   b. Receptors to maintain chronic abnormal levels
   c. Receptors capable of hormonal cessation
   d. Receptors capable of upregulation or downregulation.

2. Many hormones act as a "first messenger" to the cell, and the hormone–receptor complex activates a "second messenger," which _____ intracellular structures to produce characteristic cellular functions and products.

3. Which of the following statements is true about the endocrine and nervous systems?
   a. They function as agonists in relation to body functions.
   b. They do not work in conjunction with one another.
   c. They work to integrate and regulate body functions.
   d. They work as separate and distinct body systems.

4. Water-soluble, protein-derived hormones have a short duration of action and are inactivated by which of the following types of enzymes?
   a. Pancreatic enzymes
   b. Gastrointestinal enzymes
   c. Enzymes mainly in the liver and kidneys
   d. Enzymes mainly in the pancreas and gastrointestinal system

5. Hormones given for therapeutic purposes may be obtained from which of the following types of sources? (Select all that apply.)
   a. Individual sources
   b. Human sources
   c. Animal sources
   d. Synthetic sources

6. The physiologic use of hormones includes adrenal corticosteroid administration in _____ disease.

7. Adrenal corticosteroids are used as which of the following?
   a. Hormonal suppressants
   b. Anti-inflammatory drugs
   c. Hyperglycemic drugs
   d. Anti-seizure medications

8. Hormones are given for physiologic or pharmacologic effects and are more often given for disorders resulting from which of the following condition of an endocrine gland?
   a. Hypofunction
   b. Dysfunction
   c. Failure
   d. Hyperfunction

9. Physiologic use of hormones involves giving _____ doses as a replacement or substitute for the amount secreted by a normally functioning endocrine gland.

10. Many of the most important hormones have been synthesized. Which of the following are characteristics of synthesized hormones compared with naturally occurring hormones? (Select all that apply.)
    a. Increased potency
    b. Prolonged effects
    c. Decreased potency
    d. Short-term effects necessitating higher doses of the medication

11. Administration of one hormone may _____ effects of other hormones through complex hormone interactions.

12. Malfunction of an endocrine organ is usually associated with what type of change to secretion of its hormones? (Select all that apply.)
    a. Hyposecretion   c. Asecretion
    b. Hypersecretion   d. Inappropriate

13. Steroid hormones cross cell membranes easily because they have which of the following characteristics?
    a. They are protein soluble.
    b. They are electrolyte balanced.
    c. They are lipid soluble.
    d. They are carbohydrate soluble.

14. The lipid component of diacylglycerol is arachidonic acid, the precursor for prostaglandins and _____.

15. Phospholipids are major components of which portion of all body cells?
    a. Mitochondrial   c. Ribosomal
    b. Chromosomal   d. Cell membrane

16. The gastrointestinal mucosa produces hormones that are important in the digestive process. What hormones are they? (Select all that apply.)
    a. Gastrin   c. Cholecystokinin
    b. Secretin   d. Bromine

17. The kidneys produce a hormone that stimulates the bone marrow to produce red blood cells. What is this hormone called?
    a. Poietin   c. Phagopoietin
    b. Erythropoietin   d. Leukopoietin

18. Which of the following types of tumors may produce corticotropin (adrenocorticotropic hormone, or ACTH), antidiuretic hormone, or parathyroid hormone?
    a. Renal tumors   c. Lung tumors
    b. Brain tumors   d. Gastric tumors

19. White blood cells produce cytokines that function as messengers among _____ in inflammatory and immune processes.

20. Secretion of almost all hormones from the pituitary gland is controlled by the _____.

CHAPTER 22

Hypothalamic and Pituitary Hormones

■ Section I: Learning Objectives

1. Identify the clinical uses of selected hormones.
2. Differentiate between characteristics and functions of anterior and posterior pituitary hormones.
3. Recognize the limitations of hypothalamic and pituitary hormones as therapeutic agents.
4. Identify major nursing considerations in the care of patients receiving specific hypothalamic and pituitary hormones.

■ Section II: Assessing Your Understanding

ACTIVITY A

Fill in the Blanks

1. The hypothalamus of the brain and the pituitary gland interact to control most metabolic functions of the body and to maintain _____.
2. The hypothalamus and the pituitary gland are anatomically connected by the funnel-shaped _____ stalk.
3. The _____ controls secretions of the pituitary gland.
4. The pituitary gland regulates secretions or functions of other body tissues, called

   _____ _____.
5. The posterior pituitary is anatomically an extension of the hypothalamus and is composed mainly of _____ fibers.

ACTIVITY B

Matching

Match the term in Column A with the definition in Column B.

COLUMN A

1. _____ Thyrotropin-releasing hormone (TRH)
2. _____ Gonadotropin-releasing hormone (GnRH)
3. _____ Corticotropin
4. _____ GH
5. _____ Thyrotropin

COLUMN B

A. Also called ACTH; stimulates the adrenal cortex to produce corticosteroids
B. Also called somatotropin; stimulates growth of body tissues
C. Causes release of follicle-stimulating hormone (FSH) and luteinizing hormone (LH)
D. Also called TSH; regulates secretion of thyroid hormones
E. Causes release of TSH in response to stress, such as exposure to cold

ACTIVITY C

Short Answers

Briefly answer the following questions.

1. What is the function of FSH in the human body?
2. What is the function of LH in the human body?
3. What is the function of prolactin in the human body?
4. What is the function of the melanocyte-stimulating hormone in the human body?
5. What is the function of oxytocin in the human body?

■ Section III: Applying Your Knowledge

ACTIVITY D
Case Study
Consider the scenario and answer the questions.

Mr. Chasen is diagnosed with end-stage prostate cancer. The physician orders Lupron 1 mg subcutaneously each day. You are responsible for the client's education regarding his disease process and medication regimen.

1. You explain that leuprolide (Lupron) initially stimulates LH and FSH secretion. After chronic administration of therapeutic doses, however, what does the drug do?
2. Mr. Chasen is concerned when he is told that his medication regimen will decrease his testosterone level and asks whether this change is permanent. How would you respond?
3. Mrs. Chasen, your patient's wife, is hesitant to administer the medication by injection and asks whether her husband can take the medication by mouth. How would you respond? What other information can you give Mrs. Chasen regarding dosing?
4. What information would you give the patient regarding the adverse effects related to Lupron?

■ Section IV: Practicing for NCLEX

Answer the following questions.

1. Antidiuretic hormone (ADH), also called _____ functions to regulate water balance.

2. The posterior pituitary gland stores and releases two hormones that are synthesized by nerve cells in the hypothalamus. What are these two hormones?
   a. PTH   c. ADH
   b. MSH   d. Oxytocin

3. Mrs. Gates is diagnosed with hyperpituitarism. This condition is most often treated with which of the following? (Select all that apply.)
   a. Medication to reduce pituitary secretion
   b. Antibiotics
   c. Surgery
   d. Radiation

4. Mrs. Caster is diagnosed with a pituitary hormone deficiency. She complains that her drug dosages are modified frequently; you explain that the dosage of all pituitary hormones must be individualized. Which of the following factors determines the dosage?
   a. The responsiveness of affected tissues, which varies
   b. The age of the client
   c. The weight of the client
   d. The responsiveness of affected tissues, which is static

5. Mrs. Andrews, age 45, states that she has experienced a burst of energy since she received GH at a clinic. She presents to the physician's office with dizziness and headaches. Which of the following is a side effect of GH?
   a. Congestive heart failure
   b. Vertigo
   c. Hyperglycemia
   d. Hypertension

6. Ms. Banka, age 43, has a history of breast cancer, hyperlipidemia, and atrial fibrillation. She has heard that GH will improve her appearance and increase her energy. You understand that, based on her diagnoses, GH increases Ms. Banka's risk for which of the following conditions?
   a. Cancer
   b. Gastrointestinal disease
   c. Pancreatitis
   d. Diabetes type 2

7. Mrs. Strands, age 22, is 2 weeks after her due date for delivery of her second child. In order to induce labor, the physician orders IV _____.

8. Mrs. Strands asks how the IV medication will induce labor. Which of the following does the medication do?
   a. Promotes uterine irritability
   b. Increases oxygenation to the uterus
   c. Causes labor to continue slowly
   d. Promotes uterine contractility

9. _____ is used in the treatment of bleeding esophageal varices because of its vasoconstrictive effects.

10. Mrs. Bates is diagnosed with diabetes insipidus. The physician orders desmopressin, which is the synthetic equivalent of which of the following hormones?
    a. PTH   c. ADH
    b. ACTH   d. PTCH

11. Mr. France is diagnosed with acromegaly. His secondary diagnoses include hypertension, diabetes type 2, and a status post myocardial infarct in 1992. Based on his diagnoses, the physician would modify the dose of which of his medications?
    a. Hypoglycemic medication
    b. Antihypertensive medication
    c. Antianginal medication
    d. Nitrate medication

12. The main clinical use of GH is for children whose growth is impaired by a deficiency of _____ hormone.

13. Octreotide has pharmacologic actions similar to those of somatostatin. For which of the following diagnoses and symptoms is octreotide prescribed? (Select all that apply.)
    a. Hyperlipidemia   c. Hypertension
    b. Acromegaly   d. Diarrhea in AIDS

14. _____, a synthetic formulation, is commonly used to test for suspected adrenal insufficiency.

15. When ADH is secreted, it has which of the following effects on renal tubules?
    a. It makes them less permeable to water.
    b. It decreases potassium secretion.
    c. It increases sodium secretion.
    d. It makes them more permeable to water.

16. _____ secretion is controlled by a negative feedback mechanism in proportion to metabolic needs.

17. GH, also called *somatotropin*, performs which of the following functions? (Select all that apply.)
    a. Stimulating growth of body tissues
    b. Regulating cell division and protein synthesis
    c. Promoting an increase in cell size and number
    d. Decreasing long bone growth in young adults

18. Mr. Saks is prescribed GH. He also takes a medication to control his diabetes type 2. Which of the following conditions does GH cause?
    a. Hyperinsulinemia   c. Hypertension
    b. Hypoinsulinemia   d. Hyperglycemia

19. Levels of GH rise rapidly during adolescence, peak in the _____, and then start to decline.

20. GH stimulates protein _____ in many tissues.

CHAPTER 23

Corticosteroids

■ Section I: Learning Objectives

1. Review physiologic effects of endogenous corticosteroids.
2. Discuss clinical indications for use of exogenous corticosteroids.
3. Differentiate between physiologic and pharmacologic doses of corticosteroids.
4. Differentiate between short-term and long-term corticosteroid therapy.
5. Recognize at least 10 adverse effects of long-term corticosteroid therapy.
6. Explain the pathophysiologic basis of adverse drug effects.
7. Examine the potential benefits for administering corticosteroids topically when possible rather than systemically.
8. Analyze the use of other drugs and interventions to decrease the need for corticosteroids.
9. Discuss the use of corticosteroids in selected populations and conditions.
10. Apply the nursing process with a patient receiving long-term systemic corticosteroid therapy, including teaching needs.

■ Section II: Assessing Your Understanding

ACTIVITY A

Fill in the Blanks

1. _____, also called *glucocorticoids* or *steroids*, are hormones produced by the adrenal cortex, part of the adrenal glands.
2. _____ corticosteroids are used as drugs in a variety of disorders.
3. When plasma corticosteroid levels rise to an adequate level, secretion of corticosteroids _____ or _____.

4. The mechanism by which the hypothalamus and anterior pituitary "learn" that no more corticosteroids are needed is called a

   _____ _____ _____.
5. _____ are secreted directly into the bloodstream.

ACTIVITY B

Matching

Match the term in Column A with the definition in Column B.

COLUMN A

1. _____ Hyperaldosteronism

2. _____ Congenital adrenogenital syndromes and adrenal hyperplasia

3. _____ Secondary adrenocortical insufficiency

4. _____ Primary adrenocortical insufficiency (Addison's disease)

5. _____ Adrenocortical hyperfunction (Cushing's disease)

COLUMN B

A. Produced by inadequate secretion of corticotrophin, most often caused by prolonged administration of corticosteroids

B. Associated with destruction of the adrenal cortex by disease processes or hemorrhage and with atrophy of the adrenal cortex

C. A rare disorder caused by adenoma or hyperplasia of the adrenal cortex cells that produce aldosterone

D. Result from deficiencies in one or more enzymes required for cortisol production

E. May result from excessive corticotrophin or a primary adrenal tumor

ACTIVITY C

Short Answers

Briefly answer the following questions.

1. Discuss the process by which corticosteroid secretion is controlled.
2. How does the stress response affect the sympathetic nervous system?
3. What are glucocorticoids, and how do they affect the body's processes?
4. What are mineralocorticoids, and how do they affect the body's processes?
5. What are adrenal sex hormones, and how do they affect the body's processes?

■ Section III: Applying Your Knowledge

ACTIVITY D

Case Study

Consider the scenario and answer the questions.

You are participating in a study group of nursing students studying the indications for the various uses of corticosteroids.

1. Mr. Janis is diagnosed with a system lupus erythematosus. Where would you expect to find inflammation in this patient?
2. Name some skin disorders that may be treated with corticosteroids.
3. Corticosteroids are effective in the treatment of neoplastic diseases. What mechanism of action do they have that makes them effective?
4. Mr. Castile received a kidney transplant 6 months ago. He is not comfortable with the changes in his body related to the corticosteroids he must take. He asks why they are necessary. How would you respond?
5. In patients with asthma, what is the effect of corticosteroids? In patients with anaphylactic shock resulting from an allergic reaction, what is the effect of corticosteroids?

■ Section IV: Practicing for NCLEX

Answer the following questions.

1. Ms. Petski's physician discontinues her systemic corticosteroid using a sliding scale and orders an inhaler. Ms. Petski asks if she can begin flunisolide; her friend uses it and suggested it as Ms. Petski's next option. How should you respond?
   a. That you will ask the physician to change his original prescription
   b. That flunisolide is a safe option
   c. That flunisolide is not the primary medication to treat her disease process
   d. That the physician did not order flunisolide because it may cause death

2. Adverse effects of systemic corticosteroids may include which of the following? (Select all that apply.)
   a. Hirsutism
   b. Hypertension
   c. Glucose intolerance
   d. Premature puberty in children

3. Strategies to minimize HPA suppression and risks of acute adrenal insufficiency include which of the following?
   a. Reducing the dose of systematic corticosteroids when the client on long-term therapy experiences high-stress situations
   b. Administering a systemic corticosteroid during high-stress situations in clients on long-term systemic therapy
   c. Concurrent use of oral contraceptives and corticosteroids in women to reduce the stress on the adrenal gland
   d. Drug holidays for clients with long-term corticosteroid use

4. Mr. Spade experiences an acute exacerbation of his asthma secondary to an allergic reaction. The physician orders which of the following types of therapy to minimize HPA suppression and risks of acute adrenal insufficiency?

    a. A short course of systemic therapy

    b. Long-term systemic therapy to prevent future exacerbations of his asthma

    c. Long-term systemic therapy with drug holidays every 6 months

    d. A short course of systemic therapy with a prn prescription of corticosteroids

5. Mrs. Granit experiences weight gain secondary to her systemic steroid therapy for temporal arteritis. She calls the physician's office to ask if she can discontinue the medication for 1 week, to fit into her dress for her class reunion. Which response is appropriate?

    a. "A temporary discontinuance will not adversely affect your health."

    b. "I will ask the physician for a change in your prescription."

    c. "Your prescription must be tapered gradually with the physician's order."

    d. "Your prescription must be tapered for 2 days only with the physician's order."

6. Mr. Bates develops a mild rash secondary to sensitivity to a new laundry detergent. The physician orders a topical corticosteroid. Mr. Bates states that this medication will take too long to work and asks whether he can just take a steroid by mouth. Which of the following is an appropriate response?

    a. "Oral corticosteroids will not reduce the inflammation of contact dermatitis."

    b. "Oral corticosteroids are contraindicated for cases of contact dermatitis."

    c. "Local therapy will resolve the symptoms of the dermatitis quicker than the use of oral corticosteroids."

    d. "Using local rather than systemic corticosteroids reduces adrenal insufficiency."

7. Adrenocortical hyperfunction (Cushing's disease) may result from excessive _____ or a primary adrenal tumor.

8. Mr. Abernathy is diagnosed with Addison's disease. Which of the following daily medications would you expect to be administered?

    a. Warfarin   c. Apresoline

    b. Hydrochlorothiazide   d. Prednisone

9. Mineralocorticoid and _____ effects of exogenous corticosteroids are usually considered adverse reactions.

10. Which of the following are the most frequently desired pharmacologic effects of exogenous corticosteroids? (Select all that apply.)

    a. Anti-inflammatory   c. Anticoagulant

    b. Immunosuppressive   d. Antianxiety

11. You are working in a home care setting. Mrs. Blanc is prescribed oral corticosteroids by her physician secondary to a diagnosis of Addison's disease. Which of the following tasks is your responsibility?

    a. Supervising and monitoring the administration of the drug

    b. Administering all doses of the oral medication

    c. Administering all doses of the oral medication for the first month of use

    d. Teaching all family members to administer the medication

12. Mr. Bean is diagnosed with pneumocystosis and his physician orders corticosteroids. Which of the following is an accurate statement to include in your teaching plan for Mr. Bean?

    a. Corticosteroids may reduce his survival rate but improve his quality of life.

    b. Corticosteroids decrease risks of respiratory failure.

    c. Corticosteroids decrease cerebral edema associated with pneumocystosis.

    d. Corticosteroids decrease the white blood cell count related to pneumocystosis.

13. Mrs. Maris is diagnosed with septic shock. What would you expect a long course of low-dose corticosteroids to do?
    a. Diminish her survival secondary to impaired immunity
    b. Improve her survival without causing harm
    c. Improve her survival with long-term adrenal insufficiency
    d. Diminish her survival secondary to superinfection

14. Mr. Anspar is diagnosed with adult respiratory distress syndrome. His family asks whether corticosteroids may help him to breathe easier. Which of the following statements about corticosteroids is accurate?
    a. They are successfully used for the long-term treatment of ARDS.
    b. They are successful for the short-term treatment of ARDS.
    c. They are not used when the patient is at risk for *Pneumocystis* pneumonia.
    d. They are not a beneficial treatment for ARDS.

15. Mr. Gonzalez receives IV methylprednisolone to treat status asthmaticus. Corticosteroid use may increase the risk of which of the following conditions for Mr. Gonzalez?
    a. Pulmonary infection   c. Pulmonary edema
    b. Bronchospasm   d. Bronchoconstriction

16. Ms. Brinks is diagnosed with adrenal insufficiency. She presents to the emergency room with hypotension. Which of the following would you expect the physician to prescribe?
    a. Vasopressors   c. ACE inhibitors
    b. Corticosteroids   d. Beta-blockers

17. Metabolism of corticosteroids is _____ by severe hepatic disease.

18. Systemic corticosteroids should be used with caution because of slowed excretion, with possible accumulation and signs and symptoms of _____ .

19. The use of corticosteroids in older adults may aggravate which of the following conditions? (Select all that apply.)
    a. Congestive heart failure
    b. Gout
    c. Diabetes mellitus
    d. Arthritis

20. For children with asthma, evidence indicates that starting with a _____ dose of inhaled corticosteroid is comparable to starting with a high-dose and titrating down.

CHAPTER 24

Thyroid and Antithyroid Drugs

■ Section I: Learning Objectives

1. Recognize the physiologic effects of thyroid hormone.
2. Assess subclinical, symptomatic, and severe effects of inadequate or excessive thyroid hormone.
3. Describe characteristics, uses, and effects of thyroid drugs.
4. Identify characteristics, uses, and effects of antithyroid drugs.
5. Evaluate the influence of thyroid and antithyroid drugs on the metabolism of other drugs.
6. Teach patients effective self-care activities related to the use of thyroid and antithyroid drugs.
7. Apply the nursing process with patients receiving thyroid and antithyroid drugs.

■ Section II: Assessing Your Understanding

ACTIVITY A

Fill in the Blanks

1. The thyroid gland produces three hormones: _____, triiodothyronine, and calcitonin.
2. Production of T_3 and T_4 depends on the presence of _____ and _____ in the thyroid gland.
3. Thyroid hormones control the rate of _____ _____ and thereby influence the functioning of virtually every cell in the body.
4. _____ _____ occurs when disease or destruction of thyroid gland tissue causes inadequate production of thyroid hormones.
5. _____ _____ occurs when a child is born with a poorly functioning or absent thyroid gland.

ACTIVITY B

Matching

Match the term in Column A with the definition in Column B.

COLUMN A

1. _____ Levothyroxine (Synthroid, Levothroid)
2. _____ Sodium iodide [131]I (Iodotope)
3. _____ Strong iodine solution (Lugol's solution) and saturated solution of potassium iodide (SSKI)
4. _____ Propylthiouracil (PTU)
5. _____ Methimazole (Tapazole)

COLUMN B

A. Synthetic preparation of T_4; the drug of choice for long-term treatment of hypothyroidism and serves as the prototype
B. Prototype of the thioamide antithyroid drugs
C. Similar to PTU in actions, uses, and adverse reactions; well absorbed with oral administration, rapidly reaches peak plasma levels
D. Radioactive isotope of iodine
E. Sometimes used in short-term treatment of hyperthyroidism

ACTIVITY C

Short Answers

Briefly answer the following questions.

1. Define hyperthyroidism and the various causes of this disease process.
2. Define thyrotoxic crisis and discuss the various causes of this complication.
3. What are the mechanisms of action for both thyroid and antithyroid medications?
4. What are the indications for use for both thyroid and antithyroid medications?
5. Identify the various contraindications for the use of iodine preparations and thioamide antithyroid drugs.

■ Section III: Applying Your Knowledge

ACTIVITY D

Case Studies

Consider the scenarios and answer the questions.

Case Study 1

Ms. Davis, a nursing student, is diagnosed with subclinical hypothyroidism. You are responsible for the education care plan regarding the client's diagnosis.

1. Ms. Davis asks you to explain the difference between clinical and subclinical hypothyroidism. How would you describe subclinical hypothyroidism?
2. Ms. Davis asks you how long she will need the replacement therapy ordered by the physician. What is the standard duration of this type of therapy? How long does the patient have to be euthyroid before a change in therapy is considered?

Case Study 2

Mrs. Michelson, age 62, is diagnosed with subclinical hyperthyroidism. You are responsible for her education plan.

1. What are the laboratory values of T_3, T_4, and TSH that represent subclinical hyperthyroidism?
2. For Mrs. Michelson's age and sex, what is a risk factor associated with subclinical hyperthyroidism? If this patient has multiple cardiac diagnoses, what new diagnosis is she also at risk for?

■ Section IV: Practicing for NCLEX

Answer the following questions.

1. The FDA has issued a black box warning regarding the use of thyroid hormones for the treatment of which of the following conditions?
   a. Obesity   c. Diabetes mellitus type 1
   b. Hypotension   d. GERD

2. Sara Jones, age 25, is diagnosed with hypothyroidism. She is admitted to your hospital for acute gall bladder disease and subsequent surgical intervention. When planning postoperative opioid pain management; you must take into account the fact that the patient is at greater risk for which of the following conditions, secondary to her hypothyroidism diagnosis?
   a. Hypotension   c. Respiratory depression
   b. Hypertension   d. Atrial fibrillation

3. You are responsible for the education plan for parents of a child born with congenital hypothyroidism. When should drug therapy start for this patient?
   a. Within 72 hours after birth
   b. Within 6 weeks after birth
   c. Within 24 hours after birth
   d. Within 48 hours after birth

4. Which of the following is the rationale for lifetime drug therapy for congenital hypothyroidism (cretinism)?
   a. To prevent cardiac dysrhythmias
   b. To prevent seizure disorder
   c. To prevent chronic hypotension
   d. To prevent mental retardation

5. Thyroid replacement therapy in the patient with hypothyroidism is lifelong due to remissions and exacerbations. Replacement therapy usually continues until the patient is euthyroid for how long?
   a. 6-12 months   c. 3-6 months
   b. 18-24 months   d. 8-12 months

6. _____, a synthetic preparation of T₄, is the drug of choice for long-term treatment of hypothyroidism and serves as the prototype.

7. Mrs. Blankenship comes to the physician's office for her annual checkup. Her medications include a regimen to treat her hyperthyroidism. Which of the following symptoms or diseases processes would you be alert for at this time?
   a. Hypothyroidism   c. Dysrhythmias
   b. Hyperthyroidism   d. Hypertension

8. _____ is the prototype of the thioamide antithyroid drugs and is used alone to treat hyperthyroidism, as part of the preoperative preparation for thyroidectomy, before or after radioactive iodine therapy, and in the treatment of thyroid storm.

9. The home care nurse may be involved in a wide range of activities when caring for the client with hyperthyroidism or hypothyroidism. Which of the following would be included in the client's plan of care? (Select all that apply.)
   a. Assessing the patient's response to therapy
   b. Teaching about the disease process
   c. Modifying medication dosages based on symptomatology
   d. Preventing and managing adverse drug effects

10. Mrs. Graves is admitted to the intensive care unit in thyrotoxic crisis. What would you expect to happen to her medication dosages?
   a. They would decrease in frequency.
   b. They would increase in frequency.
   c. They would be given by the intramuscular route only.
   d. They would be given by the subcutaneous route only.

11. Mrs. Bates is diagnosed with liver disease. How would this affect the metabolism of the drugs used to treat her hypothyroidism?
   a. It would be unaffected.
   b. It would be rapid.
   c. It would be prolonged.
   d. It would be short-lived.

12. The liver plays an important role in thyroid hormone metabolism, and _____ is important for normal hepatic function and bilirubin metabolism.

13. Mr. Bartholomew, age 83, is diagnosed with hypothyroidism and cardiovascular disease. He is given levothyroxine to manage the hypothyroidism. You would be alert for which of the following symptoms or disease processes after institution of the drug?
   a. Congestive heart failure
   b. Hypertension
   c. Seizures
   d. Anaphylaxis

14. What are the potential risks for the use of PTU or methimazole in children? (Select all that apply.)
   a. Cancer caused by radioactive iodine
   b. Chromosome damage
   c. Chronic hypertension
   d. Chronic hypotension

15. Mrs. Wills' diagnoses include hyperthyroidism, congestive heart failure, and diabetes mellitus type 2. Which of the following effects will the treatment of hyperthyroidism have on her routine medications?
   a. Metabolism will be slower than normal, and the dose will be increased.
   b. Metabolism will be slower than normal, and the dose will be decreased.
   c. Metabolism will be faster than normal, and the dose will be decreased.
   d. Metabolism will be faster than normal, and the dose will be increased.

16. Mrs. Janis' physician has ordered a trial discontinuance of her thyroid medication. You are responsible for her medication education plan. When will her medication will be discontinued?
   a. With her next prescription
   b. Gradually over weeks or months
   c. Gradually over a week
   d. Gradually over 48-72 hours

17. Ms. Bates is diagnosed with both hypothyroidism and adrenal insufficiency. If the adrenal insufficiency is not treated first, which of the following conditions would administration of thyroid hormone cause?

    a. Hypertensive crisis

    b. Acute congestive heart failure

    c. Acute adrenocortical insufficiency

    d. Life-threatening dysrhythmias

18. In patients with symptomatic hypothyroidism, _____ therapy is indicated.

19. Regardless of the cause of hypothyroidism and the age at which it occurs, the specific treatment is replacement of thyroid hormone from a/an _____ source.

20. The goal of treatment with thyroid drugs is to restore the individual to a _____ state with normal metabolism.

CHAPTER 25

Hormones That Regulate Calcium and Bone Metabolism

■ Section I: Learning Objectives

1. Examine the roles of parathyroid hormone, calcitonin, and vitamin D in regulating calcium metabolism.
2. Manage individuals at risk for hypocalcemia.
3. Discuss the prevention and treatment of hypocalcemia and osteoporosis.
4. Manage individuals at risk for hypercalcemia.
5. Outline appropriate management strategies of hypercalcemia as a medical emergency.
6. Evaluate the use of calcium and vitamin D supplements, calcitonin, and bisphosphonate drugs in the treatment of osteoporosis.

■ Section II: Assessing Your Understanding

ACTIVITY A

Fill in the Blanks

1. Three hormones regulate calcium and bone metabolism: _____, calcitonin, and vitamin D.
2. _____ secretion is stimulated by low serum calcium levels and inhibited by normal or high levels (a negative feedback system).
3. The patient diagnosis related to insufficient production of PTH would be _____.
4. Excessive production of PTH usually related to removal or damage to the parathyroid glands during neck surgery is called _____.
5. Clinical manifestations and treatment of hypoparathyroidism are the same as those of _____.

ACTIVITY B

Matching

Match the term in Column A with the definition in Column B.

COLUMN A

1. _____ Vitamin D
2. _____ Calcium and vitamin D
3. _____ Calcitonin
4. _____ An intravenous (IV) calcium salt
5. _____ Calcium carbonate or citrate

COLUMN B

A. Hormone from the thyroid gland whose secretion is controlled by the concentration of ionized calcium in the blood flowing through the thyroid gland
B. Used to treat hypocalcemia and to prevent and treat osteoporosis
C. Given for acute, symptomatic hypocalcemia
D. Given for asymptomatic, less severe, or chronic hypocalcemia
E. Fat-soluble vitamin that includes both ergocalciferol and cholecalciferol

ACTIVITY C

Short Answers

Briefly answer the following questions.

1. How is the secretion of PTH regulated?
2. When the serum calcium level falls below the normal range, how does the level normalize?
3. Discuss the causes of hyperparathyroidism.
4. What is the role of calcitonin as it relates to serum calcium?
5. What is the role of vitamin D as it relates to calcium and bone metabolism?

■ Section III: Applying Your Knowledge

ACTIVITY D

Case Study

Consider the scenario and answer the questions.

Mrs. Bates, age 52, is diagnosed with osteoporosis based on bone density studies. You are responsible for the education plan for both her disease process and her medication regimen.

1. Mrs. Bates confides that her friend told her that osteoporosis is a form of cancer. How would you reply?
2. What causes osteoporosis?
3. Explain the concept of bone remodeling.
4. The physician orders Fosamax for the treatment of Mrs. Bates' osteoporosis. What is the mechanism of action for this drug? What instructions would you give Mrs. Bates about taking the drug with food?

■ Section IV: Practicing for NCLEX

Answer the following questions.

1. Mr. Gustafson is being treated with long-term corticosteroids. Which of the following effects will these drugs have?
   a. They will decrease testosterone levels.
   b. They will increase testosterone levels.
   c. They will not affect testosterone levels.
   d. They will increase fertility.

2. Both men and women who take corticosteroids are at risk for which of the following side effects?
   a. Infertility   c. Hypertension
   b. Osteoporosis   d. Paget's disease

3. Which of the following patients is at the highest risk for osteoporosis?
   a. The patient receiving diuretic therapy
   b. The patient with a diagnosis of renal hypertension
   c. The patient with frequent falls
   d. The female patient age 76

4. Calcium deficiency commonly occurs in the elderly because of which of the following factors? (Select all that apply.)
   a. Impaired absorption of calcium from the intestine
   b. Excessive exposure to ultraviolet rays
   c. Lack of exposure to sunlight
   d. Impaired liver or kidney metabolism of vitamin D

5. In general, intake of calcium should not exceed _____ mg daily, from all sources.

6. Intake of vitamin D should not exceed _____ international units daily.

7. Deficiency of vitamin D causes inadequate absorption of which of the following elements?
   a. Phosphorus
   b. Calcium
   c. Magnesium
   d. Calcium and phosphorus

8. Which of the following is a frequent cause of hyperparathyroidism? (Select all that apply.)
   a. A tumor of a parathyroid gland
   b. Hypercalcemia
   c. Hyperplasia of a parathyroid gland
   d. Hypocalcemia

9. Mr. Jenks, age 45, is scheduled for renal dialysis. He develops hypercalcemia. The physician orders a calcium-free solution for his dialysis treatments. Which of the following would the physician order to prevent hyperphosphatemia?
   a. Calcium acetate   c. Vitamin D
   b. Calcium and vitamin D   d. Magnesium

10. Which of the following is a common reason for calcium deficiency? (Select all that apply.)
    a. Long-term dietary deficiencies of calcium and vitamin D
    b. Impaired absorption of calcium from the intestine
    c. Lack of exposure to sunlight
    d. Overexposure to ultraviolet rays

11. Ms. Henderson presents to the physician's office for a routine physical examination. You assess her current over-the-counter drug history and discover that she takes vitamin D 600 international units daily. Ms. Henderson is at risk for which of the following?
    a. Paget's disease   c. Hypocalciuria
    b. Hypocalcemia   d. Hypercalcemia

12. Mrs. Pennywise, age 45, is diagnosed with osteoporosis. For 10 years she has been taking phenytoin to control her seizure disorder. Which of the following effects do anticonvulsant medications have on osteoporosis?
    a. They do not affect calcium metabolism.
    b. They decrease hepatic metabolism of vitamin D, contributing to the development of osteoporosis.
    c. They increase hepatic metabolism of vitamin D, which decreases calcium absorption in the intestine.
    d. They only marginally affect calcium metabolism and reabsorption of calcium in the bone.

13. Mr. Gonzales, age 43, takes prednisone 7.5 mg daily to treat his temporal arteritis. His dose varies from 7.5 to 10 mg based on symptoms and laboratory test analysis. His disease process has been managed successfully with this drug regimen for 7 years. To prevent osteoporosis, which of the following would his physician order? (Select all that apply.)
    a. A calcium supplement
    b. Testosterone
    c. A bisphosphonate drug
    d. Regular weight-bearing exercise

14. The laboratory test that indicates a vitamin D deficiency is serum _____.

15. Acute hypercalcemia, as evidenced by severe symptoms or a serum calcium level greater than _____ mg/dL, is a medical emergency, and rehydration is a priority.

16. Mrs. Gillis, age 54, is diagnosed with atrial fibrillation, which has been effectively controlled by digoxin for 6 years. She has also been self-administering calcium for 6 months. Which of the following conditions might the combination of digoxin and calcium preparations cause? (Select all that apply.)
    a. Dysrhythmia
    b. Hypertension
    c. Digoxin toxicity
    d. Subtherapeutic digoxin levels

17. A prolonged and painful spasm of the voluntary muscles is called _____.

18. Mrs. Niles presents to the emergency department with symptoms and laboratory values indicative of hypercalcemia. Which of the following IV solutions would the physician order to treat the hypercalcemia?
    a. Sodium chloride (0.9%)
    b. D51/2 normal saline
    c. D51/4 normal saline
    d. Lactated Ringer's solution

19. Phosphates should be given only when hypercalcemia is accompanied by hypophosphatemia. Hypophosphatemia is assumed when the serum phosphorus is less than what level?
    a. Less than 5 mg/dL
    b. Less than 10 mg/dL
    c. Less than 4 mg/dL
    d. Less than 3 mg/dL

20. Furosemide (Lasix) is a loop diuretic that increases calcium excretion in urine by preventing its reabsorption in the _____ _____.

CHAPTER 26

Antidiabetic Drugs

■ Section I: Learning Objectives

1. Describe major effects of endogenous insulin on body tissues.
2. Discuss characteristics and uses of the various types of insulins and insulin analogs.
3. Discuss the relationships among diet, exercise, and drug therapy in controlling diabetes.
4. Differentiate types of oral agents used to manage diabetes mellitus in terms of mechanisms of action, indications for use, adverse effects, and nursing process implications.
5. Discuss the indications, characteristics, and benefits of amylin analogs, incretin mimetics, and dipeptidyl peptidase-4 (DPP-4) inhibitors.
6. Explain the benefits of maintaining glycemic control in preventing complications of diabetes mellitus.
7. State reasons for combinations of insulin and oral agents or different types of oral agents.
8. Assist patients or caregivers in learning how to manage diabetes care, including administration of medication agents used to manage diabetes mellitus.
9. Collaborate with nurse diabetes educators, dietitians, pharmacists, and others in teaching self-care activities to patients with diabetes.
10. Assess and monitor patients' conditions in relation to diabetes mellitus and their compliance with prescribed management strategies.
11. Discuss dietary and herbal supplements that affect blood sugar and diabetes control.
12. Review the National Cholesterol Education Program (NCEP) Adult Treatment Panel III (ATP III) guidelines for lipid management in high-risk and/or diabetic states.

■ Section II: Assessing Your Understanding

ACTIVITY A

Fill in the Blanks

1. _____ is a protein hormone secreted by beta cells in the pancreas.
2. _____, a pancreatic hormone secreted with insulin, delays gastric emptying, increases satiety, and suppresses glucagon secretion, thus complementing the effects of insulin on the blood sugar.
3. Insulin is secreted into the portal circulation and transported to the _____, where about half is used or degraded.
4. Liver, muscle, and _____ cells have many insulin receptors and are primary tissues for insulin action.
5. In the kidneys, insulin is filtered by the _____ and reabsorbed by the tubules, which also degrade it.

ACTIVITY B

Matching

Match the term in Column A with the definition in Column B.

COLUMN A

1. _____ Exogenous insulin
2. _____ Exubera
3. _____ Sulfonylureas
4. _____ Acarbose and miglitol
5. _____ Metformin

COLUMN B

A. Oldest and largest group of oral agents

B. Inhaled insulin, approved and then removed from the market

C. Increases the use of glucose by muscle and fat cells, decreases hepatic glucose production, and decreases intestinal absorption of glucose

D. Used to replace endogenous insulin; has the same effects as the pancreatic hormone

E. Inhibits alpha-glucosidase enzymes in the GI tract; delays digestion of complex carbohydrates into simple sugars

ACTIVITY C

Short Answers

Briefly answer the following questions.

1. How does the drug Metformin help the client with type 2 diabetes manage his or her disease?
2. How do thiazolidinediones decrease insulin resistance?
3. Identify the characteristics of the drug pramlintide (Symlin) and the mechanism by which it helps the patient to control his or her blood glucose?
4. How does the drug extenatide help the patient to control his or her blood glucose?
5. Identify one supplement that may increase blood glucose levels and describe the supplement's mechanism of action.

■ Section III: Applying Your Knowledge

ACTIVITY D

Case Study

Consider the scenario and answer the questions.

Mrs. Ingles, age 45, is diagnosed with diabetes type 2. She works in an office and leads a sedentary lifestyle. Her vital signs are as follows: BP 140/84, AP101 regular, R 20, fasting glucose is 154; height 5'6" and weight 210 pounds. You are responsible for her education plan regarding both her diabetes disease process and the medication ordered by her primary physician.

1. Based on your assessment, what are two indicators that place Mrs. Ingles at high risk for diabetes?
2. What are the signs and symptoms of hyperglycemia?
3. Laboratory tests indicate that Mrs. Ingles is dehydrated. What is the relationship between uncontrolled diabetes type 2 and dehydration?
4. Mrs. Ingles is given a diet and exercise program and revisits her physician 3 months later. Her fasting glucose is 164, and she has not lost weight. She feels that there are not enough hours in the day to adhere to an exercise program and admits that she is not motivated to comply. The physician orders extenatide (Byetta). What can you teach Mrs. Ingles about this medication?

■ Section IV: Practicing for NCLEX

Answer the following questions.

1. Mr. Franks, age 43, weighs 246 pounds and is 5'10'' tall. His occupation is sedentary and he works 50-60 hours a week. His fasting glucose test results are 132 and 140 on two separate occasions. What non-medication methods would you include in your education plan to assist Mr. Franks to reduce his blood glucose? (Select all that apply.)
   a. Oral hyperglycemics
   b. Routine exercise
   c. Oral hypoglycemics
   d. Diet approved by physician

2. The parameters for a diagnosis of diabetes are a fasting plasma glucose test (FPG) greater than or equal to what level on two separate occasions?
   a. 130 mg/dL   c. 120 mg/dL
   b. 118 mg/dL   d. 126 mg/dL

3. You are part of a group of physicians and nurses who are establishing parameters for an outpatient clinic geared to diabetes testing and treatment. Which of the following is the fastest and most cost-effective test to determine a diagnosis of diabetes?
   a. Fasting plasma glucose test
   b. Preprandial and postprandial blood glucose test
   c. Urine dip test
   d. Capillary random blood glucose

4. Mrs. Dromedy visits the physician's office after routine labs are drawn. You note that her A1C is 9. Which of the following does this indicate?
   a. Normal lab result
   b. Abnormal lab result
   c. Borderline high lab result
   d. Diagnosis of hypoglycemia

5. Mrs. Smith is a newly diagnosed diabetic. She is a stay-at-home mother and responsible for meal planning and management of the home. As the home care nurse, which of the following are you responsible for? (Select all that apply.)
   a. Establishing goals and treatment modalities needed to maintain homeostasis
   b. Mobilizing and coordinating healthcare providers
   c. Teaching and supporting patients and caregivers
   d. Monitoring the patient's health status and progress in disease management

6. Mrs. Batel is admitted into your critical care unit with a diagnosis of myocardial infarct and subsequent bypass grafts. She is diabetic type 1 for 10 years. You understand that strict control of her hyperglycemia is critical to prevent which of the following outcomes? (Select all that apply.)
   a. Postoperative infections
   b. Increased mortality
   c. Decreased absorption of antibiotics
   d. Hypertensive crisis

7. Mr. Gonzalez, age 54, is diagnosed with chronic renal failure and hyperglycemia. He asks if he can be prescribed sulfonylurea because it works well for his friend. If he were to be given sulfonylurea, this patient's renal impairment may lead to which of the following effects?
   a. Accumulation and hypoglycemia
   b. Accumulation and hyperglycemic reactions
   c. Decreased absorption of the sulfonylurea
   d. Hypersensitivity to sulfonylurea

8. Treatment with thiazide diuretics, corticosteroids, and estrogens may cause which of the following conditions?
   a. hypoglycemia
   b. pulmonary hypertension
   c. congestive heart failure
   d. hyperglycemia

9. Type 2 diabetes is being increasingly identified in children. This trend is mainly attributed to which of the following?
   a. Working parents
   b. Economics
   c. Obesity and inadequate exercise
   d. Lack of after-school programs due to budget constraints

10. In young children, hypoglycemia may be manifested by which of the following signs or symptoms? (Select all that apply.)
    a. Changes in behavior
    b. Poor appetite
    c. Impaired mental functioning
    d. Flat affect

11. Recognition of hypoglycemia may be delayed in children because signs and symptoms are vague and the children may be unable to communicate them to parents or caregivers. Because of these difficulties, most pediatric diabetologists recommend maintaining blood glucose levels in what range?
    a. Between 90 and 110 mg/dL
    b. Between 100 and 200 mg/dL
    c. Between 120 and 150 mg/dL
    d. Between 110 and 150 mg/dL

12. Avoiding hypoglycemia is a major goal in infants and young children because of potentially damaging effects on growth and development. An adequate supply of glucose is needed for which of the following types of development to occur?
    a. Skeletal development
    b. Organ development
    c. Brain and spinal cord development
    d. Spatial development

13. James Elliot, age 2 months, is diagnosed with diabetes. His parents are having difficulty measuring 2 units of insulin in the U100 syringe. What would you expect the physician to order?
    a. U-50 (50 units/mL) insulin
    b. U-20 (20 units/mL) insulin
    c. U-30 (30 units/mL) insulin
    d. U-10 (10 units/mL) insulin

14. Julie Hart, age 4 years, is diabetic with a blood glucose level of 120 mg/dL. Julie's mother brings her to the physician's office with symptoms of the flu and dehydration. Which of the following would you expect the physician to order?
    a. Regular sodas, clear juices, regular gelatin desserts
    b. Diet sodas, clear juices, regular gelatin desserts
    c. IV Ringer's solution
    d. IV saline 0.9%

15. Richard Sykes, age 4 years, is diagnosed with type 1 diabetes. You are responsible for his family education plan. In addition to insulin, which of the following is needed for effective management of Richard's diabetes? (Select all that apply.)
    a. Consistent schedule of meals and snacks
    b. Limited exercise based on blood glucose monitoring
    c. Blood glucose monitoring
    d. Limited involvement in contact sports programs

16. _____ therapy is a major component of any treatment for DKA.

17. IV fluids, the first step in treating DKA, usually consist of which of the following solutions?
    a. D51/2 NS
    b. Lactated Ringer's
    c. D5
    d. 0.9% sodium chloride

18. Studies indicate that insulin is absorbed fastest from which area of injection?
    a. Deltoid   c. Abdomen
    b. Thigh   d. Hip

19. With regular insulin before meals, it is very important that the medication be injected at the correct time so that the insulin will be available when blood sugar increases after the meal. How many minutes before a meal should regular insulin be injected?

    a. 10 to 15   c. 20 to 30
    b. 30 to 45   d. 15 to 20

20. In acute situations, dosage of regular insulin needs frequent adjustments based on measurements of _____ _____.

CHAPTER 27

Estrogens, Progestins, and Hormonal Contraceptives

■ Section I: Learning Objectives

1. Discuss the effects of endogenous estrogens and progestins.
2. Outline the benefits and risks of postmenopausal hormone replacement therapy.
3. Recognize adverse effects associated with estrogens, progestins, and hormonal contraceptives.
4. Apply the nursing process with patients taking estrogens, progestins, and hormonal contraceptives.

■ Section II: Assessing Your Understanding

ACTIVITY A

Fill in the Blanks

1. _____ and _____ are female sex hormones produced primarily by the ovaries and secondarily by the adrenal cortex in nonpregnant women.
2. Small amounts of _____ are also synthesized in the liver, kidneys, brain, skeletal muscle, testes, and adipose tissue.
3. Women with anorexia nervosa, chronic disease, or malnutrition and those who are long-distance runners usually have _____.
4. With _____ _____, regaining weight and body mass usually re-establishes normal menstrual patterns.
5. As with other steroid hormones, estrogens and progestins are synthesized from _____.

ACTIVITY B

Matching

Match the term in Column A with the definition in Column B.

COLUMN A

1. _____ Desogestrel and norgestimate
2. _____ Monophasic contraceptives
3. _____ Ethinyl estradiol
4. _____ Black cohosh
5. _____ Biphasics and triphasics

COLUMN B

A. Most widely used synthetic steroidal estrogen
B. Progestins with minimal androgenic activity
C. Containing fixed amounts of both estrogen and progestin components
D. Containing either fixed amounts of estrogen and varied amounts of progestin or varied amounts of both estrogen and progestin
E. Herb used to self-treat symptoms of menopause reportedly effective in relieving vasomotor instability

ACTIVITY C

Short Answers

Briefly answer the following questions.

1. Explain the process by which estrogens and progestins are synthesized from cholesterol.
2. Discuss the function of estrogen in the female body.
3. Discuss the role of estrogen in the menstrual cycle
4. How is estrogen metabolized and excreted within the body?
5. How does progesterone affect the nonpregnant woman's body functions?

■ Section III: Applying Your Knowledge

ACTIVITY D
Case Study

Consider the scenario and answer the questions.

Mrs. Johnson, age 55, is experiencing signs and symptoms of menopause. Her physician does not prescribe hormone replacement therapy due to a history of estrogen-dependent cancer in her immediate family. He suggests the use of black cohosh, an herbal treatment, to alleviate the symptoms associated with menopause. You are responsible for the client's medication education care plan.

1. Mrs. Johnson asks you if the black cohosh will stop her periods as well as the night sweats and hot flashes. How would you respond?
2. Mrs. Johnson states that both her sister and her mother died of endometrial cancer. She is concerned that black cohosh may place her at increased risk for cancer. What information can you give her?
3. Mrs. Johnson also has a diagnosis of essential hypertension. You instruct her to return to the office frequently for blood pressure checks, because black cohosh may have an effect on blood pressure. What is the possible effect? What other adverse effects can black cohosh have?
4. Mrs. Johnson purchases Remefemin 20 mg per tablet. She states that her friend takes the same medication and has taken it without adverse side effects for years. Her friend takes one tablet three times a day because it works best for her. What can you tell Mrs. Johnson about the dosage of the medication and about how long she can safely take it?

■ Section IV: Practicing for NCLEX

Answer the following questions.

1. Mrs. Reams, an executive in an advertising firm, presents to the physician's office with symptoms of menopause. She asks the physician for hormone replacement therapy for the duration of menopause, because she does not want to experience night sweats, which interfere with her sleep patterns. The physician prescribes an herbal supplement and assigns the medication education to you. Mrs. Reams asks why she is not prescribed HRT. Which of the following is the FDA recommendation for HRT?

   a. It should be used only for women with symptoms severe enough to warrant its use.

   b. It should be used only for women who experience night sweats five or more times a week.

   c. It should be used only for women older than 55 years of age.

   d. It should be used only for women with a history of endometrial cancer.

2. Mrs. Beren, age 57, asks the physician for HRT to prevent heart disease. She states that both her mother and her sister suffered from heart attacks at her age, and she is concerned that it will happen to her. You are responsible for patient education regarding HRT. Which of the following is an appropriate response?

   a. "The physician ordered short-term HRT."

   b. "Studies have demonstrated no evidence for HRT in secondary prevention of heart disease."

   c. "Studies support HRT as an effective deterrent to heart disease and it is prescribed for the duration of menopause."

   d. "Your HMO will not cover the cost of HRT because of your family history."

3. Mrs. Vent, age 45, is admitted to the hospital with a deep vein thrombosis and subsequent pulmonary embolism. The physician ordered HRT 3 months ago for severe menopausal symptoms. Based on the information provided, when do you expect thromboembolic disorders are most likely to occur?

   a. During the first 90 days of use

   b. During the first 6 months of use

   c. There is not a documented relationship between thromboembolic events and HRT

   d. During the first year of use

4. The FDA has issued a black box warning that estrogens increase the risk for developing cancer of the _____.

5. Ms. Gretna takes oral contraceptives. She presents to the physician's office with a low-grade temperature and a sore throat. The rapid strep test verifies the physician's diagnosis of strep throat and he orders the appropriate antibiotic. Which of the following would you expect the physician's orders to include? (Select all that apply.)

   a. A larger dose of oral contraceptive

   b. An additional or alternative form of birth control

   c. Discontinuance of the oral contraceptive during the duration of the antibiotic

   d. A lower dose of oral contraceptive

6. Estrogen alone is not used for postmenopausal women because it causes which of the following conditions?

   a. Hirsutism

   b. Fibrotic breast disease

   c. Endometrial hyperplasia

   d. Stomatitis

7. Because estrogens cause _____ _____, they should be used with caution in children before completion of bone growth and attainment of adult height.

8. Ms. Jinks, age 25, smokes two packs of cigarettes per day. She asks her physician for a prescription for oral contraceptives. You are responsible for the client's education plan. The combination of cigarette smoking and oral contraceptives may lead to an increased risk for which of the following conditions?

   a. Endometrial hyperplasia

   b. Blood clots in the legs, lungs, heart, or brain

   c. Congestive heart failure

   d. Postural hypotension

9. Ms. James states that she has multiple sexual partners and wants an effective oral contraceptive to prevent pregnancy and sexually transmitted diseases. As part of your education plan, which of the following is a correct statement?

   a. "Most oral contraceptives with estrogen and progestins will prevent both pregnancy and STDs."

   b. "Most oral contraceptives with estrogen will prevent both pregnancy and STDs."

   c. "Most oral contraceptives will prevent both pregnancy and STDs."

   d. "Oral contraceptives are very effective at preventing pregnancy, but they do not prevent transmission of sexually transmitted diseases."

10. When exogenous estrogens and progestins are administered for therapeutic purposes, they produce the same effects as _____ hormones.

11. In families that include postmenopausal women, home care nurses may need to teach about nonhormonal strategies for preventing or treating which of the following conditions?

   a. Osteoporosis

   b. Endometrial cancer

   c. Cardiovascular disease

   d. Endometrial hyperplasia

12. When visiting families that include adolescent girls or young women, home care nurses may need to provide teach about which of the following?

    a. Preventing heart disease by using contraceptives

    b. Preventing osteoporosis by improving diet and exercise patterns

    c. Preventing breast cancer by using contraceptives

    d. Preventing endometrial cancer by improving diet and exercise patterns

13. Mrs. Jones has a history of hepatitis B. She visits the community clinic to obtain a prescription for oral contraceptives. The physician orders liver function tests, and the results are abnormal. He chooses not to prescribe the oral contraceptives, for which of the following reasons?

    a. Women with impaired liver function are at increased risk for the development of endometrial cancer when taking oral contraceptives.

    b. In women with impaired liver function, oral contraceptives may lead to increased estrogen metabolism and pregnancy.

    c. Women with impaired liver function are at increased risk for breast cancer.

    d. In women with impaired liver function, oral contraceptives may lead to impaired estrogen metabolism, with resultant accumulation and adverse effects.

14. When hormonal contraceptives are given to adolescent girls, as in other populations, the _____ effective doses should be used.

15. Prevention and treatment of osteoporosis may be accomplished by which treatment in place of HRT? (Select all that apply.)

    a. Calcium and vitamin D supplements

    b. Progesterone

    c. Bisphosphonate drugs

    d. Magnesium citrate

16. In ERT therapy, which of the following is the main function of the progestin?

    a. To decrease the risk of endometrial cancer

    b. To manage vasomotor symptoms

    c. To decrease the risk for cardiac disease

    d. To decrease the risk for DVT

17. _____ _____ (_____) is the only emergency contraceptive on the market used to avoid pregnancy after unprotected sexual intercourse. It should be used only as a backup method and is not for routine birth control.

18. Oral contraceptives decrease effects of which of the following drugs? (Select all that apply.)

    a. Benzodiazepines   c. Warfarin

    b. Insulin   d. Hydrochlorothiazide

19. Naturally occurring, nonconjugated estrogens (estradiol, estrone) and natural progesterone are given _____.

20. When progestins are given in the first 4 months of pregnancy, evidence suggests that which of the following may happen?

    a. Habitual abortion may be prevented.

    b. Fetal harm is possible.

    c. A dosage modification may be necessary.

    d. The mother may become hypertensive.

CHAPTER 28

Androgens and Anabolic Steroids

■ Section I: Learning Objectives

1. Examine the effects of endogenous androgens.
2. Discuss the uses and effects of exogenous androgens and anabolic steroids.
3. Identify potential consequences of abusing androgens and anabolic steroids.
4. Counsel clients about the physiologic effects of the dietary supplements androstenedione and dehydroepiandrosterone (DHEA).

■ Section II: Assessing Your Understanding

ACTIVITY A

Fill in the Blanks

1. _____ are male sex hormones secreted by the testes in men, the ovaries in women, and the adrenal cortex of both sexes.
2. Like the female sex hormones, the naturally occurring male sex hormones are steroids synthesized from _____.
3. The androgens produced by the ovaries have little androgenic activity and are used mainly as precursor substances for the production of naturally occurring _____.
4. The adrenal glands produce several androgens, including _____ and dehydroepiandrosterone (DHEA).
5. _____ is normally the only important male sex hormone.

ACTIVITY B

Matching

Match the term in Column A with the definition in Column B.

COLUMN A

1. _____ Male sex hormones
2. _____ Naturally occurring androgens
3. _____ Oral testosterone
4. _____ Intramuscular (IM) testosterone cypionate and testosterone enanthate
5. _____ Danazol

COLUMN B

A. Given to women to antagonize or reduce the effects of female sex hormones
B. Synthetic drug with weak androgenic activity
C. Extensively metabolized in its first pass through the liver
D. Given by injection because they are metabolized rapidly by the liver if given orally
E. Drugs with slow onsets of action and lasting 2 to 4 weeks

ACTIVITY C

Short Answers

Briefly answer the following questions.

1. What is the function of testosterone as it relates to the male?
2. Describe the function of anabolic steroids.
3. Why are athletes considered a high-risk group for the abuse of anabolic steroids?
4. What are the negative effects of anabolic steroids when used by adolescents?
5. Identify the liver disorders related to anabolic steroid use.

■ Section III: Applying Your Knowledge

ACTIVITY D
Case Study

Consider the scenario and answer the questions.

Your friend's son is self-administering over-the-counter DHEA to promote muscle development while he is weight training. His mother asks you about the safety and efficacy of the medication.

1. She asks you why the drugs are marketed. How would you answer this question?
2. Explain what these products do. In what kinds of situations are these products contraindicated?
3. What are the adverse effects of DHEA?
4. Your friend's son switches to androstenedione. What are the possible effects of androstenedione?
5. Your friend asks if large doses of OTC DHEA and androstenedione can produce the same adverse effects as the standard drugs. How would you respond?

■ Section IV: Practicing for NCLEX

Answer the following questions.

1. Michael Smith, age 6, is prescribed androgens for a diagnosed deficiency. You arrange for x-rays every 6 months because androgens may cause which of the following?
   a. Long bone pain
   b. Premature epiphyseal closure
   c. Premature secondary female sexual characteristics
   d. Irregular bone growth

2. Androstenedione and DHEA, androgens produced by the _____ _____, are also available as over-the-counter (OTC) dietary supplements.

3. Because of their abuse potential, androgens and anabolic steroids are classified as what type of substances?
   a. Schedule IV controlled substances
   b. Schedule II controlled substances
   c. Schedule I controlled substances
   d. Schedule III controlled substances

4. Androgens and anabolic steroids are used to enhance athletic performance and are termed *ergogenic*. Which of the following effects do they have?
   a. They cause an increase in muscular work capacity.
   b. They cause a decrease in musculature, increasing muscle mass.
   c. They cause a decrease in muscular work capacity.
   d. They increase vascularity of the muscle mass.

5. The main functions of testosterone are related to the development of male sexual characteristics, reproduction, and what other function?
   a. Catabolism   c. Metabolism
   b. Testicular atrophy   d. Production of sterols

6. The androgens produced by the ovaries have little androgenic activity and are used mainly as precursor substances for the production of which of the following?
   a. Estrogens   c. Androgens
   b. Progestin   d. Ova

7. Mr. Gardner is prescribed androgens; he develops cirrhosis of the liver. Which of the following would you expect the physician to do?
   a. Decrease the dose of the androgens
   b. Discontinue the androgens
   c. Maintain the current dose of the androgens
   d. Increase the dose of the androgens

8. Mr. Fields develops jaundice while taking androgens. The physician discontinues the drugs. Which of the following would you expect to be the effect on the drug-induced jaundice?

   a. It will reverse.

   b. It will continue due to liver impairment.

   c. It will be a precursor to liver cancer.

   d. It will increase as liver function continues to deteriorate.

9. Mr. Chandler, age 75, takes androgens he procured illegally to enhance sexual stimulation. He presents to the physician's office with urinary frequency and bladder distention. In the older male, which of the following is a possible effect of androgens?

   a. Decreasing prostate size

   b. Causing renal dysfunction

   c. Causing dysfunction of the bladder detrusor muscles

   d. Increasing prostate size

10. Mr. Porter, age 75, presents to the physician's office with exacerbation of his congestive heart failure. He takes his son's anabolic steroids to increase his muscle mass. Which of the following might be caused by anabolic steroids?

    a. Hyperkalemia

    b. Sodium and water retention

    c. Hyponatremia

    d. Hyperosmolality of the cells

11. The main indication for use of androgens is a _____ state in men.

12. Jamie, age 5, is diagnosed with an androgen deficiency. Which area of the body should be routinely x-rayed to detect bone maturation?

    a. Hands and wrists   c. Skull

    b. Femur   d. Ulna

13. Mr. Bard is prescribed androgens for a deficiency. He develops a deep vein thrombosis and is prescribed warfarin. Which of the following would you expect the physician to do?

    a. Discontinue the warfarin

    b. Monitor the INR frequently

    c. Monitor the BUN frequently

    d. Monitor the PTT frequently

14. Mr. Stagias is concurrently using androgens and a sulfonylurea antidiabetic drug. Which of the following would you expect the physician to do?

    a. Decrease the dose of the androgen

    b. Increase the dose of the antidiabetic

    c. Decrease the dose of the antidiabetic

    d. Increase the dose of the androgen

15. Danazol inhibits metabolism of carbamazepine and _____ risks of toxicity.

16. Androgens and anabolic steroids are contraindicated during pregnancy, for which of the following reasons?

    a. Because of the risk of spontaneous abortion

    b. Because of possible hormonal imbalance

    c. Because of masculinizing effects on a female fetus

    d. Because estrogen induces endometrial cancer

17. In women, danazol (Danocrine) may be used to prevent or treat _____ or fibrocystic breast disease.

18. The most clearcut indication for use of male sex hormones is to treat androgen deficiency states, such as which of the following? (Select all that apply.)

    a. Hypogonadism   c. Cryptorchidism

    b. Hyperpituitarism   d. Oligospermia

19. All synthetic anabolic steroids are weak androgens. When given to children, which of the following effects might these drugs have?

    a. Decrease muscle mass

    b. Decrease growth in the skull

    c. Cause change in sexual development

    d. Cause hypernatremia

20. Several transdermal formulations of testosterone are available. They have a rapid onset of action and last approximately _____ hours.

CHAPTER 29

General Characteristics of Antimicrobial Drugs

■ Section I: Learning Objectives

1. Identify populations who have an increased risk of infection.
2. Discuss common pathogens and methods of infection control.
3. Outline common and potentially serious adverse effects of antimicrobial drugs.
4. Identify patients at increased risk for adverse drug reactions.
5. Discuss ways to increase benefits and decrease hazards of antimicrobial drug therapy.
6. Discuss ways to minimize emergence of drug-resistant microorganisms.
7. State appropriate nursing implications for a patient receiving an antimicrobial drug.
8. Discuss important elements of using antimicrobial drugs in children, older adults, patients with renal or hepatic impairment, and patients with critical illness.

■ Section II: Assessing Your Understanding

ACTIVITY A

Fill in the Blanks

1. _____ drugs are used to prevent or treat infections caused by pathogenic (disease-producing) microorganisms.
2. In an infection, _____ initially attach to host cell receptors (i.e., proteins, carbohydrates, lipids).
3. _____ are intracellular parasites that survive only in living tissues.
4. Human pathogens include _____, herpes viruses, and retroviruses.
5. _____ are plant-like organisms that live as parasites on living tissue or as saprophytes on decaying organic matter.

ACTIVITY B

Matching

Match the term in Column A with the definition in Column B.

COLUMN A

1. _____ Opportunistic microorganisms
2. _____ Gram's stain
3. _____ Culture
4. _____ Detection of antigens
5. _____ Polymerase chain reaction (PCR)

COLUMN B

A. Involves growing a microorganism in the laboratory
B. Usually normal endogenous or environmental flora, nonpathogenic
C. Uses features of culture and serology but reduces the time required for diagnosis
D. Can detect whether DNA for a specific organism is present in a sample
E. Identifies microscopic appearance, including shape and color of the organisms

ACTIVITY C

Short Answers

Briefly answer the following questions.

1. Explain how infections occur in the human body.
2. Give an example of normal flora and discuss the role of normal flora in the human body.
3. Define colonization.
4. Describe the conditions needed for opportunistic infections to invade the human body.
5. How do broad-spectrum antibiotics affect the human body?

■ Section III: Applying Your Knowledge

ACTIVITY D

Case Study

Consider the scenario and answer the questions.

You are part of a group of nursing students who are studying the immune system. Your section to share to the group is the role of normal flora as it relates to health and illness.

1. What are the sterile areas of the body? What are some colonized areas of the body?
2. Discuss the pathogenicity of the microorganisms that are part of the normal flora. How does this normal flora protect the human host? What vitamins does the normal bowel flora synthesize?
3. What happens if the normal flora is suppressed by antimicrobial drug therapy? What happens to the normal flora when antibiotics are used? Use *Candida albicans* as an example.

■ Section IV: Practicing for NCLEX

Answer the following questions.

1. Ms. Green is treated with antibiotics for bacterial pneumonia. When obtaining a drug history you find that Ms. Green ceased her medication regimen when she no longer experienced symptoms during the first round of antibiotics. You are responsible for her education plan. In order to effectively treat the pneumonia, what must Ms. Green do?
   a. Complete a full course of antibiotics as prescribed
   b. Continue the antibiotics for 1 week after cessation of symptoms
   c. Take the antibiotics at breakfast, lunch, and supper
   d. Take the antibiotics every 3 hours during the day

2. Mrs. Beach takes an antibiotic, left over from her last bout with bronchitis, when she discovers that her child has developed strep throat. She takes the antibiotic as a preventive measure. Which of the following effects might this practice have? (Select all that apply.)
   a. Increasing adverse drug effects
   b. Increasing the risk of infections with drug-resistant microorganisms
   c. Becoming a cost-effective method to manage infectious processes
   d. Reducing healthcare costs

3. The physician orders an antibiotic for Mrs. Beach. She states that she cannot take antibiotics on an empty stomach because they make her nauseous. Which of the following instructions should you give her?
   a. Take the medication with food to reduce nausea.
   b. Take the medication three times a day with meals.
   c. Take the medication on an empty stomach.
   d. Take the antibiotic on an empty stomach until symptoms abate.

4. Antibiotics should be scheduled at _____ _____ intervals around the clock, to maintain therapeutic blood levels.

5. Mr. Ruiz is treated for urinary tract infections several times a year, secondary to urinary retention and an enlarged prostate. He also is treated for chronic renal failure, hypertension, and diabetes type 2. Which of the following might happen when Mr. Ruiz is treated with antibiotics?
   a. He may be nephrotoxic.
   b. He may be at increased risk for congestive heart failure.
   c. It may precipitate a hypertensive crisis.
   d. It may cause prostate enlargement.

6. Mrs. Lawrence is 48 hours post-op for a hip replacement. When you assess her incision line, you find redness, warmth, and drainage from the proximal section of the wound. Which of the following would you expect the physician to order?

   a. Amoxicillin   c. Bactrim

   b. Penicillin   d. Cefazolin

7. The physician orders an antibiotic for Mr. Boone three times a day for 7 days. Mr. Boone asks you if this is correct, because his son took the same antibiotic for 5 days. On which of the following factors is the amount and frequency of the antibiotic dosing based?

   a. Characteristics of the causative organism

   b. Age of the client

   c. Sex of the client

   d. Condition of the gastrointestinal system

8. Drug-resistant bacterial strains can be produced in the _____ of antimicrobial drugs.

9. Mr. Benjamin is diagnosed with osteomyelitis secondary to an untreated bone fracture. You understand that IV therapy for this disease process is which of the following?

   a. Short term

   b. Long term

   c. Modified based on the client's age

   d. Modified based on the client's home environment

10. You are Mr. Benjamin's home care nurse. Your role will include teaching the patient and the family about which of the following? (Select all that apply.)

    a. How to acquire the equipment and medication

    b. How to store and administer the medication

    c. How to monitor the IV site

    d. How to report patient responses

11. Mr. Johnson is diagnosed with a drug-resistant infection in his wound. As his home care nurse, which of the following should you teach Mr. Johnson and his family?

    a. To avoid social contact while the infection is treated

    b. To avoid using the same bathroom until the infection abates

    c. To use gloves when handling drainage from the wound

    d. To use bleach when washing all laundry

12. Mr. Treetman is admitted to your critical care unit from a trauma center. He is status post surgery after a fall from a roof in a construction site. He has multiple fractures and internal injuries. The dosage of his IV antibiotic will change based on which of the following factors?

    a. Cardiovascular assessment of the critically ill patient

    b. Neurovascular assessment of the critically ill patient

    c. Changing physiology of the critically ill patient

    d. Altered mentation of the critically ill patient

13. On his second day in the unit, Mr. Treetman develops a left lower lobe infiltrate and is diagnosed with nosocomial pneumonia. Which of the following do you expect is the cause of the pneumonia?

    a. *Pseudomonas*   c. *Clostridium difficile*

    b. *Streptococcus*   d. *Staphylococcus aureus*

14. Mr. Treetman's pneumonia is diagnosed as bacterial. Pending culture results, what would you expect the physician to order?

    a. Broad-spectrum antibiotics

    b. Short-term oral antibiotic therapy

    c. Short-term IV antibiotic therapy

    d. Long-term oral antibiotic therapy

15. Mr. Diemen is placed on a ventilator. To reduce the rate of ventilator-associated pneumonia and mortality, which of the following would you expect the physician to order?
    a. Antibiotic rotation
    b. IV antibiotics in intervals of 4-6 weeks
    c. Oral antibiotics in intervals of 4-6 weeks
    d. An antifungal alternated with an antibiotic

16. Mr. Gaines is diagnosed with hepatitis and bronchitis. Which of the following medications will probably *not* be ordered by the physician? (Select all that apply.)
    a. Tetracycline   c. Isoniazid
    b. Penicillin   d. Rifampin

17. Which laboratory value of CrCl indicates severe renal impairment?
    a. Greater than 15-30 mL/minute
    b. Less than 45-60 mL/minute
    c. Less than 15-30 mL/minute
    d. Greater than 45-60 mL/minute

18. Mr. King is diagnosed with severe renal failure and an infection. You know that, unless the organism causing his infection is sensitive only to this class of drugs, the _____ and _____ should be avoided.

19. Mrs. Gibbs is receiving hemodialysis three times weekly. The physician orders an antibiotic. Which of the following do you expect will happen with the dosage of the antibiotic related to the dialysis?
    a. The dosage may be decreased on dialysis days.
    b. An extra dose may be needed on dialysis days.
    c. A double dose may be needed on dialysis days.
    d. It is not necessary to modify the dose of the antibiotic on dialysis days.

20. _____ and cephalosporins are considered safe for most age groups, including children.

CHAPTER 30

Beta-Lactam Antibacterials: Penicillins, Cephalosporins, and Other Drugs

■ Section I: Learning Objectives

1. Describe the general characteristics of beta-lactam antibiotics.
2. Discuss penicillins in relation to effectiveness, safety, spectrum of antibacterial activity, mechanism of action, indications for use, administration, observation of patient response, and teaching of patients.
3. Differentiate among extended-spectrum penicillins.
4. Question patients about allergies before the initial dose of a penicillin.
5. Describe the characteristics of beta-lactamase inhibitor drugs.
6. State the rationale for combining a penicillin and a beta-lactamase inhibitor drug.
7. Discuss similarities and differences between cephalosporins and penicillins.
8. Differentiate cephalosporins in relation to antibacterial spectrum, indications for use, and adverse effects.
9. Describe major characteristics of carbapenem and monobactam drugs.
10. Apply principles of using beta-lactam antibacterials in selected patient situations.

■ Section II: Assessing Your Understanding

ACTIVITY A

Fill in the Blanks

1. When _____ was introduced, it was effective against many organisms; it had to be given parenterally because it was destroyed by gastric acid; and injections were painful.

2. As a class, _____ usually are more effective in infections caused by gram-positive bacteria than in those caused by gram-negative bacteria.
3. Allergy to a drug of another class with similar chemical structure is called _____.
4. _____, _____, and _____ are the drugs of choice for methicillin-susceptible *Staphylococcus aureus*.
5. _____, _____, and _____ have a broad spectrum of antimicrobial activity, especially against gram-negative organisms such as *Pseudomonas* and *Proteus* species and *Escherichia coli*.

ACTIVITY B

Matching

Match the term in Column A with the definition in Column B.

COLUMN A

1. _____ Augmentin

2. _____ Unasyn

3. _____ Carbapenems

4. _____ Cephalosporins

5. _____ Meropenem (Merrem)

COLUMN B

A. Combination of ampicillin and sulbactam
B. Broad-spectrum, bactericidal beta-lactam antimicrobials
C. Widely used group of drugs that are derived from a fungus
D. Contains amoxicillin and clavulanate
E. Has a broad spectrum of antibacterial activity and may be used as a single drug for empiric therapy before causative microorganisms are identified

ACTIVITY C

Short Answers

Briefly answer the following questions.

1. How should the dose of penicillins be modified if a client is on hemodialysis?
2. What impact does Augmentin have on the liver? Should it be used in clients with hepatic disease?
3. What is the role of the home care nurse when the client receives beta-lactam antibiotics?
4. What metabolic and electrolyte imbalances may occur in patients receiving penicillins who have renal impairment or congestive heart failure?
5. When are beta-lactam antimicrobials commonly used?

■ Section III: Applying Your Knowledge

ACTIVITY D

Case Studies

Consider the scenarios and answer the questions.

Case Study 1

Mrs. Spades developed an intra-abdominal infection after hernia surgery. She presents to the physician's office with a temperature of 102.4 orally, BP 180/78, AP 97 regular and respirations 32. Her skin is cold and clammy, and pallor of the skin is evident. The physician orders hospitalization to manage the infectious process. Initial orders include a course of ertapenem IM.

1. After collecting the patient's history, you discover that the patient's current medical diagnoses include asthma and a seizure disorder; her allergies include prednisone and sulfonamides. Why would you need to call the physician prior to medication administration?
2. The physician confirms the order for ertapenem. What kind of preparation does this medication need before administration? If Mrs. Spade's culture results include the bacteria *P. aeruginosa*, what would you expect the physician to do with the ertapenem order?

Case Study 2

Mrs. Spade is now going home. You are responsible for her discharge teaching. One of her discharge medications is aztreonam.

1. Mrs. Spade asks you if she might take the penicillin that she has instead of the aztreonam, because it is cheaper. What is an appropriate response?
2. Mrs. Spade's daughter is a nurse and states that in her experience aminoglycosides are just as effective for her mother's infectious processes. How would you respond?

■ Section IV: Practicing for NCLEX

Answer the following questions.

1. Which of the following medications blocks renal excretion of the penicillins and can be given concurrently with penicillins to increase serum drug levels?
   a. Probenecid (Benemid)   c. Augmentin
   b. Piperacillin-tazobactam   d. Gentamicin

2. In the rare instance in which penicillin is considered essential, which of the following procedures may be helpful in assessing hypersensitivity?
   a. Administering the medication in a controlled environment
   b. Administering a loading dose of the medication
   c. Administering a skin test
   d. Administering the medication by the intravenous route only

3. As a class, penicillins usually are more effective in infections caused by which of the following types of bacteria?
   a. Gram-negative   c. Anaerobic
   b. Gram-positive   d. Aerobic

4. Choice of a beta-lactam antibacterial depends on which of the following factors? (Select all that apply.)

   a. The organism causing the infection

   b. Severity of the infection

   c. Age of the patient

   d. Sex of the patient

5. Which of the following are beta-lactam antibiotics? (Select all that apply.)

   a. Penicillins   c. Monobactams

   b. Cephalosporins   d. Sulfonamides

6. Mrs. Konas is admitted to the critical care unit with sepsis related to a contaminated central line. The physician orders intravenous beta-lactam antimicrobials. The patient's current laboratory report reflects renal impairment. Which of the following would you expect the physician to do?

   a. Maintain the drug dose

   b. Increase the drug dose

   c. Decrease the drug dose

   d. Administer the drug via an intramuscular route

7. The beta-lactam drugs are frequently given concomitantly with other antimicrobial drugs in critically ill patients. Why?

   a. They often have drug-resistant organisms.

   b. Their immune systems are impaired.

   c. They are susceptible to drug-resistant organisms.

   d. They often have multiorganism or nosocomial infections.

8. Mr. Anza is placed on an IV regimen of aztreonam. You would expect the physician to order which of the following laboratory tests?

   a. CBC   c. Serum albumin

   b. Hematocrit   d. Liver function

9. Mrs. Ponds is hospitalized for sepsis. She also receives hemodialysis three times a week. How much of the initial dose of monobactam should be administered after each hemodialysis session, in addition to the maintenance doses?

   a. 12.5%   c. 10%

   b. 25%   d. 50%

10. Mr. Bates received the initial loading dose of aztreonam this morning. You receive his laboratory results, and his CrCl is 28 mL/minute. You call the physician regarding the laboratory results. Which of the following would you expect the physician to do?

    a. Increase the dose of aztreonam

    b. Decrease the dose of aztreonam by 50%

    c. Maintain the current dose of aztreonam

    d. Discontinue the aztreonam

11. Unless hemodialysis is started within 48 hours, imipenem is contraindicated for clients with severe renal impairment. Which of the following laboratory measurements would indicate renal impairment?

    a. Hematocrit   c. Serum albumin

    b. White blood count   d. Creatinine clearance

12. Penicillins and cephalosporins are used cautiously in neonates due to which of the following factors?

    a. Immature liver function

    b. Immature immune function

    c. Immature kidney function

    d. Immature pancreatic function

13. Mr. Watts is admitted to your unit for a total hip replacement. The surgeon orders a first-generation cephalosporin as a surgical prophylaxis because of the nature of the organisms associated postoperatively with this type of procedure. What type of bacteria are they?

    a. Gram-negative   c. Gram-positive

    b. Anaerobic   d. Aerobic

14. Mr. Ganes is admitted to your unit with *P. aeruginosa* sepsis. The physician orders aminoglycoside to be given concomitantly with penicillin intravenously. How do you administer these drugs?

    a. You mix both drugs in normal saline solution.

    b. You administer the drug in separate IV bags.

    c. You administer the drugs dextrose 5% and 0.9% normal saline.

    d. You administer the drugs every other day.

15. Probenecid (Benemid) can be given concurrently with _____ to increase serum drug levels.

16. Ms. Slate demonstrates symptoms of shock after a single intravenous does of penicillin. Treatment of the shock would include which of the following? (Select all that apply.)

    a. Epinephrine   c. Oxygen

    b. A tongue blade   d. Tracheostomy

17. _____ is the most common cause of drug-induced anaphylaxis, a life-threatening hypersensitivity (allergic) reaction, and a person known to be hypersensitive should be given another type of antibiotic.

18. Most _____ must be given every 4 to 6 hours to maintain therapeutic blood levels, because the kidneys rapidly excrete them.

19. When given alone, the antibiotic imipenem is rapidly broken down by an enzyme, _____, in renal tubules and therefore reaches only low concentrations in the urine.

20. A client with sepsis is reading material given to him on the drug imipenem. He asks you why it is formulated with cilastatin and cannot be taken alone. Which of the following is the appropriate response?

    a. "Cilastatin prevents destruction of imipenem by an enzyme created by the renal tubules."

    b. "Cilastatin is a preservative and prevents the destruction of the imipenem in the gastrointestinal tract."

    c. "Cilastatin helps the imipenem to cross the blood–brain barrier."

    d. "Cilastatin prevents the destruction of the imipenem in the liver."

CHAPTER 31

Aminoglycosides and Fluoroquinolones

■ Section I: Learning Objectives

1. Identify characteristics of aminoglycosides and fluoroquinolones in relation to effectiveness, safety, spectrum of antimicrobial activity, indications for use, administration, and observation of patient responses.
2. Recognize factors influencing selection and dosage of aminoglycosides and fluoroquinolones.
3. State the rationale for the increasing use of single daily doses of aminoglycosides.
4. Discuss the importance of measuring serum drug levels during aminoglycoside therapy.
5. Describe measures used to decrease nephrotoxicity and ototoxicity with aminoglycosides.
6. Describe the characteristics, uses, adverse effects, and nursing process implications of fluoroquinolones.
7. Discuss principles of using aminoglycosides and fluoroquinolones in renal impairment and critical illness.

■ Section II: Assessing Your Understanding

ACTIVITY A

Fill in the Blanks

1. The _____ have been widely used to treat serious gram-negative infections for many years.
2. The _____ are older drugs originally used only for treatment of urinary tract infections.
3. The _____ are synthesized by adding a fluorine molecule to the quinolone structure.
4. Aminoglycosides are _____ agents with similar pharmacologic, antimicrobial, and toxicologic characteristics.

5. After _____ administration, aminoglycosides are widely distributed in extracellular fluid and reach therapeutic levels in blood, urine, bone, inflamed joints, and pleural and ascitic fluids.

ACTIVITY B

Matching

Match the term in Column A with the definition in Column B.

COLUMN A

1. _____ Neomycin and kanamycin

2. _____ Gatifloxacin

3. _____ Trovafloxacin

4. _____ Kanamycin

5. _____ Neomycin

COLUMN B

A. Has been associated with hypoglycemic and hyperglycemic events more commonly than other fluoroquinolones

B. May be given to suppress intestinal bacteria before bowel surgery and to treat hepatic coma

C. Is associated with severe liver injury leading to liver transplantation or death and should be reserved for serious infections only

D. Is not recommended for use in infants and children

E. Is associated with increased risk for ototoxicity in older adults

ACTIVITY C

Short Answers

Briefly answer the following questions.

1. The fluoroquinolones are synthesized by adding a fluorine molecule to the quinolone structure. Explain how this addition changes the drug activity of this antibiotic.
2. Give examples of the microorganisms that aminoglycosides are used to treat.
3. Explain how aminoglycosides are absorbed, including IV peaks.
4. After parenteral administration, aminoglycosides are widely distributed throughout the body. Discuss the areas in the body where aminoglycosides are accumulated and the impact on body systems.
5. Where are aminoglycosides excreted in the body?

■ Section III: Applying Your Knowledge

ACTIVITY D

Case Study

Consider the scenario and answer the questions.

While hospitalized for multiple trauma associated with a motor vehicle accident, Ms. Blanchard develops nosocomial pneumonia. She required surgery for fractures and serious internal injuries. You are the primary nurse assigned to Ms. Blanchard's case.

1. What is the cause of most nosocomial respiratory infections?
2. What part of Ms. Bouchard's current condition or situation puts her at risk for nosocomial infection?
3. Based on a sputum culture positive for *Pseudomonas,* the physician orders an aminoglycoside concurrently with piperacillin. Why do you think the physician ordered this combination of medications? What therapeutic effect does the combination have, and what is its target?
4. Ms. Blanchard fears that the pneumonia will cause her death because her body's reserves are limited. What effect is this combination antibiotic therapy expected to have on the patient's prognosis? If Ms. Blanchard's infection was not related to *Pseudomonas,* but to another gram-negative infection, what effect might this combination therapy have?

■ Section IV: Practicing for NCLEX

Answer the following questions.

1. Mr. Smith, age 75, is diagnosed with an infection. He is currently being treated for type 2 diabetes, hypertension, benign prostatic hypertrophy, and chronic congestive heart failure. The physician orders a fluoroquinolone to treat the infection. Fluoroquinolones are associated with which of the following?

   a. Hypoglycemia and hyperglycemia
   b. Atrial fibrillation
   c. Exacerbation of congestive heart failure
   d. Hypertensive crisis

2. Mr. Bates is prescribed aminoglycosides for a bladder infection secondary to benign prostatic hypertrophy. These drugs reach higher concentrations in which organs? (Select all that apply.)

   a. Kidneys   c. Pericardium
   b. Inner ears d. Peritoneum

3. Mr. Johnson develops a wound infection, and the physician orders once-daily intravenous multiple-dose regimens of aminoglycosides. Which of the following kinds of monitoring do you expect the physician to order?

   a. Peak and trough serum levels
   b. A complete blood count every 48 hours
   c. A serum albumin determination every 48 hours
   d. Measurement of electrolytes every 48 hours

4. Mr. Gonzalez is scheduled for a bowel resection secondary to an exacerbation of his Crohn's disease, which did not respond to medical management. You would expect the physician to order _____ or _____ before surgery to suppress intestinal bacteria.

5. The major clinical use of parenteral aminoglycosides is to treat serious systemic infections caused by susceptible _____ gram-negative organisms.

6. Before the selection of an aminoglycoside to treat Mr. Jones' wound infection, which of the following would you expect the physician to order?

   a. White blood count

   b. Electrolyte panel

   c. Complete blood count

   d. Culture and sensitivity

7. Mr. Adams is concerned that he cannot afford to have his wife's community-acquired pneumonia (CAP) treated in the hospital. He has limited health insurance, and the cost of intravenous antibiotic therapy is prohibitive. According to the American College of Chest Physicians' position statement, where will Mr. Adam's wife be treated?

   a. In the hospital using intravenous therapy

   b. In the home using oral drugs

   c. In the hospital using oral medications

   d. In the home using intravenous therapy

8. Mrs. Harrison, age 80, is a type 2 diabetic whose condition is controlled by glyburide. She develops an infection, and the physician orders fluoroquinolones as a treatment. With this combination of medications, Mrs. Harrison is at risk for which of the following?

   a. Hyperglycemia

   b. Diabetic ketoacidosis

   c. Severe hypoglycemia

   d. Diabetic shock

9. You call a covering physician with the results of a culture and sensitivity test for Mrs. Harrison (as addressed in question #8). The physician orders gatifloxacin. Gatifloxacin increases Mrs. Harrison's risk for which of the following conditions?

   a. Hyperglycemia

   b. Diabetic ketoacidosis

   c. Severe hypoglycemia

   d. Diabetic shock

10. Mr. Giles is NPO as a consequence of a cerebrovascular accident sustained 3 years ago. His care is managed at home by his wife, and he receives all medications via gastrostomy tube. The physician orders a fluoroquinolone for Mr. Giles to treat an infection. You would instruct Mrs. Giles to administer the medication in which of the following ways?

    a. With the enteral feeding

    b. On a full stomach

    c. With antacids

    d. On an empty stomach

11. Mr. Walsh is a patient in your critical care unit. He is receiving aminoglycosides for an infectious process. Which of the following do you need to monitor?

    a. Complete blood count

    b. Liver function tests

    c. Serum albumin concentration

    d. White blood count

12. Aminoglycosides and fluoroquinolones are often used in _____ _____ patients, because this population has a high incidence of serious and difficult-to-treat infections.

13. A black box warning reports that _____ is associated with severe liver injury leading to liver transplantation or death and should be reserved for serious infections only. Clinical manifestations range from abnormalities in liver enzyme test results to hepatitis, liver necrosis, and hepatic failure.

14. Mr. Wallace, a ventilator-dependent patient, is admitted to your critical care unit. His current diagnoses include respiratory arrest, diabetes type 2, hepatitis C, and chronic obstructive pulmonary disease. The physician orders aminoglycosides. Which of the following statements is true in this case?

    a. Risk for hepatic impairment is significant, because the drug is metabolized in the liver.

    b. Risk for hepatic impairment is significant because of a higher risk for toxicity.

    c. Risk for hepatic impairment is not significant, because the drug is excreted through the kidneys.

    d. Risk for hypertensive crisis is increased.

15. With fluoroquinolones, reported renal effects include which of the following? (Select all that apply.)
    a. Glycosuria   c. Crystalluria
    b. Azotemia   d. Hematuria

16. Aminoglycosides are _____ and must be used very cautiously in patients with renal impairment.

17. Aminoglycosides must be used cautiously in children as in adults. Dosage must be accurately calculated according to which of the following factors?
    a. Weight and renal function
    b. Height and weight
    c. Age and weight
    d. Weight and leukocytosis

18. A patient who is receiving aminoglycosides must be kept well hydrated, for which of the following reasons?
    a. Hydration increases drug concentration in serum and body tissues.
    b. Hydration decreases drug concentration in serum and body tissues.
    c. Hydration stabilizes peak serum levels.
    d. Hydration stabilizes trough serum levels.

19. With impaired renal function, dosage of aminoglycosides must be _____.

20. _____ doses are based on serum drug concentrations.

CHAPTER 32

Tetracyclines, Sulfonamides, and Urinary Agents

■ Section I: Learning Objectives

1. Discuss the major characteristics and clinical uses of tetracyclines.
2. Recognize doxycycline as the tetracycline of choice in renal failure.
3. Discuss the characteristics, clinical uses, adverse effects, and nursing implications of selected sulfonamides.
4. Recognize trimethoprim-sulfamethoxazole as a combination drug that is commonly used for urinary tract and systemic infections.
5. Describe the use of urinary antiseptics in the treatment of urinary tract infections.
6. Teach patients strategies for preventing, recognizing, and treating urinary tract infections.

■ Section II: Assessing Your Understanding

ACTIVITY A

Fill in the Blanks

1. Urinary _____ are used only in urinary tract infections (UTI).
2. Urinary antiseptics may be bactericidal for sensitive organisms in the urinary tract because these drugs are concentrated in _____ _____ and reach high levels in urine.
3. Tetracyclines penetrate microbial cells by _____ diffusion and an active transport system.
4. All tetracyclines (except doxycycline) and sulfonamides are contraindicated in patients with _____ _____.
5. Tetracyclines decompose with _____, exposure to light, and extreme heat and humidity.

ACTIVITY B

Matching

Match the term in Column A with the definition in Column B.

COLUMN A

1. _____ Tetracyclines and sulfonamides
2. _____ Tetracyclines
3. _____ Doxycycline (Vibramycin)
4. _____ Trimethoprim-sulfamethoxazole (Bactrim, Septra)
5. _____ Phenazopyridine (Pyridium)

COLUMN B

A. Older, broad-spectrum, bacteriostatic drugs; rarely used for systemic infections because of microbial resistance and development of more effective or less toxic drugs
B. Useful in the treatment of bronchitis
C. Still used to treat bacterial infections caused by *Brucella* and *Vibrio cholerae*
D. One of the drugs of choice for *Bacillus anthracis* (anthrax) and *Chlamydia trachomatis*
E. Given to relieve pain associated with UTI

ACTIVITY C

Short Answers

Briefly answer the following questions.

1. Name two organisms/disease processes that are still treated with tetracyclines.
2. Explain how tetracyclines are excreted.
3. Name two organisms or disease processes in which sulfonamides may be an effective treatment.
4. Describe the mechanism of action used by tetracyclines.
5. For what types of UTIs are sulfonamides prescribed?

■ Section III: Applying Your Knowledge

ACTIVITY D
Case Study
Consider the scenario and answer the questions.

Mrs. Banks calls the physician's office with symptoms of burning on urination, left flank pain, and urinary frequency. The physician asks you to make an appointment for Mrs. Banks for an assessment. You are responsible for Mrs. Banks' medication education and treatment plan.

1. Mrs. Banks asks if the physician can just call in a prescription for her. How would you respond? Why are urine cultures and susceptibility tests needed?
2. Mrs. Banks is diagnosed with a urinary tract infection that is susceptible to sulfonamides. The physician prescribes a loading dose before the maintenance dose. What can you tell the patient about a loading dose?
3. Why is the urine pH important in drug therapy? Is alkalinization needed for this patient?

■ Section IV: Practicing for NCLEX

Answer the following questions.

1. Urinary antiseptics may be bactericidal for sensitive organisms in the urinary tract because these drugs are concentrated in which of the following structures?
   a. Renal tubules   c. Nephrons
   b. Bladder   d. Renal calculi

2. Urinary antiseptics are not used in systemic infections, for which of the following reasons?
   a. They do not sustain therapeutic plasma levels.
   b. They do not attain therapeutic plasma levels.
   c. They are not effective against systemic infections in general.
   d. They attain therapeutic blood levels rapidly.

3. Sulfasalazine (Azulfidine) is contraindicated in people who are allergic to which of the following?
   a. Salicylates   c. Nonopioid analgesics
   b. Diuretics   d. NSAIDs

4. Sulfonamides are bacteriostatic against a wide range of gram-positive and gram-negative bacteria, but they are becoming less useful, for which of the following reasons?
   a. Decreased resistance
   b. Increased susceptibility
   c. Intermittent resistance
   d. Increasing resistance

5. The tetracyclines are effective against a wide range of which of the following types of organisms?
   a. Gram-positive organisms
   b. Gram-negative organisms
   c. Gram-positive and gram-negative organisms
   d. Beta-lactamase–positive organisms

6. Mr. Jay presents to the emergency department in pain. He is diagnosed with mild to moderate burns on his forearms secondary to exposure to hot pipes in his home. The physician orders which of the following topical medications?
   a. Penicillin   c. Tetracycline
   b. Amoxicillin   d. Sulfadiazine

7. The treatment of choice for *P. jiroveci* pneumonia is which of the following?
   a. Trimethoprim-sulfamethoxazole
   b. Tetracycline
   c. Amoxicillin
   d. Sulfadiazine

8. Tetracyclines may be used to treat sepsis caused by which of the following? (Select all that apply.)
   a. Rickettsial organisms
   b. Chlamydial organisms
   c. Streptococcal organisms
   d. *Legionella pneumophila*

9. Tetracyclines are generally contraindicated in pregnant women because they may do which of the following? (Select all that apply.)
   a. Cause fatal hepatic necrosis in the mother
   b. Cause renal impairment in the mother
   c. Cause renal impairment in the fetus
   d. Interfere with bone and tooth development in the fetus

10. Ms. Dagistino is diagnosed with hepatitis C as well as a urinary tract infection. The organism is sensitive to tetracycline. The physician is reluctant to order tetracycline, because hepatic impairment does which of the following?
    a. Slows drug elimination
    b. Increases drug elimination
    c. Causes intermittent drug elimination
    d. Eliminates absorption of the medication

11. In patients with renal impairment, which of the following IV doses of tetracycline has been associated with death from liver failure?
    a. >1.5 g/day   c. >3 g/day
    b. >2 g/day   d. <5 g/day

12. Sulfonamides cause _____ jaundice in a small percentage of patients and should be used with caution in patients with hepatic impairment.

13. A fluid intake of _____ liters daily is needed to reduce formation of crystals and stones in the urinary tract when taking tetracyclines.

14. With the combination of trimethoprim-sulfamethoxazole, older adults are at increased risk for severe adverse effects, including which of the following?
    a. Severe skin reactions
    b. Bone marrow depression
    c. GI bleed
    d. Leukocytosis

15. High concentrations of tetracyclines _____ protein synthesis in human cells.

16. Tetracyclines should not be used in children younger than 8 years of age because of their effects on which of the following?
    a. Teeth and bones   c. Blood
    b. Kidneys   d. Liver

17. If a fetus or young infant receives a sulfonamide by placental transfer, in breast milk, or by direct administration, the drug displaces bilirubin from binding sites on albumin. As a result, the fetus experiences which of the following?
    a. Hyperbilirubinemia   c. Hypernatremia
    b. Hyperkalemia   d. Kernicterus

18. With sulfonamide therapy, alkaline urine increases drug solubility and helps prevent _____.

19. Sulfonamides are often used to treat UTI in children older than what age?
    a. 6 months   c. 2 months
    b. 4 months   d. 12 months

20. Tetracyclines must be used cautiously in the presence of which of the following?
    a. Cerebral vascular accident
    b. Liver impairment
    c. Cardiovascular disease
    d. Kidney impairment

CHAPTER 33

Macrolides and Miscellaneous Antibacterials

■ Section I: Learning Objectives

1. Identify the characteristics and specific uses of macrolide and ketolide antibacterials.
2. Compare and contrast macrolides and ketolides with other commonly used antibacterial drugs.
3. Apply the principles of using macrolides and ketolides in selected patient situations.
4. Discuss the characteristics and clinical indications for using chloramphenicol, clindamycin, daptomycin, linezolid, metronidazole, quinupristin-dalfopristin, rifaximin, spectinomycin, and vancomycin.
5. Discuss the roles of metronidazole and oral vancomycin in the treatment of pseudomembranous colitis.

■ Section II: Assessing Your Understanding

ACTIVITY A

Fill in the Blanks

1. Macrolides are widely distributed into body tissues and fluids and may be _____ or bactericidal, depending on drug concentration in infected tissues.
2. *Mycobacterium avium* complex (MAC) disease is an opportunistic infection that occurs mainly in people with advanced _____ _____ _____ infection.
3. *Helicobacter pylori,* a pathogen implicated in peptic ulcer disease, is treated by _____ or clarithromycin as part of a combination regimen.
4. Telithromycin is excreted by the _____ and kidneys.
5. The macrolides and ketolides enter microbial cells and reversibly bind to the 50S subunits of _____, thereby inhibiting microbial protein synthesis.

ACTIVITY B

Matching

Match the term in Column A with the definition in Column B.

COLUMN A

1. _____ Telithromycin (Ketek)
2. _____ Chloramphenicol (Chloromycetin)
3. _____ Clindamycin (Cleocin)
4. _____ Daptomycin (Cubicin)
5. _____ Tigecycline (Tygacil)

COLUMN B

A. Broad-spectrum, bacteriostatic antibiotic, active against most gram-positive and gram-negative bacteria, rickettsiae, chlamydiae, and treponemes
B. A lincosamide, similar to the macrolides in its mechanism of action and antimicrobial spectrum
C. The first member of the ketolide class
D. A member of the glycylcline class, currently the only member in its class
E. Belongs to the lipopeptide class, a new class of antibiotics

ACTIVITY C

Short Answers

Briefly answer the following questions.

1. Discuss how erythromycin is metabolized and excreted in the body. Does food have an effect on the absorption of erythromycin?
2. What is the mechanism of action of macrolides and ketolides?
3. Identify two contraindications related to the administration of macrolides and ketolides.
4. What are the clinical indications for the use of metronidazole?
5. Name two categories of drugs that should not be administered with quinupristin-dalfopristin. Explain how quinupristin-dalfopristin interferes with the identified medication's absorption.

■ Section III: Applying Your Knowledge

ACTIVITY D

Case Study

Consider the scenario and answer the questions.

Mr. Gresham presents to physician's office with chest pain and shortness of breath. He is taking his second course of antibiotics for pneumonia. The physician orders sputum for culture and sensitivity. The sputum culture results indicate that Mr. Gresham has methicillin-resistant *Staphylococcus aureus* pneumonia. Mr. Gresham is hospitalized and IV vancomycin is ordered.

1. Vancomycin is effective against MRSA. What is the mechanism of action of the drug?
2. Mr. Gresham develops antibiotic-induced diarrhea (*C. difficile*) secondary to the use of the antibiotics prior to his diagnosis of MRSA pneumonia. He states that the vancomycin he is receiving should also treat the *C. difficile*. What information can you give Mr. Gresham? What medication would you expect the physician to order for the initial treatment of Mr. Gresham's *C. difficile*?
3. Discuss the limitations to the use of vancomycin.
4. During the second dose of parental vancomycin, Mr. Gresham develops "red man syndrome." What is the syndrome attributed to?
5. If Mr. Gresham were to develop kidney impairment during his hospitalization, what do you expect would happen to his vancomycin dose?

■ Section IV: Practicing for NCLEX

Answer the following questions.

1. Mr. Costello presents to the emergency department with an abdominal dehiscence. He states he had a hernia repair 18 days earlier, and the physician removed his wound staples 5 days ago. Mr. Costello states that the dehiscence occurred when he lifted a box this morning for his wife. The wound is red, and there is evidence of foul-smelling drainage. The wound is cultured, and an anaerobic bacterium is identified. The physician orders metronidazole because it is effective against which of the following organisms?
   a. All gram-positive bacteria
   b. All gram-negative bacteria
   c. *Staphylococcus*
   d. Anaerobic bacteria

2. Ms. Robinson is noncompliant with the medication treatment plan for her gonococcal infection. She failed to complete the second course of antibiotics because she felt better after 5 days and states that she experienced unpleasant side effects. You would expect the physician to order medication education and which of the following drugs?
   a. Spectinomycin   c. Erythromycin
   b. Streptomycin   d. Zithromax

3. Mr. and Mrs. Williams return from a vacation with traveler's diarrhea. What is the treatment of choice?
   a. Robaxin   c. Rifampin
   b. Rifaximin   d. Relafen

4. Vancomycin is effective against: gram-_____ organisms only, including MRSA and SSNA.

5. Mr. Gustafson, who underwent abdominal surgery 6 weeks ago, is diagnosed with VREF. The physician orders which of the following medications?
   a. Vancomycin   c. Quinupristin-dalfopristin
   b. Rifampin   d. Rifaximin

6. Ms. Seinfeld presents to the physician's office with a skin infection on her forearm. The infection is resistant to over-the-counter antibiotics. After receiving the culture and sensitivity results, the physician orders tigecycline. What is the patient's diagnosis?

    a. *C. difficile*   c. MRSA

    b. VRE   d. VREF

7. Daptomycin belongs to the lipopeptide class of antibiotics that kills gram-positive bacteria. What is the mechanism of action for this antibiotic?

    a. Inhibition of synthesis of bacterial proteins

    b. Inhibition of synthesis of DNA only

    c. Inhibition of mitochondrial reproduction

    d. Inhibition of cell wall osmosis

8. Mrs. Benz is taking clindamycin for an infectious process. She presents to the physician's office with symptoms of dehydration. What adverse reaction is she experiencing from the administration of clindamycin?

    a. Diuresis   c. Dysphasia

    b. Diaphoresis   d. Diarrhea

9. Ms. Gains is diagnosed with VRE. The physician orders chloramphenicol. Ms. Gains should be monitored for the development of which of the following side effects?

    a. Dizziness   c. Nausea

    b. Blood dyscrasias   d. Vomiting

10. Mr. Bethel is diagnosed with myasthenia gravis. He develops an infectious process that is sensitive to telithromycin. Telithromycin is contradicted for Mr. Bethel because of the risk of which of the following conditions?

    a. Respiratory failure

    b. Congestive heart failure

    c. Myocardial infarct

    d. Renal failure

11. The ketolide telithromycin and a macrolide, erythromycin estolate, can cause severe _____ injury.

12. Mrs. Gonzalez is diagnosed with community-acquired pneumonia. The physician orders telithromycin. What is the mechanism of action for this antibiotic?

    a. Inhibition of microbial cell wall synthesis

    b. Destruction of the microbial cell wall

    c. Prevention of osmosis within the microbial cell

    d. Inhibition of microbial protein synthesis

13. Mr. Amie is diagnosed with an infectious process that is sensitive to penicillin. He is allergic to penicillin, so the physician orders a drug with a similar antibacterial spectrum. Which of the following medications will the physician order?

    a. Streptomycin   c. Vancomycin

    b. Erythromycin   d. Dicloxacillin

14. Ms. Cushing is diagnosed with acute bacterial sinusitis. The physician orders azithromycin. How long a course of this drug do you expect the physician to order?

    a. 5 days   c. 7 days

    b. 10 days   d. 3 days

15. Mr. Quinn is given linezolid for a diagnosis of VREF. The drug will be administered for a period that extends beyond 2 weeks. Which of the following laboratory tests would you expect the physician to order on a regular basis because of the length of administration of the drug?

    a. Electrolytes

    b. Complete blood count

    c. Potassium

    d. Serum albumin

16. Mr. Quinn is taking digoxin, SSRIs, and aspirin as part of his daily drug regimen. A patient with Mr. Quinn's drug history who is also receiving linezolid would be at risk for which of the following?

    a. Serotonin syndrome

    b. Diabetes type 2

    c. Congestive heart failure

    d. Renal failure

17. Because linezolid is a weak monoamine oxidase (MAO) inhibitor, patients should avoid foods high in tyramine content, such as which of the following? (Select all that apply.)

    a. Aged cheeses   c. Red wine

    b. Milk   d. Tap beers

18. Mrs. Goldman's medical history includes diabetes type 2, CVA, dysphasia, and chronic renal failure. She develops an infectious process. The physician orders erythromycin. Based on the client's medical history, why is erythromycin the drug of choice?

    a. It is metabolized in the liver.

    b. It is metabolized in the kidneys.

    c. It is excreted into the bloodstream.

    d. It is excreted into the GI tract.

19. Chloramphenicol concentrations may _____ in patients with impaired renal function.

20. Erythromycin inhibits liver metabolism and may _____ elimination of several other drugs.

CHAPTER 34

Drugs for Tuberculosis and *Mycobacterium avium* Complex (MAC) Disease

■ Section I: Learning Objectives

1. Describe the characteristics of latent, active, and drug-resistant tuberculosis infections.
2. Identify populations at high risk for developing tuberculosis.
3. List characteristics, uses, effects, and nursing implications of primary antitubercular drugs.
4. Describe the rationale for multiple-drug therapy in the treatment of tuberculosis.
5. Discuss ways to increase adherence to antitubercular drug therapy regimens.
6. Discuss circumstances in which directly observed therapy (DOT) is needed.
7. Describe factors that affect drug therapy in multidrug-resistant tuberculosis (MDR-TB) and extensively drug-resistant tuberculosis (XDR-TB).
8. Describe *Mycobacterium avium* complex disease and the drugs used to prevent or treat it.

■ Section II: Assessing Your Understanding

ACTIVITY A
Fill in the Blanks

1. Tuberculosis (TB) is an infectious disease that usually affects the lungs but may affect lymph nodes, pleurae, bones, joints, _____, and the gastrointestinal tract.
2. Tuberculosis is caused by _____ _____, the tubercle bacillus.
3. In general, the tubercle bacilli multiply slowly; they may lie dormant in the body for many years; they resist _____ and survive in phagocytic cells.
4. Tubercle bacilli may develop resistance to _____ drugs.

5. Authorities estimate that _____ of the world's population is infected with tuberculosis organisms and that tuberculosis is the cause of death in almost 2 million people every year.

ACTIVITY B
Matching

Match the term in Column A with the definition in Column B.

COLUMN A

1. _____ Isoniazid (also called INH)
2. _____ Rifampin (Rifadin)
3. _____ Rifabutin (Mycobutin)
4. _____ Ethambutol (Myambutol)
5. _____ Pyrazinamide

COLUMN B

A. A rifamycin that is bactericidal for both intracellular and extracellular TB organisms
B. A rifamycin that is active against mycobacteria
C. Used with INH and rifampin for the first 2 months of treating active TB
D. The most commonly used antitubercular drug and prototype; bactericidal, relatively inexpensive, and nontoxic; can be given orally or by injection
E. A tuberculostatic drug that inhibits synthesis of RNA and thus interferes with mycobacterial protein metabolism

ACTIVITY C

Short Answers

Briefly answer the following questions.

1. Explain how tuberculosis is transmitted.
2. What is *primary infection* as it relates to tuberculosis?
3. How does latent tuberculosis infection (LTBI) affect the diagnosed individual?
4. What are the causes of active tuberculosis?
5. What are the signs and symptoms of latent tuberculosis infection?

■ Section III: Applying Your Knowledge

ACTIVITY D

Case Study

Consider the scenario and answer the questions.

Mr. White is diagnosed with drug-resistant *M. tuberculosis*. He recently completed 3 months of treatment for latent tuberculosis infection.

1. Mr. White states that he maintains strict compliance regarding his treatment regimen and asks how his disease became drug resistant. How would you respond? Why wasn't the mutant strain of the bacteria killed or weakened by his current drug regimen?
2. Mr. White asks you whether his family is safe from this strain of TB. Once a drug-resistant strain of TB develops, how is it transmitted to other people?
3. MDR-TB stands for *multiple-drug-resistant tuberculosis*. What are these organisms resistant to? What factors contribute to the development of drug-resistant disease?
4. Mr. White states that he wishes to delay treatment until he consults with his son who lives out of state. He informs you that his treatment will be delayed for only a few weeks while he discusses his condition with his son. Why would this be cause for concern?

■ Section IV: Practicing for NCLEX

Answer the following questions.

1. Mr. Vento is concerned because his drug regimen for drug-resistant TB is different from that of his friends. Which of the following explanations is accurate?
   a. "Treatment varies based on the length of time you are ill."
   b. "Treatment is based on the amount of sputum production."
   c. "Treatment is based on drug susceptibility reports."
   d. "There is a standardized treatment regimen."

2. In drug-susceptible active TB, the treatment of choice is 2 months of INH, rifampin, and pyrazinamide, followed by 4 months of INH and _____.

3. Mr. Steiner is diagnosed with latent tuberculosis infection. You expect that the treatment plan will include which of the following drugs?
   a. Ethambutol   c. INH
   b. Pyrazinamide   d. Cyclosporine

4. As a public heath nurse, you are required to be present for each administered dose of antitubercular therapy administered to the clients on your caseload. Which of the following is the reason for this practice?
   a. It causes clients to resent and become noncompliant with therapy.
   b. It prevents inadequate drug therapy.
   c. It promotes safety within the home.
   d. It prevents adverse reactions to the drugs administered.

5. Multidrug-resistant and _____ _____ _____ tuberculosis are of increasing concern.

6. Your state is considering budget cuts to the public health department in the coming fiscal year. Because TB is rarely diagnosed, the fiscal cutbacks will include elimination of the team responsible for diagnosing and treating tuberculosis. What can you do as a taxpayer?

   a. Support the decision based on tuberculosis statistics in your state.

   b. Suggest a modified platform that will discontinue DOT.

   c. Suggest a modified platform that will limit diagnosis to private physicians.

   d. Suggest that the program be supported without change.

7. With individual patients receiving antitubercular drugs for latent or active infection, which of the following does the home care nurse need to do? (Select all that apply.)

   a. Assist the patient in taking the drugs as directed.

   b. Teach about the importance of taking the drugs and the possible consequences of not taking them.

   c. Report drug resistance.

   d. Arrange and monitor compliance regarding follow-up appointments.

8. The responsibility of the home care nurse in relation to TB within the community includes which of the following? (Select all that apply.)

   a. Being active in identifying cases

   b. Investigating contacts of newly diagnosed cases

   c. Suggesting isolation within the community setting

   d. Promoting efforts to manage tuberculosis effectively

9. Mr. Jenks, an alcoholic, is diagnosed with tuberculosis. You are responsible for his education plan as well as administering his medication. Before administration of the medication regimen, which of the following tests do you expect the physician to order?

   a. Serum ALT and AST

   b. CBC

   c. Electrolytes

   d. Serum albumin and potassium

10. Mrs. Gonzales' treatment regimen includes rifampin. After a brief hospitalization, she is diagnosed with chronic renal insufficiency. Because the rifampin is an integral part of her tuberculosis treatment regimen, which of the following actions would you expect the physician to take?

    a. Increase the dose of rifampin

    b. Decrease the dose of rifampin

    c. Discontinue the rifampin

    d. Maintain the current dose of rifampin

11. Mr. Adams, age 80, is diagnosed with latent tuberculosis infection. Which of the following is a risk for the elderly population when being treated with INH?

    a. Hypovolemia   c. Hepatotoxicity

    b. Hypoxemia   d. Renal failure

12. For treatment of LTBI, only one of the four regimens currently recommended for adults is recommended for patients younger than 18 years of age. Which treatment is recommended?

    a. INH and rifampin for 9 months

    b. INH for 9 months

    c. INH for 12 months

    d. INH and rifabutin for 9 months

13. Ms. Sterling is treated for HIV with NNRTIs. She develops tuberculosis, and the physician includes rifampin in her treatment regimen. Why would this be cause for concern?

    a. Rifampin decreases blood levels of anti-HIV drugs.

    b. Rifampin increases adverse side effects of anti-HIV drugs.

    c. Rifampin causes exacerbation of HIV infections.

    d. Rifampin causes critical anemias in clients with HIV.

14. Mr. Hall is HIV positive and develops tuberculosis. You would expect his treatment regimen to be which of the following?

    a. Longer than a client who does not have HIV

    b. Similar to a patient who does not have HIV

    c. Of shorter duration than a patient who does not have HIV

    d. Contraindicated due to his HIV status

15. Mr. Stall's treatment regimen includes pyrazinamide and he develops gout. Pyrazinamide interacts with the gout medication allopurinol in which of the following ways?

    a. It may cause allopurinol toxicity.

    b. It does not affect therapeutic levels of allopurinol.

    c. It is contraindicated for use concomitantly with allopurinol.

    d. It may decrease the effects of allopurinol.

16. Mrs. Bates is prescribed rifampin as part of her antitubercular regimen. She also takes oral contraceptives. Why would this be cause for concern?

    a. She is at risk for blood clots.

    b. She is at risk for stroke.

    c. She is at risk for pregnancy.

    d. She is at risk for DVT.

17. Mr. Velasquez takes phenytoin for a seizure disorder. Before prescribing isoniazid for the patient's tuberculosis, what would you expect the physician to do?

    a. Decrease the dose of phenytoin and monitor drug levels closely.

    b. Increase the dose of INH secondary to phenytoin administration.

    c. Increase the dose of phenytoin and add Tegretol to the drug regimen.

    d. Increase the dose of phenytoin and monitor drug levels closely.

18. There are two main methods of monitoring patient responses to treatment: clinical and _____.

19. To ensure patient compliance with drug regimens, which of the following tactics might the physician take?

    a. Prescribe the medications Monday through Friday, with weekends off.

    b. Prescribe the medications, alternating the regimen weekly.

    c. Prescribe fixed-dose combinations of drugs.

    d. Prescribe medications for longer durations with fewer drugs to be administered.

20. Sputum culture and susceptibility reports require _____ to _____ weeks, because the tubercle bacillus multiplies slowly.

CHAPTER 35

Antiviral Drugs

■ Section I: Learning Objectives

1. Describe the characteristics of viruses and common viral infections.
2. Discuss difficulties in developing and using antiviral drugs.
3. Identify patients at risk for development of systemic viral infections.
4. Differentiate types of antiviral drugs used for various viral infections.
5. Describe selected antiviral drugs in terms of indications for use, adverse effects, and nursing process implications.
6. Discuss the rationale for using combinations of drugs in treating HIV infection.
7. Discuss the guidelines for using antiviral drugs in special populations.
8. Teach patients strategies to prevent viral infections.

■ Section II: Assessing Your Understanding

ACTIVITY A
Fill in the Blanks

1. Viruses cause acquired immunodeficiency syndrome (AIDS), hepatitis, _____, and other disorders that affect almost every body system.
2. Viruses can be spread by secretions from infected people, ingestion of contaminated food or water, _____ in skin or mucous membrane, sexual contact, pregnancy, breastfeeding, and organ transplantation.
3. Viruses are _____ parasites that gain entry to human host cells by binding to receptors on cell membranes.
4. The locations and _____ of the receptors determine which host cells can be infected by a virus.

5. The mucous membranes lining the tracheobronchial tree have receptors for the influenza A virus; helper T lymphocytes and other white blood cells have CD4 molecules, which are the receptors for the _____ _____ _____.

ACTIVITY B
Matching

Match the term in Column A with the definition in Column B.

COLUMN A

1. _____ Acyclovir, famciclovir, and valacyclovir

2. _____ Foscarnet, ganciclovir, and valganciclovir

3. _____ Trifluridine

4. _____ Tenofovir (Viread)

5. _____ Indinavir, ritonavir, and saquinavir

COLUMN B

A. Applied topically to treat keratoconjunctivitis and corneal ulcers caused by the herpes simplex virus (herpetic keratitis)

B. Similar to the NRTIs in that it inhibits the reverse transcriptase enzyme

C. Inhibits viral reproduction after the drugs are activated by a viral enzyme found in virus-infected cells

D. The oldest PIs

E. Penetrate virus-infected cells, become activated by an enzyme, and inhibit viral DNA reproduction

ACTIVITY C

Short Answers

Briefly answer the following.

1. Describe how viruses use cellular metabolic activities for their own survival and replication.
2. How do viruses transmit their infection to other host cells?
3. Describe symptoms usually associated with acute viral infections.
4. How do herpesviruses differ from other viruses?
5. Describe how viruses induce antibodies and immunity.

■ Section III: Applying Your Knowledge

ACTIVITY D

Case Study

Consider the scenario and answer the questions.

Mr. Grant presents to the physician's office with complaints of a recurrent rash in his genital area. He is diagnosed with genital herpes. The physician prescribes acyclovir. You are responsible for the education plan.

1. Mr. Grant asks you how acyclovir works and whether it will treat his genital herpes. How do you respond? What effect does acyclovir have? What may prolonged or repeated courses of acyclovir result in?
2. Mr. Grant returns for a physician visit 1 year later. He is compliant with the prescribed acyclovir regimen and experiences few outbreaks. He asks if he can discontinue the medication regimen for a while. What will happen if drug therapy is discontinued?
3. Mr. Grant asks you how long will it take for the acyclovir to remove the virus from his body. What can you tell him?
4. Mr. Grant asks if there is an ointment that may be applied to the lesions during outbreaks in addition to taking his oral acyclovir. What do you think the physician will order?

■ Section IV: Practicing for NCLEX

Answer the following questions:

1. Mrs. Waters' physician orders a combination of antiretroviral drugs to treat her illness. She states that she is concerned because she fears increased adverse effects. Which of the following is the reason for using combination antiretroviral medications?
   a. To increase effectiveness
   b. To prevent the emergence of drug-resistant viruses
   c. To decrease adverse effects
   d. To cure the virus in less than 6 weeks

2. Mr. Willis is concerned about how the antiviral drugs he is taking will affect his cells. Viruses are intracellular parasites and have which of the following effects on human cells?
   a. They travel from cell to cell without causing damage.
   b. They do not affect the human cell.
   c. They incapacitate the cell for a short time before moving on.
   d. They are relatively toxic to human cells.

3. For which of the following viral infections is drug therapy available? (Select all that apply.)
   a. Asthmatic bronchitis   c. HIV infection
   b. Hepatitis B and C   d. Influenza

4. To prevent viral infections, which of the following precautions should the general public take?
   a. Use intermittent hand hygiene
   b. Become vaccinated against prevalent virus infections
   c. Wear masks
   d. Wear personal protective equipment

5. Viral infections commonly occur in which of the following age groups?
   a. Young children   c. All age groups
   b. Older adults   d. Infants

6. The role of the home care nurse caring for patients with HIV includes which of the following tasks? (Select all that apply.)
   a. Teaching neighborhood groups about the disease and its treatment
   b. Assisting with drug therapy for HIV or opportunistic infections
   c. Coordinating medical and social services
   d. Preventing or minimizing opportunistic infections

7. Mrs. Leblanc is diagnosed with HIV and hepatitis C, and the physician orders antiviral therapy. You would expect the physician to order monitoring of which of the following laboratory values?
   a. CBC   c. LFTs
   b. Electrolytes   d. Serum albumin

8. The physician prescribes nevirapine for the treatment of Mr. Bryant's HIV infection. Based on moderately abnormal LFTs 3 months later, you would expect the physician to do which of the following?
   a. Discontinue the drug until LFTs return to baseline
   b. Reduce the amount of drug prescribed
   c. Recheck the laboratory values
   d. Increase the amount of drug prescribed

9. Ms. Jordan is diagnosed with HIV and hepatitis B. The physician prescribes zidovudine. When her LFTs become moderately elevated, the physician can be expected to reduce the dose of zidovudine by how much?
   a. 20%   c. 40%
   b. 25%   d. 50%

10. Mr. Canfield is prescribed amantadine as part of the treatment regimen for his Parkinson's disease. Because the patient also is diagnosed with renal disease, the physician titrates the dose of amantadine based on which of the following factors?
    a. White blood cell count
    b. Potassium
    c. Creatinine clearance
    d. Calcium

11. Ms. Billings is diagnosed with CMV retinitis. The physician orders foscarnet. Renal impairment is most likely to occur within which period of time?
    a. First 72 hours of therapy
    b. First week of therapy
    c. Second week of therapy
    d. First month of therapy

12. When foscarnet is administered, renal impairment may be minimized by doing which of the following?
    a. Monitoring renal function two or three times weekly during induction
    b. Monitoring renal function at least every 2 to 3 months during maintenance therapy
    c. Stopping the drug if creatinine clearance drops to less than 0.2 mL/minute/kg
    d. Placing the client on fluid restriction

13. Mrs. Clark is prescribed indinavir for her HIV infection. To avoid nephrolithiasis, you should teach the client to do which of the following?
    a. Maintain a fluid restriction of 800 mL daily
    b. Maintain a fluid restriction of 1000 mL daily
    c. Consume 48 to 64 oz of fluid a day
    d. Consume 64 to 82 oz of fluid a day

14. Mr. Wallace is prescribed amantadine to prevent influenza A. As the nurse on the unit, you should monitor the patient for which of the following? (Select all that apply.)
    a. CNS effects
    b. Gastrointestinal bleeding
    c. Cardiovascular effects
    d. Orthostatic hypotension

15. Jason B., age 10, is prescribed oseltamivir to treat influenza A. Which of the following is an adverse effect of this drug?
    a. Dizziness   c. Difficulty breathing
    b. Hallucinations   d. Diarrhea

16. Ms. Butler is HIV positive and pregnant with her first child. At 14 to 34 weeks of gestation, the physician orders zidovudine. Which of the following dosages is correct?

    a. 75 mg PO five times a day

    b. 50 mg PO five times a day

    c. 25 mg PO five times a day

    d. 100 mg PO five times a day

17. What constitutes viral load?

    a. Viral levels in the tissues

    b. HIV DNA particles within the blood

    c. HIV RNA particles within the blood

    d. All sites of viral reproduction

18. Patients should be assessed for signs and symptoms of adverse drug effects approximately every _____ months during antiviral therapy.

19. Viral vaccines are used to control epidemics of viral disease in a community or to produce which of the following types of immunity in patients who have not yet been exposed?

    a. Passive immunity

    b. Intermittent immunity

    c. Immunity to all viruses

    d. Active immunity

20. Which of the following are two methods to prevent sexually transmitted viral infections such as genital herpes? (Select two.)

    a. Complete abstinence

    b. Avoiding sex when skin lesions are present

    c. Use of a diaphragm when lesions are present

    d. Using condoms

CHAPTER 36

Antifungal Drugs

■ Section I: Learning Objectives

1. Describe the characteristics of fungi and fungal infections.
2. Discuss antibacterial drug therapy and immunosuppression as risk factors for development of fungal infections.
3. Describe commonly used antifungal drugs in terms of indications for use, adverse effects, and nursing process implications.
4. Differentiate between adverse effects associated with systemic and topical antifungal drugs.
5. Teach patients about prevention and treatment of fungal infections.

■ Section II: Assessing Your Understanding

ACTIVITY A
Fill in the Blanks

1. _____ are molds and yeasts that are widely dispersed in the environment and are either saprophytic or parasitic.
2. Molds are _____ organisms comprised of colonies of tangled strands.
3. Some fungi, called _____, can grow only at the cooler temperatures of body surfaces.
4. _____ fungi can grow as molds outside the body and as yeasts in the warm temperatures of the body.
5. Dimorphic fungi include a number of human pathogens such as those that cause blastomycosis, histoplasmosis, and _____.

ACTIVITY B
Matching

Match the term in Column A with the definition in Column B.

COLUMN A

1. _____ Amphotericin B
2. _____ Nystatin
3. _____ Fluconazole (Diflucan)
4. _____ Posaconazole (Noxafil)
5. _____ Caspofungin

COLUMN B

A. Has the same mechanism of action as amphotericin B; used only for topical therapy of oral, intestinal, and vaginal candidiasis because it is too toxic for systemic use

B. A second-generation azole with activity against *Candida* and *Aspergillus* species

C. Is active against most types of pathogenic fungi and is fungicidal or fungistatic, depending on the concentration in body fluids and the susceptibility of the causative fungus

D. Is often the drug of choice for localized candidal infections (e.g., urinary tract infections, thrush) and is useful for systemic candidiasis

E. Is used for systemic *Candida* and *Aspergillus* infections. It is highly bound to plasma albumin; metabolized slowly; and excreted in feces and urine

ACTIVITY C

Short Answers

Briefly answer the following.

1. Identify the areas of the body in which *Candida albicans* is part of the normal flora.
2. What conditions alter the body's natural restraining forces and cause fungal overgrowth and opportunistic infections?
3. Identify the enzyme produced by *Aspergillus* organisms that allows them to destroy structural proteins and penetrate body tissues.
4. How do *Cryptococcus neoformans* organisms invade the normal defense mechanism of phagocytosis?

■ Section III: Applying Your Knowledge

ACTIVITY D

Case Study

Consider the scenario and answer the questions.

Mrs. Franks is diagnosed with a systemic fungal infection. She is hospitalized for management of her infection and will eventually be discharged to continue treatment at home. The physician orders IV amphotericin B.

1. Amphotericin B is only used for serious fungal infections. Why?
2. Mrs. Franks has a preexisting renal impairment. Which formulation of amphotericin B would you expect the physician to prescribe?
3. Mrs. Franks is concerned because her HMO will not cover the formulation that the physician ordered, and she asks whether another form of amphotericin B may be used. The HMO suggested an alternative. How should you respond?
4. Mrs. Franks asks how the drug will help her if the particular site of her infection is unknown. What explanation can you give?
5. Discuss two of the tactics used to decrease nephrotoxicity when amphotericin B is prescribed.
6. Mrs. Franks is concerned when her peripheral IV is discontinued and the physician orders the insertion of a central line. She asks if this is really necessary. What can you tell her about peripheral sites?

■ Section IV: Practicing for NCLEX

Answer the following questions.

1. Laboratory monitoring for clients on all systemic antifungal drugs should include which of the following?
   a. CBC
   b. BUN and creatinine
   c. Electrolytes
   d. LFTs (liver function tests)

2. Which of the following serious adverse effects is associated with amphotericin B?
   a. Nephrotoxicity   c. Cardiogenic shock
   b. Hypovolemia   d. Septic shock

3. Mr. Bates presents to the physician's office with complaints of a fungal infection on his foot. He informs you that when the itching gets too bad, he applies fungal foot powder. Which of the following statements is true about this patient's approach to self-care?
   a. "Intermittent treatment will eventually cure the fungal infection."
   b. "Fungal infections such as the one you have require lifelong treatment."
   c. "Fungal infections often require long-term drug therapy."
   d. "Fungal infections may be healed with a short course of antibiotics and antifungals."

4. Mr. Hanes, who is HIV positive, is being treated for recurrent fungal infections. Clients whose immune systems are suppressed are at risk for which of the following?
   a. Failure to thrive and therefore increased fungal infections
   b. Recurrent bacterial infections
   c. Impaired healing
   d. Development of serious fungal infections

5. Serious fungal infections and infections with _____ *Candida* strains are increasing.

6. With IV antifungal drugs for serious infections, which of the following might the home care nurse need to do? (Select all that apply.)

   a. Assist in managing the environment

   b. Facilitate reverse isolation precautions

   c. Administer the drug

   d. Monitoring for adverse effects

7. Mr. Gains is receiving intravenous antifungal therapy at home to treat his pneumonia. Five weeks ago, he completed a 6-week course of therapy. He feels fine and asks if he can begin woodworking projects around the home to keep himself busy. Which of the following is an appropriate response?

   a. "Yes, as long as you don't overexert yourself."

   b. "No, because of risk for infection."

   c. "I will have to consult the physician."

   d. "Yes, as long as you complete most of the project outdoors."

8. When itraconazole is used in critically ill patients, a loading dose of 200 mg three times daily may be given for what period of time?

   a. 3 days   c. 2 days

   b. 48 hours   d. 5 days

9. Mrs. Bette receives hemodialysis three times a week. She is diagnosed with a severe fungal infection, but the physician is reluctant to order amphotericin B. The patient asks if the hemodialysis could be used to remove any excess drug. Which of the following is the appropriate response?

   a. Blood levels cannot be maintained if the patient is receiving hemodialysis.

   b. Hemodialysis should not be used to manage blood levels.

   c. Hemodialysis will not remove the drug.

   d. Hemodialysis is an effective method to manage blood levels in this case.

10. Mr. Murray's fungal infection extends to his cerebral spinal fluid. Which of the following medications do you expect the physician to order?

    a. Amphotericin B   c. Nystatin

    b. Fluconazole   d. Itraconazole

11. The azole antifungals are relatively contraindicated in patients with which of the following conditions?

    a. Hypovolemia

    b. Pancreatitis

    c. HIV

    d. Increased liver enzymes or active liver disease

12. Mr. Mitchell is diagnosed with cancer. The physician prescribes cytotoxic cancer drugs. Fungal infections related to these drugs include *Candida* and _____ organisms.

13. Mr. Davis, age 75, develops a systemic fungal infection. His current diagnoses include diabetes mellitus type 2, chronic congestive heart failure, hypertension, and mild renal impairment. For which of the following conditions should he be monitored? (Select all that apply.)

    a. Renal impairment   c. Hypovolemia

    b. Hypokalemia   d. Hypotension

14. Terbinafine may increase the effects of which of the following drugs? (Select all that apply.)

    a. Metoprolol   c. Desipramine

    b. Digoxin   d. Nortriptyline

15. To reduce fever and chills related to the administration of amphotericin IV, the client may be premedicated with a combination of medications including which of the following?

    a. An NSAID and diphenhydramine

    b. An NSAID and a corticosteroid

    c. Acetaminophen, diphenhydramine, and a corticosteroid

    d. Acetaminophen, antifungal, and an NSAID

16. To reduce phlebitis caused by the administration of amphotericin IV, the nurse may implement which of the following prevention techniques? (Select all that apply.)

    a. Administer medication on alternate days

    b. Add 500 to 2000 units of heparin to the infusion

    c. Administer via heparin lock

    d. Removing the needle after infusion

17. Mr. Armstrong is prescribed Fungizone. His physician informs him that his maintenance dose may be doubled and infused on alternate days and establishes the medication protocol. You should be concerned when a single dose exceeds which of the following amounts?
    a. 1.5 mg/kg   c. 1.0 mg/kg
    b. 2.0 mg/kg   d. 3.0 mg/kg

18. Mr. Smith is diagnosed with localized lympho-cutaneous infection. Which of the following is the drug of choice for this infection?
    a. Fluconazole   c. Amphotericin B
    b. Nystatin   d. Itraconazole

19. Predisposing factors for fungal infections include which of the following types of medications?
    a. Antihistamines   c. Antibacterials
    b. Anticoagulants   d. Antihypertensives

20. _____ is a broad-spectrum antifungal that inhibits an enzyme needed for synthesis of ergosterol, a structural component of fungal cell membranes.

CHAPTER 37

Antiparasitics

■ Section I: Learning Objectives

1. Describe environmental and other major factors in prevention and recognition of selected parasitic diseases.
2. Discuss assessment and treatment of pinworm infestations and pediculosis in school-age children.
3. Teach preventive interventions to patients planning travel to a malarious area.

■ Section II: Assessing Your Understanding

ACTIVITY A

Fill in the Blanks

1. A _____ is a living organism that survives at the expense of another organism, called the host.
2. Amebiasis is caused by the pathogenic protozoan, _____ _____.
3. Amebiasis is transmitted by ingestion of food or water contaminated with human feces containing _____ _____.
4. _____ are active amebae that feed, multiply, move about, and produce clinical manifestations of amebiasis.
5. Trophozoites produce a/an _____ that allows them to invade body tissues.

ACTIVITY B

Matching

Match the term in Column A with the definition in Column B.

COLUMN A

1. _____ Chloroquine (Aralen)
2. _____ Iodoquinol (Yodoxin)
3. _____ Metronidazole (Flagyl)
4. _____ Tinidazole (Tindamax)
5. _____ Mefloquine (Lariam)

COLUMN B

A. An iodine compound that acts against active amebae (trophozoites) in the intestinal lumen
B. Effective against protozoa that cause amebiasis, giardiasis, and trichomoniasis and against anaerobic bacilli
C. Used to prevent *P. falciparum* malaria, including chloroquine-resistant strains, and to treat acute malaria caused by *P. falciparum* or *P. vivax*
D. Used mainly for its antimalarial effects
E. A chemical relative of metronidazole approved for the treatment of amebiasis, giardiasis, and trichomoniasis

ACTIVITY C

Short Answers

Briefly answer the following questions.

1. Identify the populations that are most likely to contract amebiasis.
2. Describe how toxoplasmosis is transmitted.
3. Describe how trichomoniasis is transmitted.
4. Describe how scabies is transmitted.
5. How is pediculosis capitis diagnosed?

■ Section III: Applying Your Knowledge

ACTIVITY D
Case Study

Consider the scenario and answer the questions.

Mr. and Mrs. Bean returned from a trip to Central America about 1 week ago. They present to the physician's office with symptoms consistent with giardiasis. You are responsible for the clients' education plan.

1. Mr. Bean states that he didn't drink the water while on vacation. Which method or action on the Beans' part may have caused transmission of the disease?
2. Mrs. Bean asks why they didn't get sick while on vacation. What explanation can you give them? How does giardial infection manifest?
3. Mrs. Bean is embarrassed to pick up the prescription at the pharmacy for her treatment. She states, "What if people find out what we have?" What kind of education can you give these patients concerning their treatment? What symptoms may develop later, and what is the cause of these later symptoms?
4. The Beans' son, age 9, presents to the pediatrician's office with symptoms of giardiasis. What would you expect the physician to order for this patient, given his age?

■ Section IV: Practicing for NCLEX

Answer the following questions.

1. The physician orders an antiparasitic drug for your client. The drug is prescribed for treatment of local effects in the skin and which other area?
   a. GI tract   c. Oral mucosa
   b. Lungs   d. Ocular cavity

2. Which of the following is one method that you can teach to prevent many parasitic infections?
   a. Avoidance of campgrounds
   b. Personal and public hygiene practices
   c. Avoidance of specific vacation spots
   d. Avoidance of nonbottled water

3. Mr. Cheshire is traveling to a country where malaria is endemic. You suggest that he visit his physician and receive which of the following medications?
   a. Tinidazole   c. Iodoquinol
   b. Metronidazole   d. Chloroquine

4. Parasitic infestations _____ host tissues.

5. You visit Mrs. Waite for a wound treatment. While you are preparing to leave, her child comes home from school with complaints related to a parasitic infection. Which of the following is one of the responsibilities of the home care nurse in this situation?
   a. Suggest a treatment modality to the mother
   b. Collaborate with the school to prevent or control outbreaks
   c. Tell the mother that her child's poor hygiene is the cause of the infection
   d. Tell the child not to return to school for 48 to 72 hours

6. A treatment is ordered for Mrs. Waite's son. Which of the following are the responsibilities of the home care nurse? (Select all that apply.)
   a. Examine close contacts of the child and assess their need for treatment
   b. Assist the parents so that drugs are used appropriately
   c. Provide treatments for the parasitic illness
   d. Teach personal and environmental hygiene measures to prevent reinfection

7. Mrs. Bates treats her three children for head lice after they come home from school with a note from the school nurse. She complains that this is the third time that she treated them in a month. Which of the following is an appropriate action for you to take?
   a. Review the directions for the product ordered by the physician
   b. Inform her that some children are carriers of the parasite
   c. Inform her that sometimes treatment must be done several times before it is effective
   d. Tell the client that she is "doing it all wrong"

8. Which of the following medications, used to treat malaria, should not be given to children younger than 8 years of age?

   a. Tetracycline   c. Primaquine

   b. Mefloquine   d. Quinine

9. Antiparasitic drugs should be used along with _____ and public health control measures to prevent the spread of parasitic infestations.

10. The physician orders a pyrethrin preparation for Mr. Ford's children, who came home from school with head lice. You tell Mr. Ford that the medication is available over-the-counter and that the initial treatment should be repeated in what period of time?

   a. In 5 days   c. In 48 hours

   b. In 10 days   d. In 72 hours

11. Mr. Walker finds that his child developed a sensitivity reaction to permethrin during treatment for head lice. The physician orders _____ as an alternative treatment modality.

12. _____ is the drug of choice for both pediculosis and scabies.

13. How does mebendazole (Vermox) kill helminths?

   a. It prevents hydration of the helminths by preventing fluid absorption.

   b. It prevents uptake of the glucose necessary for parasitic metabolism.

   c. It reduces circulation and oxygenation to the helminths.

   d. It prevents reproduction of the organism.

14. Mrs. Child's son is diagnosed with cryptosporidiosis. She is concerned because he is also being treated for HIV. Which of the following drugs would you expect the physician to order?

   a. Nitazoxanide (Alinia)

   b. Ivermectin (Stromectol)

   c. Mebendazole (Vermox)

   d. Pyrantel (Pin-Rid)

15. In addition to its use as an antimalarial, quinine may also be used to treat which of the following conditions?

   a. Amebiasis   c. CNS symptoms

   b. Pinworms   d. Cramped skeletal muscles

16. The physician orders primaquine to prevent an initial occurrence of malaria. After the client returns from the malarious area, what would you expect the physician to order?

   a. A repetition of the current order

   b. A proliferative agent

   c. A suppressive agent

   d. A causal prophylaxis

17. Chloroquine acts against erythrocytic forms of plasmodial parasites to prevent or treat which of the following conditions?

   a. Pinworm infestation

   b. Helminth infestation

   c. Pediculosis

   d. Malaria

18. Which of the following are antibiotics that act against amebae in the intestinal lumen by altering the bacterial flora required for amebic viability? (Select all the apply.)

   a. Tetracycline   c. Doxycycline

   b. Penicillin   d. Rifampin

19. Metronidazole should be used with caution in which of the following types of patients?

   a. Those with central nervous system disorders

   b. Those with diabetes type 1

   c. Those with cardiac dysrhythmia

   d. Those with a history of myocardial infarction

20. Drugs used for treatment of _____ are called *anthelmintics*.

CHAPTER 38

Physiology of the Hematopoietic and Immune Systems

■ Section I: Learning Objectives

1. Review hematopoiesis, body defense mechanisms, and immune mechanisms.
2. Differentiate between cellular and humoral types of immunity.
3. Describe the antigen–antibody reaction.
4. Discuss roles of various white blood cells in the immune response.
5. Describe the functions and roles of cytokines and hematopoietic growth factors.
6. Discuss selected factors that affect hematopoietic and immune system functions.
7. Discuss selected connections between the immune system and cancer.

■ Section II: Assessing Your Understanding

ACTIVITY A
Fill in the Blanks

1. Hematopoietic and immune blood cells originate in bone marrow in stem cells, which are often called _____ stem cells because they are capable of becoming different types of cells.
2. As these stem cells reproduce, some cells are exactly like the original cells and are retained in _____ _____ to maintain a continuing supply.
3. Hematopoietic growth factors or _____ control the reproduction, growth, and differentiation of stem cells and CFUs.
4. Cytokines are involved in numerous physiologic responses, including _____ cellular proliferation and differentiation, inflammation, wound healing, and cellular and humoral immunity.
5. Cytokines act by binding to _____ on target cells.

ACTIVITY B
Matching

Match the term in Column A with the definition in Column B.

COLUMN A

1. _____ Adaptive or acquired immunity
2. _____ Active immunity
3. _____ Passive immunity
4. _____ Innate or natural immunity
5. _____ Memory

COLUMN B

A. Is produced by the person's own immune system in response to a disease caused by a specific antigen or administration of an antigen (e.g., a vaccine) from a source outside the body, usually by injection

B. Is not produced by the immune system; includes general protective mechanisms

C. Develops during gestation or after birth and may be active or passive

D. Unique characteristic of long-term active immunity

E. Occurs when antibodies are formed by the immune system of another person or animal and transferred to the host

ACTIVITY C

Short Answers

Briefly answer the following questions.

1. What is the function of the immune system?
2. Define the term *epitopes*.
3. What occurs when the immune system is hypoactive?
4. What occurs when the immune system is hyperactive?
5. What happens when the immune system is inappropriately activated?

■ Section III: Applying Your Knowledge

ACTIVITY D

Case Study

Consider the scenario and answer the questions.

You are participating in a study group of student nurses studying cellular and humoral immunity.

1. Explain the difference between cellular and humoral immunity, including the role of antigens.
2. Discuss the part of humoral immunity known as the secretory, or mucosal, immune system. How do cells in this system migrate? Discuss the antibodies involved.
3. Explain how local protection combats foreign substances that are inhaled, are swallowed, or come in contact with external body substances.

■ Section IV: Practicing for NCLEX

Answer the following questions.

1. Mr. Gates is diagnosed with an autoimmune disorder. You are responsible for his education plan. You explain that autoimmune disorders occur when the body erroneously perceives its own tissues as which of the following?
   a. As antibodies and initiates an autoimmune response
   b. As antigens and initiates an immune response
   c. As immune assays and initiates an immune response
   d. As antigens and prohibits an immune response

2. B cells produce antibodies in response to antigens; _____ (IGs) A, D, G, E, and M, are important in immune responses, including allergic disorders.

3. Which of the following are the major regulators of both humoral and cellular immunity?
   a. B lymphocytes   c. M lymphocytes
   b. NK lymphocytes   d. T lymphocytes

4. _____ are important regulators of immune and inflammatory responses.

5. Which of the following interferons have antiviral and immunomodulating effects? (Select all that apply.)
   a. Alfa   c. Beta
   b. Theta   d. Gamma

6. Hematopoietic growth factors include which of the following? (Select all that apply.)
   a. Erythropoietin   c. Epipoietin
   b. Thrombopoietin   d. Gammopoietin

7. All hematopoietic and immune blood cells are derived from which cells in the bone marrow?
   a. Stem cells   c. Alfa cells
   b. Beta cells   d. Theta cells

8. Drugs that modify the immune system can enhance or _____ immune responses to various disease processes.

9. HIV decreases the numbers and almost all functions of T lymphocytes and which other type?
   a. A lymphocytes   c. NK lymphocytes
   b. B lymphocytes   d. M lymphocytes

10. Which of the following are considered to be autoimmune disorders? (Select all that apply.)
    a. Asthmatic bronchitis
    b. Gallbladder disease
    c. Rheumatoid arthritis
    d. Type 1 diabetes mellitus

11. In allergic disorders, IgE binds to antigen on the surface of mast cells and causes the release of chemical mediators. What are these mediators called?
    a. Antihistamines
    c. Basophils
    b. Histamines
    d. T lymphocytes

12. Mr. Philips is employed as the financial officer of a company at risk for bankruptcy. He presents to the physician's office with complaints of constant colds and headaches. Here is evidence that which of the following statements is true?
    a. Stress causes the common cold.
    b. Stress depresses immune function.
    c. Stress causes a hyperactive immune system.
    d. Stress increases immunity.

13. Vitamin deficiencies may also depress T- and B-cell function. Which of the following is an enzyme cofactor in lymphocytes?
    a. Vitamin K
    c. Vitamin B_{12}
    b. Vitamin C
    d. Vitamin A

14. Older adults have impaired immune responses to antigens. They may require which of the following changes in dosing?
    a. Higher doses of immunizing antigens
    b. Lower doses of immunizing antigens
    c. The same dose of immunizing antigens as younger adults
    d. Multiple injections of low dose immunizing antigens

15. At birth, the neonatal immune system is still immature. Which of the following immunoglobulins is present at near-adult levels in umbilical cord blood?
    a. Immunoglobulin A (IgA)
    b. Immunoglobulin D (IgD)
    c. Immunoglobulin G (IgG)
    d. Immunoglobulin M (IgM)

16. Antibody titers in infants decrease as maternal antibodies are catabolized. This occurs over approximately how long a period of time?
    a. Six months
    c. Three months
    b. Four months
    d. Two months

17. Cytokines regulate the immune response by stimulating or inhibiting the activation, proliferation, and differentiation of various cells and by which of the following other actions?
    a. Inhibiting the secretion of cytokines
    b. Inhibiting the secretion of antibodies
    c. Regulating the secretion of antibodies
    d. Regulating the secretion of M lymphocytes

18. IgM acts only in the bloodstream, for which of the following reasons?
    a. Its small molecular size
    b. Its large molecular size
    c. It fosters capillary permeability.
    d. It binds with hemoglobin.

19. IgG protects against bacteria, toxins, and viruses as it circulates in the bloodstream. Molecules of IgG combine with molecules of antigen, and the antigen–antibody complex activates which of the following processes?
    a. Phagocytosis
    b. The inflammatory reaction
    c. Inactivation of the antigen
    d. Complement

20. Cytotoxic T cells are recruited and activated by helper _____ cells.

CHAPTER 39

Immunizing Agents

■ Section I: Learning Objectives

1. Discuss the common characteristics of immunizations.
2. Discuss the importance of immunizations in promoting health and preventing disease.
3. Identify authoritative sources for immunization information.
4. Identify immunizations recommended for children.
5. Identify immunizations recommended for adults.
6. Discuss ways to promote immunization of all age groups.
7. Teach parents about recommended immunizations and record keeping.

■ Section II: Assessing Your Understanding

ACTIVITY A

Fill in the Blanks

1. _____ involves administration of an antigen to induce antibody formation (for active immunity) or administration of serum from immune people (for passive immunity).
2. _____ are suspensions of microorganisms or their antigenic products that have been killed or attenuated (weakened or reduced in virulence) so that they can induce antibody formation while preventing or causing very mild forms of the disease.
3. _____ live vaccines produce immunity, usually lifelong, that is similar to that produced by natural infection.
4. _____ are bacterial toxins or products that have been modified to destroy toxicity while retaining antigenic properties.
5. Immunization with toxoids is not permanent; scheduled repeat doses called _____ are required to maintain immunity.

ACTIVITY B

Matching

Match the vaccine in Column A with its use in Column B.

COLUMN A

1. _____ *Haemophilus influenzae* b
2. _____ *Haemophilus influenzae* b (Hib) with hepatitis B (Comvax)
3. _____ Human papillomavirus (HPV) (Gardisil)
4. _____ Measles, mumps, rubella, and varicella vaccine (Proquad)
5. _____ Meningitis/meningococcal disease (Menactra; Menomune)

COLUMN B

A. Prevention of diseases caused by HPV types 6, 11, 16, and 18 (cervical, vaginal, and vulvar cancer; genital warts) in girls and women aged 9 to 26 years
B. Routine immunization of children 12 months to 12 years of age
C. Prevention of infection with Hib, a common cause of serious bacterial infections, including meningitis, in children younger than 5 years of age
D. Recommended for college students living in dormitories
E. Routine immunization of children 6 weeks to 15 months of age born to HbsAg-negative mothers

ACTIVITY C

Short Answers

Briefly answer the following questions.

1. Some vaccines may include aluminum. What method should be used to administer these medications, and what may occur if this method is not used?
2. Why are additives included in the creation of vaccines?
3. What is the impact of widespread use of vaccines on populations?
4. Why are single doses of the measles, mumps, and rubella vaccines rarely used?
5. Why is it important to immunize prepubertal girls against rubella?

■ Section III: Applying Your Knowledge

ACTIVITY D

Case Study

Consider the scenario and answer the questions.

Ms. Banks, a nurse assistant, experiences a blood exposure when caring for a client with hepatitis B. She presents to the occupational health department and explains to the nurse what happened. The physician orders immune globulin. You are responsible for the education plan for Ms. Banks.

1. The physician informs Ms. Banks that the immune globulin is given to foster passive immunity. She asks you what this means and how long it will last. How would you respond? Ms. Banks expresses concern that immune globulin may cause hepatitis B. How would you address this concern?
2. What is the goal of therapy in this case?
3. Explain why immunoglobulin fractions are preferred over serum. What type of plasma is used to prepare these products?
4. Ms. Banks asks whether there are hyperimmune serums available if she is exposed to other diseases. What other serums are available?

■ Section IV: Practicing for NCLEX

Answer the following questions.

1. When you obtain a history from a new client, you should also do which of the following?
   a. Offer all available new immunizations
   b. Assess the client's immunization status
   c. Inform the client that immunizations will be administered
   d. Inform the client that a new immunization schedule will begin

2. Mr. Clark is treated for his cancer of the colon with a combination of chemotherapy and radiation therapy. During a routine physician's visit, you determine that he is behind in his immunizations. For when should you schedule immunizations?
   a. This appointment
   b. Three months after his cancer treatment is completed
   c. The next routine appointment
   d. 30 days after his cancer treatment is completed

3. For children with HIV infection, which of the following is true about most routine immunizations?
   a. They are determined by the client's T-cell count.
   b. They are determined by the WBC.
   c. They are recommended.
   d. They are not recommended.

4. Pneumococcal vaccine is recommended for HIV-infected persons older than _____ years of age.

5. Mr. James is diagnosed with HIV. He also is diagnosed with mild bladder cancer. The physician does not prescribe BCG, for which of the following reasons?
   a. It is not effective when the client is diagnosed with HIV.
   b. It is an attenuated vaccine.
   c. It is a live vaccine.
   d. It will further impair the client's immune system.

6. Mrs. Phyllis is living with HIV. She is exposed to measles. Which of the following is the treatment of choice in this case?

    a. Live vaccine

    b. No vaccine and presumptive treatment of the disease

    c. Varicella-zoster immune globulin for active immunization.

    d. Immune globulin

7. Patients receiving a systemic corticosteroid in high doses or for longer than 2 weeks should wait at least _____ _____ before being given a live-virus vaccine.

8. Mrs. Morgan presents to the physician's office with shoulder pain and is diagnosed with bursitis. The physician administers an intra-articular injection of a corticosteroid. You discover that the client requires a tetanus booster. Which of the following would you expect the physician to do?

    a. Postpone the booster for 1 week

    b. Postpone the booster until the next physician's visit

    c. State that the booster is contraindicated at this time

    d. Order the booster

9. Mr. Crete presents to the emergency room with an asthma attack. He is treated and sent home with prednisone 10 mg on a taper and is encouraged to see his physician within 1 week. During an assessment of the chart, you notice that Mr. Crete is overdue for his tetanus booster. Which of the following would you expect the physician to do?

    a. Postpone the booster until the next physician's visit

    b. State that the booster is contraindicated at this time

    c. Order the booster

    d. Postpone the booster for 1 week

10. Which of the following types of vaccine is contraindicated in clients who have active malignant disease?

    a. Killed vaccines   c. Attenuated vaccines

    b. Toxoids   d. Live vaccines

11. Ms. Whitney is receiving chemotherapy for breast cancer. She requires a vaccine booster. For when would the physician order the administration of the vaccine?

    a. 1 year after chemotherapy is completed

    b. 3 months after chemotherapy is completed

    c. 30 days after chemotherapy is completed

    d. 6 months after chemotherapy is completed

12. Clients diagnosed with diabetes mellitus or chronic pulmonary, renal, or hepatic disorders who are not receiving immunosuppressant drugs may be given which of the following types of vaccine? (Select all that apply.)

    a. Live attenuated vaccines

    b. Killed vaccines

    c. Toxoids

    d. Conjugated vaccines

13. Mr. Reed, age 65, lives in a long-term care facility. The infection control nurse identifies a cluster of clients on his unit diagnosed with shingles. Which of the following would she expect the client's physician to order?

    a. Isolation of the client

    b. Shingles vaccine

    c. Isolation of the client's peers

    d. HBV vaccine

14. A newer tetanus-diphtheria-pertussis vaccine is recommended to replace the Td booster dose in adults up to _____ years of age.

15. The _____-_____ virus, the same virus that causes chickenpox, causes shingles.

16. Recommended immunizations for older adults include which of the following? (Select all that apply.)

    a. A tetanus-diphtheria (Td) booster every 10 years

    b. An MMR every 7 to 10 years

    c. An annual influenza vaccine

    d. A one-time administration of pneumococcal vaccine at 65 years of age

17. Mr. Victor received a dose of pneumococcal vaccine during a physician's visit at the age of 60. Which of the following would you recommend?

    a. A second dose when he turns 65

    b. A second dose when he turns 70

    c. That he maintain his healthy lifestyle; a second dose is not needed

    d. That he receive a booster in 6 months

18. Bryant, age 15, presents to the physician's office with his mother. Assuming that he received all of his primary immunizations as an infant and young child, which of the following immunizations would you expect the physician to order? (Select all that apply.)

    a. A second dose of varicella vaccine

    b. A tetanus-diphtheria-pertussis booster

    c. An MMR booster

    d. A hepatitis B booster

19. Which of the following is a contraindication to an MMR booster for an adolescent female?

    a. Menses   c. A positive titer

    b. Pregnancy   d. History of rubeola

20. Which of the following is the best source of information for current recommendations regarding immunizations and immunization schedules?

    a. Department of public health

    b. Department of epidemiology

    c. Local physician's office

    d. Centers for Disease Control and Prevention

CHAPTER 40

Hematopoietic and Immunostimulant Drugs

■ Section I: Learning Objectives

1. Describe the goals and methods of enhancing hematopoietic and immune functions.
2. Discuss the use of hematopoietic agents in the treatment of anemia.
3. Discuss the use of filgrastim and sargramostim in neutropenia and bone marrow transplantation.
4. Describe the adverse effects and nursing process implications of administering filgrastim and sargramostim.
5. Discuss interferons in terms of clinical uses, adverse effects, and nursing process implications.

■ Section II: Assessing Your Understanding

ACTIVITY A
Fill in the Blanks

1. Adequate blood cell production and development are defined as _____.
2. Immune system function is defined as _____.
3. Efforts to enhance a person's own body systems to fight disease include the development of drugs to stimulate _____ and immune function.
4. Drugs that stimulate immune function are called _____, biologic response modifiers, and immunomodulators.
5. Antiviral drugs are more accurately called _____, because they help a compromised immune system regain normal function rather than stimulating "supranormal" function.

ACTIVITY B
Matching

Match the term in Column A with the definition in Column B.

COLUMN A

1. _____ Darbepoetin alfa (Aranesp) and epoetin alfa (Epogen, Procrit)
2. _____ Bacillus Calmette-Guérin vaccine
3. _____ Oprelvekin (Neumega)
4. _____ Aldesleukin (Proleukin)
5. _____ Interferon alfa-n1 and alfacon-1

COLUMN B

A. A suspension of weakened *Mycobacterium bovis*, long used as an immunizing agent against tuberculosis
B. A recombinant DNA version of interleukin-2 (IL-2); activates cellular immunity; produces tumor necrosis factor, interleukin-1 (IL-1), and interferon gamma; and inhibits tumor growth
C. Approved for treatment of chronic hepatitis C, a condition that can lead to liver failure and liver cancer
D. Drug formulations of *erythropoietin*, a hormone from the kidney that stimulates bone marrow production of red blood cells
E. Recombinant IL-11, which stimulates platelet production; used to prevent thrombocytopenia and to reduce the need for platelet transfusions in patients with cancer who are receiving myelosuppressive chemotherapy

ACTIVITY C

Short Answers

Briefly answer the following questions.

1. Exogenous drug preparations have the same mechanisms of action as the endogenous products. Describe the mechanism of action.
2. Describe the antiproliferative and immunoregulatory activities of interferons.
3. Why are exogenous cytokines given only by a subcutaneous (Sub-Q) or intravenous (IV) injection?
4. What is the function of erythropoietin in the human body?
5. How do antiviral drugs improve the health of clients with the diagnosis of AIDS?

■ Section III: Applying Your Knowledge

ACTIVITY D

Case Study

Consider the scenario and answer the questions.

Mrs. Cantos is diagnosed with chronic renal failure and subsequent anemia. The physician orders epoetin alfa (Epogen). You are responsible for the education plan.

1. How does epoetin alfa work? How long will the patient have to take it?
2. Mrs. Cantos' insurance does not cover home care, and she will be administering her own medication. What must you teach Mrs. Cantos about administering Epogen at home?
3. Mrs. Cantos' last hemoglobin level was 14 grams per deciliter (g/dL). What might this indicate?

■ Section IV: Practicing for NCLEX

Answer the following questions.

1. Filgrastim and some interferons are conjugated with polyethylene glycol, in a process called _____, to prolong drug actions.

2. Mr. Adler is prescribed interferon. Which of the following is his diagnosis?
   a. Hypertension   c. Sepsis
   b. Viral hepatitis   d. Bacteremia

3. Mr. Smith is diagnosed with severe neutropenia. The physician prescribes filgrastim. Which of the following is the desired effect?
   a. To increase white blood cells
   b. To increase red blood cells
   c. To increase electrolytes
   d. To decrease leukocytes

4. Adverse effects of epoetin and darbepoetin include increased risks of which of the following conditions?
   a. Hyperlipidemia
   b. Diabetes mellitus type 2
   c. Myocardial infarction
   d. Cirrhosis of the liver

5. Mr. Caisse is receiving anticancer drug therapy that damaged his bone marrow. Which of the following medications would you expect his physician to order?
   a. Oprelvekin
   b. Epoetin
   c. Bacillus Calmette-Guérin vaccine
   d. Simvastatin

6. Mr. Bartholomew is self-administering epoetin in the home. You encourage him to include which of the following supplements as part of his daily medication regimen?
   a. Iron   c. Vitamin A
   b. Vitamin C   d. Folic acid

7. You are caring for Ms. Smith in the home. She is prescribed filgrastim. Which of the following would be included in your education plan?
   a. Dietary restrictions
   b. Exercise restrictions
   c. Fall prevention
   d. Techniques to reduce exposure to infection

8. Mr. Brown is prescribed sargramostim. He is diagnosed with liver impairment. Which of the following would you expect the physician to do?
   a. Monitor LFTs every 2 weeks
   b. Monitor BUN and creatinine every week
   c. Monitor CBC every other day
   d. Monitor electrolytes weekly

9. Mr. Cheshire is diagnosed with hepatitis B. The physician orders interferon alfa. Mr. Cheshire is at risk of developing which of the following?
   a. Drug tolerance
   b. Chronic flank pain
   c. Drug resistance
   d. Subclinical hepatitis B

10. Because _____ can be given once per week and maintains constant blood levels, it has largely replaced other interferons for both monotherapy and combination therapy for hepatitis C.

11. Before receiving a bone marrow transplant, the patient's immune system is _____ by anticancer drugs or irradiation.

12. Mr. Edwards is diagnosed with superficial bladder cancer. The physician orders bacillus Calmette-Guérin. This drug is administered in which of the following ways?
   a. Intravenously
   b. Instilled into the urinary bladder
   c. Orally
   d. Intramuscularly

13. Mr. Black is diagnosed with multiple myeloma. You would expect the physician to order a treatment regimen that includes which of the following?
   a. Interferon alfa
   b. Bacillus Calmette-Guérin
   c. Filgrastim
   d. Epoetin

14. Mr. Carter is diagnosed with hairy-cell leukemia. The physician orders interferon therapy to normalize his WBC. How long does therapy last with this drug?
   a. 4 to 6 weeks
   b. Indefinitely
   c. Until the WBC count is normal for 3 months
   d. 6 to 12 months

15. After Mr. Gordon undergoes bone marrow transfusion, his physician administers sargramostim. When would you expect the first dose to be administered?
   a. 30 minutes after the bone marrow infusion
   b. 1 hour after the bone marrow infusion
   c. Immediately after the bone marrow infusion
   d. 2 to 4 hours after the bone marrow infusion

16. When filgrastim is given to prevent infection in neutropenic patients with cancer, the drug should be started at least _____ hours after the last dose of the antineoplastic agent and continued during the period of bone marrow suppression and recovery.

17. Mrs. Crumb is beginning darbepoetin therapy. How often will the hemoglobin be measured?
   a. Weekly until stabilized
   b. Twice weekly until stabilized
   c. Monthly until stabilized
   d. Every other day until stabilized

18. Mr. Wilson is receiving darbepoetin. The laboratory report indicates that his hemoglobin level increased 2 g/dL in 2 weeks. You would expect the physician to do which of the following?
   a. Increase the medication
   b. Reduce the medication
   c. Maintain the current dose
   d. Discontinue the medication

19. For patients who experience severe adverse reactions with interferon alfa, dosage should be reduced by _____ or administration stopped until the reaction subsides.

20. With most of the hematopoietic and immunostimulant drugs, a CBC with WBC differential and _____ _____ should be done before and during treatment to monitor response and prevent avoidable adverse reactions.

CHAPTER 41

Immunosuppressants

■ Section I: Learning Objectives

1. Describe the characteristics and consequences of immunosuppression.
2. Discuss the characteristics and uses of major immunosuppressant drugs in autoimmune disorders and organ transplantation.
3. Identify adverse effects of immunosuppressant drugs.
4. Discuss nursing interventions to decrease adverse effects of immunosuppressant drugs.
5. Teach patients, family members, and caregivers about safe and effective immunosuppressant drug therapy.
6. Assist patients and family members to identify potential sources of infection in the home care environment.

■ Section II: Assessing Your Understanding

ACTIVITY A

Fill in the Blanks

1. Immunosuppressant drugs interfere with the production or function of immune cells and _____.
2. Autoimmune disorders occur when a person's immune system loses its ability to differentiate between _____ and its own cells.
3. Autoantigens for some disorders have been identified as specific _____ and are found in affected tissues.
4. Allergic asthma, Crohn's disease, psoriasis, psoriatic arthritis, and RA are inflammatory disorders that may be treated with _____ drugs.
5. Although many factors affect graft survival, including the degree of matching between donor tissues and recipient tissues, drug-induced _____ is a major part of transplantation protocols.

ACTIVITY B

Matching

Match the term in Column A with the definition in Column B.

COLUMN A

1. _____ Azathioprine
2. _____ Methotrexate
3. _____ Mycophenolate
4. _____ Cyclosporine
5. _____ Sirolimus

COLUMN B

A. Folate antagonist that inhibits dihydrofolate reductase, the enzyme that converts dihydrofolate to the tetrahydrofolate required for biosynthesis of DNA and cell reproduction

B. Used to prevent rejection reactions and prolong graft survival after solid organ transplantation (e.g., kidney, liver, heart, lung) or to treat chronic rejection in patients previously treated with other immunosuppressive agents

C. Used for prevention and treatment of rejection reactions with renal, cardiac, and hepatic transplantation

D. Antimetabolite that interferes with production of DNA and RNA and thus blocks cellular reproduction, growth, and development

E. Used to prevent renal transplant rejection; inhibits T-cell activation and is given concomitantly with a corticosteroid and cyclosporine

160

ACTIVITY C

Short Answers

Briefly answer the following questions.

1. How does the body react when foreign tissue is transplanted into the body?
2. What role does tumor necrosis factor (TNF)-alpha play in the response to infection?
3. Identify two factors that prevent the immune system from "turning off" an abnormal immune or inflammatory process.
4. Discuss the mechanism that causes rejection reaction.
5. What are the characteristics of acute organ reactions?

▪ Section III: Applying Your Knowledge

ACTIVITY D

Case Study

Consider the scenario and answer the questions.

Mr. Wallace received a bone marrow transplant 6 weeks ago. He presents to the physician's office for a scheduled visit. He is in distress, and the physician requests that you initiate an education plan regarding his disease process, drugs, and symptomatology.

1. The physician diagnoses Mr. Wallace with graft-versus-host disease (GVHD). How would you explain this disease to the patient?
2. What symptom would you look for that indicates that Mr. Wallace has acute GVHD? If Mr. Wallace's symptoms persist for 3 months after transplantation, the physician would diagnose him with chronic GVHD. What are the characteristics of chronic GVHD?
3. After transplantation, the physician prescribed a combination of methotrexate and cyclosporine to prevent GVHD. The dose of methotrexate ordered was lower than doses you have administered for chemotherapeutic purposes. What consequence does the lower dose have? Organ damage is possible with this combination of drugs. What should you monitor?

▪ Section IV: Practicing for NCLEX

Answer the following questions.

1. The physician changes Mrs. Gain's immunosuppressant to a newer drug. She asks the physician why this is necessary. Which of the following is true about the newer immunosuppressants?
   a. They have fewer severe adverse effects.
   b. They are less expensive.
   c. They will prolong her life.
   d. They will enhance her health and well-being.

2. Mr. Wilkes, a recent transplant client, is prescribed enzyme-inhibiting drugs by his physician. He is also prescribed tacrolimus. This drug combination may cause which of the following?
   a. Increased blood levels
   b. Decreased blood levels
   c. Drug-induced diabetes mellitus
   d. Drug-induced liver failure

3. Six months after undergoing transplantation, Mrs. Howe asks her physician if it would be all right for her to volunteer at the local children's health clinic. She has limited adverse effects from her immunosuppressant drugs and is beginning to feel healthy again. The physician suggests alternate volunteer options; he is most likely concerned about which of the following?
   a. She may not have the stamina to work at the clinic.
   b. It is too soon to volunteer in a clinic setting.
   c. She may develop an infectious process at the clinic.
   d. It will increase the risk of rejection.

4. Mr. Grant received a kidney transplant 2 years ago. He asks the physician if he may begin to wean himself off of the immunosuppressive drug therapy. He is healthy and works as an engineer full time, and he finds the cost of the medication prohibitive. Which of the following would you expect the physician to do?

a. Discontinue the medication

b. Titrate the medication and discontinue the medication

c. Use an alternative, less expensive medication and then titrate the new medication

d. Continue the medication, because it is lifelong therapy

5. Immunosuppressants are used to decrease the _____ response with allergic and autoimmune disorders and to avoid graft rejection after transplantation.

6. You are the home care nurse for Mrs. Fig. She underwent renal transplantation 8 weeks ago and is self-administering immunosuppressant drugs. Which of the following situations in the patient's life is the greatest cause for concern?

a. She runs a secretarial business from home.

b. She runs a sick child day care.

c. She is a vegetarian.

d. She likes to walk ½ mile a day.

7. Mrs. Banff's physician prescribes leflunomide for her rheumatoid arthritis. Six months later, she presents for routine laboratory testing. The physician would discontinue the medication if which of the following laboratory tests were abnormal?

a. Serum albumin   c. LDL

b. HDL   d. LFT

8. If a client who is prescribed tacrolimus has impaired liver function, what would you expect the physician to do?

a. Increase the dose

b. Discontinue the medication

c. Decrease the dose

d. Continue the current dose

9. Mr. Whitmore is status post kidney transplantation; he also has impaired liver function. Which of the following would you expect the physician to order regarding the loading dose of sirolimus?

a. Reduce it

b. Increase it

c. Keep it the same as for someone without liver impairment

d. Titrate it over 48 hours

10. Mr. Crumb is prescribed cyclosporine after renal transplantation to prevent rejection. Initially, his BUN and creatine levels were elevated; they diminished with medication adjustment and 3 weeks later are elevated again. What would you expect the physician to do?

a. Evaluate the client for transplant rejection

b. Repeat the laboratory tests

c. Evaluate the CBC

d. Order an electrolyte panel

11. Mr. Whitmore, age 78, begins an immunosuppressant therapy for his rheumatoid arthritis. You are concerned because this patient is at greater risk for which of the following complications, compared with younger adults using the same treatment modality?

a. Falls   c. Mental status changes

b. Infections   d. Self-care deficit

12. For children age 12 and older with allergic asthma, _____ is the only immunosuppressant drug approved for use.

13. Mrs. Gonzales asks the physician why her son Marco, age 4, is not receiving corticosteroids. She read in an article that they are more effective to prevent transplant rejection than the medication that is currently prescribed. Which of the following is the appropriate response?

a. Corticosteroids impair the child's mental status.

b. Corticosteroids impair growth in children.

c. Corticosteroids increase the risk for childhood illness.

d. Corticosteroids increase the risk for rejection in children younger than 6 years of age.

14. Cardiac transplant recipients are usually given cyclosporine, _____, and mycophenolate.

15. Mr. White researches his diagnosis and treatment modalities and compares the information with his current treatment. The dose of the immunosuppressant medication that he receives is different than the doses in the article he read. The rationale that the physician gives the client for the dosage choice is that the dosage is individualized according to which of the following factors? (Select all that apply.)

a. Clinical response

b. Patient's serum drug levels

c. Occurrence of adverse effects

d. Height and weight of the client

16. Immunosuppressant drugs are used to prevent rejection of transplanted tissues, a reaction involving _____ and _____ lymphocytes and multiple inflammatory cytokines.

17. Jane Ross, a nursing student, is diagnosed with rheumatoid arthritis. What is the probable cause of her rheumatoid arthritis?

a. Injury

b. Abnormal immune response

c. Overuse of NSAIDs

d. Overuse of acetaminophen

18. Psoriatic arthritis is a type of arthritis associated with psoriasis that is similar to RA. Which TNF-alpha inhibitor is used for the treatment of psoriatic arthritis?

a. Cyclosporine   c. Lithium

b. Methotrexate   d. Etanercept

19. Mr. Bates is diagnosed with Crohn's disease. You explain that Crohn's is a chronic, recurrent, inflammatory bowel disorder. Which organ can it affect?

a. The large intestine

b. The small intestine

c. The duodenum

d. Any area of the GI tract

20. The most common malignancies among transplant recipients are skin cancers and _____.

Drugs Used in Oncologic Disorders

■ Section I: Learning Objectives

1. Contrast normal and malignant cells.
2. Describe major types of antineoplastic drugs in terms of mechanism of action, indications for use, administration, and nursing process implications.
3. Discuss the rationales for using antineoplastic drugs in combination with each other, with surgical treatment, and with radiation therapy.
4. Discuss adverse drug effects and their prevention or management.
5. Assist patients/caregivers in preventing or managing symptoms associated with chemotherapy regimens.
6. Teach, promote, and practice reduction of risk factors for development of cancer, early recognition of cancer signs and symptoms, and early implementation of effective treatment measures.

■ Section II: Assessing Your Understanding

ACTIVITY A

Fill in the Blanks

1. _____ is the study of malignant neoplasms and their treatment.
2. _____ drug therapy is a major treatment modality for cancer, along with surgery and radiation therapy.
3. The term _____ is used to describe many disease processes with the common characteristics of uncontrolled cell growth, invasiveness, and metastasis, as well as numerous etiologies, clinical manifestations, and treatments.
4. _____ cells reproduce in response to a need for tissue growth or repair and stop reproduction when the need has been met.

5. The normal _____ _____ is the interval between the "birth" of a cell and its division into two daughter cells.

ACTIVITY B

Matching

Match the term in Column A with the definition in Column B.

COLUMN A

1. _____ Alkylating agents
2. _____ Pemetrexed
3. _____ Antitumor antibiotics (e.g., doxorubicin)
4. _____ Camptothecins (also called DNA topoisomerase inhibitors)
5. _____ L-Asparaginase (Elspar)

COLUMN B

A. Bind to DNA so that DNA and RNA transcription is blocked
B. Includes nitrogen mustard derivatives, nitrosoureas, and platinum compounds
C. Enzyme that inhibits protein synthesis and reproduction by depriving cells of required amino acids
D. Blocks folate and enzymes essential for cancer cell reproduction and may increase blood levels of homocysteine
E. Inhibit an enzyme required for DNA replication and repair

ACTIVITY C

Short Answers

Briefly answer the following questions.

1. Describe the mechanism used by antimetabolites to interfere with cell reproduction.
2. What does the term *cell cycle–specific* mean in relation to the action of antimetabolites on cancer cells?
3. What is homocysteine, and what are the treatments used to manage homocysteine levels?
4. Describe the toxic effects related to the use of folic acid antagonists.
5. What types of cancers are treated with folic acid antagonists, purine antagonists, and pyrimidine antagonists?

■ Section III: Applying Your Knowledge

ACTIVITY D

Case Study

Consider the scenario and answer the questions.

Mr. Caisse, a microbiologist, discovers a lump in the region of the clavicle. Biopsy reveals lymphoma stage IIIB, and the treatment modality chosen is surgery and cytotoxic antineoplastic drugs. You are responsible for the treatment plan.

1. Mr. Caisse states that he is having difficulty absorbing the information that he needs to cope with his diagnosis. He feels overwhelmed. He asks you to review how the drugs kill malignant cells. How can you explain to this patient how the cytotoxic antineoplastic drugs work?
2. The physician prescribes daunorubicin in a liposomal preparation. What are the advantages of liposomal preparations? What can you tell this patient about the risks for tumor lysis syndrome?
3. Mr. Caisse states that he understands that the symptoms of tumor lysis syndrome depend on the severity of metabolic imbalances. He develops a mild anemia and is concerned that he is beginning to experience the syndrome. Based on the patient's comment, would you say that he needs more teaching or not? What else might you be able to tell him?
4. What can be done to help prevent tumor lysis syndrome?

■ Section IV: Practicing for NCLEX

Answer the following questions.

1. Mr. Quint, age 75, is diagnosed with cancer. His current treatment modality is only minimally successful. He asks his physician to research clinical trials of drugs that may be successful for his type of cancer. The physician agrees, for which of the following reasons?
   a. Clinical trials and their subsequent costs will be covered by Medicare.
   b. The physician anticipates that no clinical trials are available for the patient's cancer.
   c. Physicians are legally permitted to present patients for clinical trials.
   d. The patient's age will no longer prevent his acceptance for a clinical trial.

2. Mr. Bates is diagnosed with prostate cancer. The treatment modality of choice includes both surgery and chemotherapy. Which of the following does the chemotherapeutic option include?
   a. Hemoglobin replacement therapy
   b. Diuretics
   c. Hormonal therapies
   d. Antidiuretic hormone

3. Biologic targeted antineoplastic agents are designed to specifically attack a target that is expressed exclusively, or disproportionally, in the _____ cell.

4. Mrs. Matson is ending an extensive chemotherapeutic regimen that included cytotoxic antineoplastic drugs. You are concerned when she begins to experience bone marrow toxicity, for which of the following reasons?
   a. It is a common adverse effect of her treatment.
   b. It is a rare side effect of the chemotherapy.
   c. It will cause the physician to increase the dose of chemotherapeutic medications.
   d. It will ultimately lead to death.

5. Mr. Smith is receiving parenteral cytotoxic medications in the home. Adjunct therapy may include which of the following substances?

a. Erythropoietin

b. Heparin

c. Normal saline 0.9% intravenously

d. Antidiuretic hormone

6. Mrs. Janis develops hepatotoxicity from the antineoplastic drugs that she is receiving. She has abnormal levels of AST, ALT, and bilirubin. The physician may not decrease the drugs, for which of the following reasons?

a. These findings do not indicate hepatotoxicity.

b. These findings may indicate renal dysfunction.

c. These findings do not indicate decreased ability to metabolize drugs.

d. These findings may indicate cardiac dysfunction.

7. Ms. Smith is receiving L-asparaginase. She is at the end of her chemotherapeutic course and is concerned because her liver function tests are abnormal. Which of the following is an appropriate response?

a. "Liver damage is an outcome of chemotherapy; a transplant may be advised after you recover."

b. "The liver damage is an acceptable consequence to chemotherapy."

c. "Liver impairment usually subsides when chemotherapy is complete."

d. "You are correct to worry; the chemotherapy may be cancelled and your cancer will recur."

8. Mr. Jackson is informed by his physician that the latest tests indicate that his cancer has spread to his liver. The patient receives capecitabine as part of his treatment regimen. Which of the following would you expect the physician to do?

a. Increase the dose of capecitabine

b. Discontinue the capecitabine

c. Add routine blood transfusions to the patient's treatment regimen

d. Monitor the patient closely and repeat LFTs routinely

9. Mr. Taber is receiving cisplatin as part of his cancer therapy and develops renal impairment. The physician chooses to titrate the dose of the cisplatin based on which of the following laboratory values?

a. BUN   c. CBC

b. LFTs   d. CrCl levels

10. Carmustine and lomustine are toxic to the kidney and are associated with azotemia and _____ _____, usually after long-term IV administration and large cumulative doses.

11. In addition to comorbidities, what other issues affect treatment for older adults? (Select all that apply.)

a. Access to care

b. Social service

c. Financial and transportation issues

d. Functional status

12. Mr. Benjamin, age 71, is receiving chemotherapy as part of the treatment regimen for his cancer. To monitor renal function, which of the following laboratory measurements would you expect the physician to order?

a. BUN   c. Electrolytes

b. Serum creatinine   d. Creatinine clearance

13. In recent years, there have been rapid advances in cancer care for children and high cure rates for many pediatric malignancies. Which of the following is the reason behind many of these advances?

a. The sensitivity of the child's immune system to chemotherapeutic agents

b. Prolonged radiation therapy

c. The systematic enrollment of children in well-designed clinical trials

d. Compliance with treatment regimens

14. Chemotherapy in children should be designed, ordered, and supervised by pediatric _____.

15. Dosage of cytotoxic drugs for children is based on which of the following factors?
    a. Weight
    b. Body surface area
    c. Height
    d. Disease process

16. Chris B. is prescribed an anthracycline drug. You would teach the parents to observe for signs and symptoms of which of the following adverse effects?
    a. Cardiotoxicity
    b. Dehydration
    c. Gallbladder disease
    d. Esophageal varices

17. Mr. Taylor is prescribed cytotoxic antineoplastic drugs as part of his cancer treatment regimen. His wife is 2 months pregnant. You teach both the patient and his wife that she should avoid contact with the drug, for which of the following reasons? (Select all that apply.)
    a. It is carcinogenic
    b. It is mutagenic
    c. It is teratogenic
    d. It is hepatogenic

18. You are teaching the handling of cytotoxic antineoplastic drugs to the wife of a patient receiving them. Which of the following should you teach her to do?
    a. Wear personal protective equipment when handling the drug.
    b. Dispose of the drug in the regular trash.
    c. Store the drug in the cellar of the home.
    d. Save the medications on the kitchen counter, so the home care nurse may dispose of them.

19. When caring for clients receiving cytotoxic antineoplastic drugs, you understand that blood and body fluids are contaminated with drugs or metabolites for how long?
    a. About 72 hours after a dose
    b. About 24 hours after a dose
    c. About 12 hours after a dose
    d. About 48 hours after a dose

20. When both hormone inhibitor and cytotoxic drug therapies are needed, how are they administered?
    a. Given concurrently
    b. Not given concurrently
    c. Administered 3 hours apart
    d. Administered 2 hours apart

CHAPTER 43

Physiology of the Respiratory System

■ Section I: Learning Objectives

1. Review the roles and functions of the main respiratory tract structures in oxygenation of body tissues.
2. Describe the role of carbon dioxide in respiration.
3. List common signs and symptoms affecting respiratory function.
4. Identify general categories of drugs used to treat respiratory disorders.

■ Section II: Assessing Your Understanding

ACTIVITY A

Fill in the Blanks

1. Oxygen is necessary for energy for _____ metabolism.
2. Permanent brain damage occurs within 4 to 6 minutes of _____.
3. In addition to providing oxygen to all body cells, the respiratory system also removes _____ _____, a major waste product of cell metabolism.
4. Excessive accumulation of CO_2 damages or kills body cells and produces respiratory _____.
5. The efficiency of the respiratory system depends on the quality and quantity of air inhaled, the patency of air passages, the ability of the lungs to expand and contract, and the ability of O_2 and CO_2 to cross the _____-_____ membrane.

ACTIVITY B

Matching

Match the term in Column A with the definition in Column B.

COLUMN A

1. _____ Ventilation
2. _____ Perfusion
3. _____ Diffusion
4. _____ Carbon dioxide
5. _____ Musculoskeletal system

COLUMN B

A. The process by which O_2 and CO_2 are transferred between alveoli and blood and between blood and body cells
B. The movement of air between the atmosphere and the alveoli of the lungs
C. Participates in chest expansion and contraction
D. Combines with hemoglobin in the cells for return to the lungs and elimination from the body
E. Blood flow through the lungs

ACTIVITY C

Short Answers

Briefly answer the following questions.

1. Explain the process of respiration.
2. What is the function of cilia within the respiratory system?
3. What is the function of the pharynx within the respiratory system?
4. Describe the structure and function of the larynx.
5. Describe the structure and function of alveoli.

▪ Section III: Applying Your Knowledge

ACTIVITY D
Case Study

Consider the scenario and answer the questions.

You are a student nurse participating in a study group discussing the structure and function of the respiratory system. You are responsible for the topic titled, "Lung Circulation."

1. What is the primary function of the pulmonary circulatory system? What is the primary purpose of the pulmonary circulation?
2. When a client develops a pulmonary embolism, what happens with the bronchial circulation?
3. What are the functions of capillary epithelial cells?
4. What may injure pulmonary endothelium? What happens when pulmonary endothelium is injured?

▪ Section IV: Practicing for NCLEX

1. Which of the following major drug groups are used to treat respiratory symptoms?
   a. Proton pump inhibitors
   b. Anxiolytics
   c. Anti-inflammatory agents
   d. H_2 antagonists

2. The respiratory system is subject to many disorders that interfere with respiration and other lung functions, including which of the following? (Select all that apply.)
   a. Respiratory tract infections
   b. Allergic disorders
   c. Inflammatory disorders
   d. Conditions that facilitate airflow

3. The nervous system regulates the rate and depth of respiration by the respiratory center in which of the following? (Select all that apply.)
   a. Medulla oblongata
   b. Pneumotaxic center in the pons.
   c. Apneustic center in the reticular formation.
   d. Pneumonic center in the corpus callosum

4. The efficiency of the respiratory system depends on which of the following? (Select all that apply.)
   a. Quality and quantity of air inhaled
   b. Vasoconstriction of air passages
   c. Ability of the lungs to expand and contract
   d. Ability of O_2 and CO_2 to cross the alveolar–capillary membrane

5. Mrs. Lynx is diagnosed with chronic obstructive lung disease. She is confused and exhibits perioral cyanosis, and you find her oxygen tubing on the floor of her room. You are concerned, for which of the following reasons?
   a. Her oxygen supply is inadequate.
   b. Her alveolar oxygenation exceeds pulmonary oxygenation.
   c. Her cardiac function is impaired.
   d. Her metabolic acidosis is exacerbated.

6. Mrs. Blaze presents to the physician's office with symptoms diagnosed as asthma. She asks whether the medications prescribed will cure her condition. You explain that the therapy prescribed will do which of the following?
   a. Heal the damage to her lungs
   b. Cure the asthma
   c. Relieve her symptoms
   d. Resolve her allergies that cause the symptoms

7. Mr. Rabinowitz is noncompliant with his medication regimen for the diagnosis of asthma. He frequently presents to the emergency department with symptoms of respiratory distress. As part of patient education, the patient should understand that noncompliance can lead to which of the following situations?
   a. Medication resistance
   b. Cancellation of his health insurance
   c. Respiratory failure
   d. Metabolic alkalosis

8. Overall, normal respiration requires atmospheric air containing at least what percentage of oxygen?
   a. 21%   c. 30%
   b. 20%   d. 41%

9. The diaphragm and external muscles produce which phase of respiration?

    a. Inspiration   c. Oxygenation

    b. Expiration   d. CO_2 retention

10. The abdominal and internal intercostal muscles are the muscles of which phase of respiration?

    a. Inspiration   c. Inhalation

    b. Oxygenation   d. Expiration

11. Which of the following does the nervous system stimulate the cough reflex to do?

    a. Stimulate respiration in the presence of respiratory disease

    b. Protect the lungs from harmful particles

    c. Increase oxygenation to alveoli

    d. Decrease carbon dioxide in the presence of COPD

12. You are caring for a patient with chronic obstructive pulmonary disease. When you review his laboratory results, you find that his CO_2 level is abnormally high. An elevated CO_2 level in this patient may lead to which of the following conditions?

    a. Increased O_2 absorption

    b. Decreased need for supplemental O_2

    c. Respiratory failure

    d. Increased need for supplemental O_2

13. In addition to exchanging O_2 and CO_2, the lungs synthesize, store, release, remove, metabolize, or inactivate a variety of _____ active substances.

14. Amines are important in regulating smooth muscle tone (i.e., constriction or dilation) in the airways and _____ _____.

15. Angiotensin-converting enzyme converts angiotensin I to angiotensin II, which is important in regulating which of the following?

    a. Respiratory rate   c. Renal function

    b. Heart rate   d. Blood pressure

16. Which area of the respiratory tract is not comprised of ciliated membranes?

    a. Nose   c. Pharynx

    b. Bronchi   d. Trachea

17. The bronchioles give rise to the _____, which are grape-like clusters of air sacs surrounded by capillaries.

18. What is the inner layer of the pleura called?

    a. Parietal pleura   c. Thoracic pleura

    b. Visceral pleura   d. Pleural cavity

19. What is the outer layer of the pleura, which lines the thoracic cavity, called?

    a. Parietal pleura   c. Thoracic pleura

    b. Visceral pleura   d. Pleural cavity

20. Elastic tissue in the bronchioles and alveoli allows the lungs to stretch or expand to accommodate incoming air. This ability is called _____.

CHAPTER 44

Drugs for Asthma and Other Bronchoconstrictive Disorders

■ Section I: Learning Objectives

1. Describe the main pathophysiologic characteristics of asthma and other bronchoconstrictive disorders.
2. Discuss the uses and effects of bronchodilating drugs, including adrenergics, anticholinergics, and xanthines.
3. Differentiate between short-acting and long-acting inhaled beta$_2$-adrenergic agonists in terms of uses and nursing process implications.
4. Discuss the uses of anti-inflammatory drugs, including corticosteroids, leukotriene modifiers, and mast cell stabilizers.
5. Discuss reasons for using inhaled drugs when possible.
6. Differentiate between "quick relief" and long-term control of asthma symptoms.
7. Discuss the use of antiasthmatic drugs in special populations.
8. Teach clients self-care and long-term control measures.

■ Section II: Assessing Your Understanding

ACTIVITY A
Fill in the Blanks

1. _____ _____ is defined as asthma resulting from repeated and prolonged exposure to industrial inhalants.
2. Asthma is an airway disorder characterized by bronchoconstriction, inflammation, and _____ to various stimuli.
3. _____ is a high-pitched, whistling sound caused by turbulent airflow through an obstructed airway.

4. Acute symptoms of asthma may be precipitated by numerous stimuli, and hyperreactivity to such stimuli may initiate both inflammation and _____.
5. Some clients are allergic to _____ and may experience life-threatening asthma attacks if they ingest foods processed with these preservatives (e.g., beer, wine, dried fruit).

ACTIVITY B
Matching

Match the term in Column A with the definition in Column B.

COLUMN A

1. _____ Albuterol and levalbuterol

2. _____ Formoterol and salmeterol

3. _____ Beclomethasone, budesonide, flunisolide, fluticasone, mometasone, and triamcinolone

4. _____ Leukotrienes

5. _____ Theophylline

COLUMN B

A. Topical corticosteroids for inhalation
B. Strong chemical mediators of bronchoconstriction and inflammation
C. Short-acting beta$_2$-adrenergic agonists
D. The main xanthine used clinically
E. Used only for prophylaxis of acute bronchoconstriction

ACTIVITY C

Short Answers

Briefly answer the following questions.

1. Describe the symptoms associated with asthma.
2. Discuss the variance in incidence and severity of asthma symptoms.
3. What impact do viral infections have on the development of asthma?
4. What instructions regarding dietary restrictions should be discussed with patients diagnosed with severe asthma?
5. What symptoms related to GERD may be associated with asthma?

■ Section III: Applying Your Knowledge

ACTIVITY D

Case Study

Consider the scenario and answer the questions.

Mrs. Livingston presents to the emergency department with status asthmaticus. She is diagnosed with an exacerbation of serious respiratory disease, not controlled by her current treatment regimen. Once her condition has stabilized, she is sent home. In addition to the first-line antiasthmatic, the physician orders theophylline. You are responsible for the patient's discharge teaching.

1. Discuss what you know about the mechanism of action for theophylline.
2. Mrs. Livingston is diagnosed with mild to moderate congestive heart failure in addition to her respiratory disease. What would you expect the physician to do?
3. Mrs. Livingston complains that she has a more productive cough since she began using theophylline. She finds this annoying and states that the medication is not working as it should. How would you explain this development to the patient?
4. What should you include in your teaching plan for Mrs. Livingston?
5. If you were to discover that Mrs. Livingston is an alcoholic, what concerns would you have about her drug prescription? Patients with alcohol addiction are at risk for development of acute gastritis. How would this development affect the prescription of theophylline?

■ Section IV: Practicing for NCLEX

Answer the following questions.

1. Mrs. Gomez presents to the emergency room with acutely deteriorating asthma. Her husband shows you salmeterol when you ask what medications his wife takes at home. He then tells you that he gave her three extra puffs when she became ill. Which of the following statements in correct in this situation?
   a. The husband made the correct decision in giving the extra doses.
   b. The extra doses facilitated bronchodilation and probably saved her life.
   c. Salmeterol is contraindicated based on his wife's condition.
   d. The physician will most likely order continuation of the salmeterol with increased dosage.

2. Because of the risk of _____, the FDA has issued a black box warning for omalizumab.

3. Mr. Benedict presents to the emergency department in bronchospasm. He has a history of smoking two packs per day for 20 years and is prescribed phenytoin to control a seizure disorder that developed after a head injury 3 years ago. Based on the client's history, which of the following would you expect the physician to order?
   a. A modified dose of aminophylline
   b. The standard dose of aminophylline
   c. A drug other than aminophylline
   d. Phenytoin intravenously

4. Mrs. Anderson's diagnoses include diabetes type 2, atrial fibrillation, asthma, and hyperlipidemia. You are concerned because the over-the-counter aerosol product she uses to control her asthma most likely contains which of the following substances?
   a. Corticosteroids   c. A glucose base
   b. Aspirin   d. Epinephrine

5. Mr. Belliveau is concerned because ever since he began his antiasthma medication his GERD symptoms are worse. You explain that his symptoms are worse because his asthma medications have which of the following effects?

   a. They cause acid indigestion.

   b. They tighten the gastroesophageal sphincter.

   c. They relax the gastroesophageal sphincter.

   d. They stimulate peristalsis.

6. Aerosols are often the drugs of choice to treat asthma because of which of the following characteristics? (Select all that apply.)

   a. They act directly on the airways.

   b. They can usually be given in smaller doses.

   c. They produce fewer adverse effects than oral or parenteral drugs.

   d. They may be given less frequently.

7. Mr. Gateau presents with symptoms of bronchospasm that occurred during a birthday party for his grandson. Which of the following medications would you expect the physician to give him?

   a. Albuterol   c. Theophylline

   b. Asthmacort   d. Omalizumab

8. Two major groups of drugs used to treat asthma, acute and chronic bronchitis, and emphysema are bronchodilators and _____ drugs.

9. During the summer, Ms. Dennis experiences increased periods of acute symptoms of her asthma. The physician increases the dose frequency of which of her medications?

   a. Epinephrine   c. Salmeterol

   b. Omalizumab   d. Albuterol

10. Which of the following is one method used to monitor clients with asthma?

    a. Incentive spirometer

    b. Monometer

    c. Peak-flow monitor

    d. Trough-flow monitor

11. With theophylline, the home care nurse needs to assess the client and the environment for substances that may do which of the following? (Select all that apply.)

    a. Affect metabolism of theophylline

    b. Decrease therapeutic effects

    c. Increase therapeutic effects

    d. Increase adverse effects

12. Mr. Banks is experiencing dysphasia secondary to a mild stroke that he had 3 weeks ago. He states that his asthma medications are not working as well or as long as they did in the past. Which of the following do you suspect is the reason for this?

    a. He is crushing the medication.

    b. He is administering the wrong medication.

    c. He is experiencing confusion.

    d. He is experiencing postural hypotension.

13. In children, high doses of nebulized albuterol have been associated with which of the following conditions? (Select all that apply.)

    a. Hyperkalemia   c. Hypokalemia

    b. Tachycardia   d. Hyperglycemia

14. Mr. Grant is prescribed montelukast and uses it successfully to manage his asthma. He develops hepatitis C. Which of the following would you expect the physician to do?

    a. Lower the dose of the montelukast

    b. Discontinue the medication and prescribe another

    c. Increase the dose of the montelukast

    d. Maintain the same dose of the montelukast

15. Mr. Bart is prescribed cromolyn and uses it successfully to manage his exercise-induced asthma. He develops chronic renal insufficiency. Which of the following would you expect the physician to do?

    a. Reduce the dosage of the medication

    b. Increase the dosage of the medication

    c. Maintain the current dose of the medication

    d. Titrate the dosage of the medication upward

16. Mr. Bronson, age 75, is diagnosed with COPD. His physician orders an adrenergic bronchodilator via inhaler and a spacer. Which of the following are the main risks associated with the drug for this patient? (Select all that apply.)
    a. Excessive cardiac stimulation
    b. Bradycardia
    c. Hypotension
    d. CNS stimulation

17. Mr. Smith, age 45, is 6 feet tall and weights 300 pounds. He is diagnosed with asthma, and the physician orders a combination of an antiasthmatic and theophylline. On which factor is the dose of theophylline based?
    a. The client's weight
    b. The client's ideal body weight
    c. The client's symptomatology
    d. The client's comorbidities

18. Cromolyn aerosol solution may be used in children 5 years of age and older, and the nebulizer solution is used in children _____ years and older.

19. Mrs. Jones is prescribed systemic corticosteroids for her asthma. For which of the following is she at risk?
    a. Pituitary insufficiency
    b. Pancreatic insufficiency
    c. Adrenal insufficiency
    d. Renal insufficiency

20. Mr. Reese is brought to the emergency department by his son with alteration in consciousness. The physician suspects theophylline overdose. Which of the following would you expect the physician to order?
    a. Dextrose and water intravenously
    b. Gastric lavage
    c. Antiemetic
    d. Saline 0.9% intravenously

CHAPTER 45

Antihistamines and Allergic Disorders

■ Section I: Learning Objectives

1. Delineate the effects of histamine on selected body tissues.
2. Describe the types of hypersensitivity or allergic reactions.
3. Discuss allergic rhinitis, allergic contact dermatitis, and drug allergies as conditions for which antihistamines are commonly used.
4. Identify the effects of histamine that are blocked by histamine1 (H_1) receptor antagonist drugs.
5. Differentiate first- and second-generation antihistamines.
6. Describe antihistamines in terms of indications for use, adverse effects, and nursing process implications.
7. Discuss the use of antihistamines in special populations.

■ Section II: Assessing Your Understanding

ACTIVITY A

Fill in the Blanks

1. _____ are drugs that antagonize the action of histamine.
2. _____ is the first chemical mediator to be released in immune and inflammatory responses.
3. Histamine is discharged from _____ _____ and basophils in response to certain stimuli (e.g., allergic reactions, cellular injury, extreme cold).
4. _____ or allergic reactions are exaggerated responses by the immune system that produce tissue injury and may cause serious disease.
5. _____ receptors are located mainly on smooth muscle cells in blood vessels and the respiratory and GI tracts.

ACTIVITY B

Matching

Match the term in Column A with the definition in Column B.

COLUMN A

1. _____ Diphenhydramine (Benadryl)
2. _____ Hydroxyzine (Vistaril) and promethazine (Phenergan)
3. _____ Loratadine (Claritin) and cetirizine (Zyrtec)
4. _____ Azelastine (Astelin)
5. _____ Desloratadine (Clarinex)

COLUMN B

A. Second-generation H_1 antagonists
B. The only antihistamine formulated as a nasal spray for topical use
C. The prototype of first-generation antihistamines
D. An active metabolite of loratadine
E. Strong CNS depressants causing extensive drowsiness

ACTIVITY C

Short Answers

Briefly answer the following questions.

1. Where is histamine located in the human body?
2. What happens to the human body when H_2 receptors are stimulated?
3. Define hypersensitivity or allergic reactions.
4. What is the cause of type I immune response (also called immediate hypersensitivity)?
5. Give an example of a type II immune response.

■ Section III: Applying Your Knowledge

ACTIVITY D

Case Study

Consider the scenario and answer the questions.

Mr. Eden presents to the physician's office with complaints of epistaxis secondary to inflamed nasal mucosa. After evaluation by the physician, Mr. Eden is diagnosed with allergic rhinitis. You are responsible for his education plan.

1. Mr. Eden is upset because the physician did not prescribe antibiotics for his rhinitis. How would you respond?
2. Mr. Eden is referred to an allergist for an analysis of the causes of his symptoms. He is diagnosed with seasonal disease (hay fever). Explain the difference between seasonal disease and perennial disease that is seasonal.
3. Explain allergic rhinitis in terms of an immune response.
4. In people with allergies, mast cells and basophils are increased in both number and reactivity. What type of response would you expect to occur due to the increase?
5. Based on his diagnosis of allergic rhinitis, what other conditions is Mr. Eden at risk for?

■ Section IV: Practicing for NCLEX

Answer the following questions.

1. Mr. Pearson's son Michael is diagnosed with an allergy to peanuts. It is important for his child's health and well being that Mr. Pearson do which of the following?
   a. Provide his son with an emergency contact in case of exposure
   b. Provide those in contact with his son with an emergency plan
   c. Avoid situations in which his son may be exposed to peanuts
   d. Give all who are in contact with his son azelastine in case of exposure

2. Patients with drug allergies should wear a _____ _____ bracelet identifying the drug.

3. Mr. Boudreau presents to the physician's office with allergy-related symptoms that interfere with his job as a car salesman. He requests a nasal spray for topical use, you would expect the physician to order which of the following?
   a. Azelastine (Astelin)
   b. Loratadine (Claritin)
   c. Cetirizine (Zyrtec)
   d. Desloratadine (Clarinex)

4. Second-generation H_1 antagonists cause less CNS depression because they are selective for peripheral H_1 receptors and because of which other property?
   a. They are excreted by the renal system.
   b. They are metabolized by the liver.
   c. They cross the blood–brain barrier.
   d. They do not cross the blood–brain barrier.

5. Mrs. Kost is prescribed a first-generation antihistamine for her allergies. You would expect her to experience which of the following adverse effects?
   a. Diarrhea   c. Dry mouth
   b. Incontinence   d. Slurred speech

6. Mrs. Lawson administers diphenhydramine to her child, who experiences seasonal allergies, before his first baseball game. Her child may experience which of the following?
   a. Hyperactivity
   b. Exacerbation of allergic symptoms
   c. Decreased mental alertness
   d. Poor reflexes

7. Some food allergens have a higher inherent risk for triggering anaphylaxis than others; these higher-risk allergens include which of the following? (Select all that apply.)
   a. Shellfish   c. Milk
   b. Egg   d. Butter

8. Allergic rhinitis is inflammation of nasal mucosa caused by which of the following?

    a. Type III hypersensitivity reaction to inhaled allergens

    b. Type II hypersensitivity reaction to inhaled allergens

    c. Type IV hypersensitivity reaction to inhaled allergens

    d. Type I hypersensitivity reaction to inhaled allergens

9. Virtually any drug may induce an immunologic response in susceptible people, and any body _____ may be affected.

10. You are visiting Mrs. O'Connor in her home for treatment of a wound. She is concerned that her husband, a truck driver, is bothered by his seasonal allergies. A friend suggested diphenhydramine. Which of the following is your response?

    a. "The drug may cause drowsiness and make driving unsafe."

    b. "The drug is safe in small doses."

    c. "The drug is safe if it is purchased over the counter."

    d. "The drug may exacerbate the allergies if used routinely."

11. Mr. Cobb presents to the emergency department with symptoms of a gastrointestinal bleed. The physician orders a blood transfusion. The client has a history of anaphylaxis. The physician orders the administration of which of the following drugs before the blood transfusion?

    a. Cetirizine   c. Azelastine

    b. Desloratadine   d. Diphenhydramine

12. Mrs. Hastings is diagnosed with diabetes mellitus type 2, hyperlipidemia, and mild hepatic impairment. She presents to the emergency department after taking promethazine, obtained from a friend, for motion sickness. You would expect which of the following adverse effects?

    a. Hypotension   c. Cholestatic jaundice

    b. Cholecystitis d. Abnormal hemoglobin

13. Mrs. Cheshire is diagnosed with severe kidney failure. You would expect the physician to order diphenhydramine with which of the following dosing intervals?

    a. 12 to 18 hours   c. 4 to 6 hours

    b. 2 to 4 hours   d. 24 to 48 hours

14. Which of the following is one of the benefits related to second-generation antihistamine administration in older adults?

    a. They do not impair thinking.

    b. They reduce the number of falls in clients diagnosed with osteoporosis.

    c. They increase the ability of clients with dementia to perform ADLs.

    d. They do not affect oxygenation.

15. Mr. Mitchell, age 74, is diagnosed with hypertension, hyperlipidemia, angina, and gout. He presents to the physician's office with complaints of seasonal allergies. His daughter has diphenhydramine at home, and he asks if it is safe for him to take it. You are concerned, because first-generation antihistamines may cause which of the following? (Select all that apply.)

    a. Hypotension   c. Syncope

    b. Hypertension   d. Myocardial hypoxia

16. Mr. Armstrong presents to the emergency room with his 4-year-old child. The child self-administered diphenhydramine of an unknown quantity. In overdosage of diphenhydramine, children may experience which of the following?

    a. Hallucinations   c. Dizziness

    b. Hypotension   d. Convulsions

17. Mr. Ames asks you whether antihistamines will help him cope with the symptoms of the common cold. Which of the following is your response?

    a. "Antihistamines are recommended."

    b. "Antihistamines do not relieve symptoms."

    c. "Antihistamines should be taken only before bed."

    d. "Antihistamines should be taken only if you are not driving."

18. Mrs. Sheffield is concerned that the antihistamine ordered by the physician is not relieving her symptoms and she will not find a medication to meet her needs. Which of the following is your response?

    a. "Antihistamines may not be the answer to your allergic symptoms."

    b. "A client who doesn't respond to one antihistamine is usually resistant to others."

    c. "A client may respond better to one antihistamine than another."

    d. "I will ask the physician to order another type of drug."

19. For treatment of acute allergic reactions, a rapid-acting agent of _____ duration is preferred.

20. An antihistamine is chosen based on the desired effect, duration of action, adverse effects, and other characteristics of available drugs. For most people, a _____-generation drug is the first drug of choice.

CHAPTER 46

Nasal Decongestants, Antitussives, and Cold Remedies

■ Section I: Learning Objectives

1. Describe the characteristics of selected upper respiratory disorders and symptoms.
2. Review decongestants and adverse effects of adrenergic drugs.
3. Describe the general characteristics and effects of antitussive agents.
4. Discuss the advantages and disadvantages of using combination products to treat the common cold.
5. Evaluate over-the-counter allergy, cold, cough, and sinus remedies for personal or patient use.
6. Use the nursing process in the care of individuals with the common cold.

■ Section II: Assessing Your Understanding

ACTIVITY A

Fill in the Blanks

1. The _____ _____, a viral infection of the upper respiratory tract, is the most common respiratory tract infection.
2. Colds can be caused by many types of viruses, most often the _____.
3. _____ is inflammation of the paranasal sinuses, air cells that connect with the nasal cavity and are lined by similar mucosa.
4. _____ (inflammation and congestion of nasal mucosa) and upper respiratory tract infections are the most common causes of sinusitis.
5. _____ _____ results from dilation of the blood vessels in the nasal mucosa and engorgement of the mucous membranes with blood.

ACTIVITY B

Matching

Match the term in Column A with the definition in Column B.

COLUMN A

1. _____ Nasal decongestants
2. _____ Antitussive agents
3. _____ Expectorants
4. _____ Mucolytics
5. _____ Vitamin C

COLUMN B

A. Agents given orally to liquefy respiratory secretions and allow for their easier removal
B. Used to reduce the incidence and severity of colds and influenza
C. Administered by inhalation to liquefy mucus in the respiratory tract
D. Suppress a cough by depressing the cough center in the medulla oblongata or the cough receptors in the throat, trachea, or lungs
E. Used to relieve nasal obstruction and discharge

ACTIVITY C

Short Answers

Briefly answer the following questions.

1. How is the common cold transmitted from one individual to another?
2. What is the primary cause of sinusitis?
3. Define rhinorrhea.
4. Define rhinitis.
5. What effect does a cough have on the respiratory tract?

■ Section III: Applying Your Knowledge

ACTIVITY D

Case Study

Consider the scenario and answer the questions.

Mrs. Hoyer develops signs and symptoms of the common cold. The purpose of the client's visit is to request a medication to shorten the cold and alleviate the symptoms. The physician suggests over-the-counter treatments. You are responsible for the education plan.

1. What do over-the-counter medications commonly include?
2. Mrs. Hoyer wishes to purchase antihistamines to inhibit her rhinitis. You suggest that she avoid antihistamines because, although they dry nasal secretions, they can have other effects. What are these effects? What other information can you give Mrs. Hoyer about OTC cold medications, especially those that are advertised as "maximum strength"?
3. If Mrs. Hoyer wants a product with pseudo-ephedrine in it, how would you advise her?
4. The ingredients in multisystem cold and allergy remedies are often difficult to identify. Why is this?
5. Mrs. Hoyer's friend received an antiviral drug from her physician for the treatment of her viral respiratory tract infection. She asks why the physician won't prescribe it for her. How would you respond?

■ Section IV: Practicing for NCLEX

Answer the following questions.

1. Mrs. Elwood calls the pediatrician's office for a suggestion regarding the best over-the-counter cough and cold medicine for her 6-month-old child. The physician advises against the medication, for which of the following reasons?
   a. The medication is not effective for croup.
   b. Misuse could result in overdose.
   c. The medication is contraindicated for the child's symptoms.
   d. The medication is contraindicated for viral infections.

2. Mr. Whitmore presents to the physician's office for his annual visit. When questioned about over-the-counter medication use, he states that he uses echinacea to prevent colds. Which of the following statements is true about echinacea?
   a. He is healthier because he uses the echinacea.
   b. Echinacea is the OTC drug of choice for prevention of viral infections.
   c. To be effective, echinacea must be taken daily regardless of symptoms.
   d. There is limited or no support for the use of echinacea to prevent or treat symptoms of the common cold.

3. First-generation antihistamines may be effective against which of the following symptoms? (Select all that apply.)
   a. Sneezing   c. Cough
   b. Rhinorrhea   d. Congestion

4. Mr. Peat presents to the physician's office with complaints of inability to breathe freely. When you review his use of over-the-counter medications, you discover that he routinely uses nasal spray three times a day and has for 1 year. The client's nasal swelling may be caused by which of the following?
   a. Chronic nasal polyps
   b. Burning of the nares secondary to chronic use of nasal sprays
   c. Rebound nasal swelling
   d. Damage of the nasal concha

5. Which of the following home remedies are effective for mouth dryness and cough? (Select all that apply.)
   a. Administration of over-the-counter antihistamine
   b. Adequate fluid intake
   c. Humidification of the environment
   d. Sucking on hard candy or throat lozenges

6. Mr. Green presents to the physician's office with a chronic cough. Which of the following conditions predisposes the client to secretion retention?
   a. Chronic lozenge use
   b. Chronic use of antihistamines
   c. Intermittent use of exercise equipment
   d. Debilitation

7. Mr. Royce is diagnosed with chronic bronchitis. Which of the following would you expect to be one of his physical complaints?

 a. Rhinitis

 b. Rhinorrhea

 c. Retention of secretions

 d. Chronic nasal swelling

8. Mr. Devon's physician will not prescribe antibiotics for his upper respiratory tract infection, for which of the following reasons?

 a. Most upper respiratory tract infections are viral in origin.

 b. The infection is resistant to antibiotics.

 c. Culture of sputum is inconclusive.

 d. The infection is multibacterial.

9. Mr. Fergusson presents to the physician's office with symptoms of a common cold. He asks you to suggest over-the-counter drugs to alleviate his symptoms. Before recommending an over-the-counter medication, which of the following actions should you take?

 a. Obtain a prescription from the physician

 b. Obtain a complete drug history

 c. Consult your pharmacist

 d. Research medications covered by the client's HMO

10. Mr. Gains, age 75, is self-administering an oral nasal decongestant. You are concerned that he is at risk for which of the following conditions? (Select all that apply.)

 a. Somnolence

 b. Hypertension

 c. Nervousness

 d. Impaired gastric motility

11. Mrs. Salter calls the pediatrician's office because her child is experiencing cold symptoms and has an oral temperature of 99.9. Which of the following would you expect the physician to do?

 a. Treat the fever only if it exceeds 100.3

 b. Treat the fever only if it exceeds 101

 c. Treat the fever only if the child is restless

 d. Treat the fever only if the child develops nasal drainage

12. Mrs. Macdowell calls the pediatrician because her baby is experiencing nasal congestion and cannot nurse. You would expect the physician to order which of the following drugs to be given just before feeding time?

 a. Saline nasal solution

 b. Diphenhydramine nasal solution

 c. Phenylephrine nasal solution

 d. Chlorpheniramine nasal solution

13. Mr. Bell calls the physician because his baby cannot sleep. When asked what medications his baby takes, he responds that the only drug is a topical agent to prevent nasal congestion just before breastfeeding. Which of the following conditions do you suspect?

 a. Central nervous stimulation

 b. Insufficient breast milk intake

 c. Irritable baby syndrome

 d. Child abuse or neglect

14. Mrs. Collins calls the pediatrician's office because her child is complaining of a sore throat. Which of the following actions would you expect the physician to take?

 a. Order an antibiotic

 b. Order an antitussive

 c. Request a list of drug allergies

 d. Request a throat culture

15. Mrs. Silver's four children, ages 12 through 18, have symptoms of a common cold. She calls the physician's office regarding advice for the most economical over-the-counter cold remedy. You respond that it is less expensive to purchase which of the following?

 a. Combination products

 b. Single-drug formulations

 c. Nasal formulas

 d. Cough and cold formulas

16. Why are nasal decongestants effective?

 a. They are absorbed systemically.

 b. They treat multiple symptoms in a cost-effective manner.

 c. They come into direct contact with nasal mucosa.

 d. Their effects last for 48 to 72 hours.

17. Which of the following medications relieves cold symptoms and aids sleep?

    a. Diphenhydramine   c. Epinephrine

    b. Phenergan   d. Antihistamine

18. Cough associated with the common cold usually stems from _____ _____ and throat irritation.

19. Cough syrups serve as vehicles for antitussive drugs and also may exert antitussive effects of their own by doing which of the following?

    a. Precipitating an anticholinergic reaction

    b. Reducing the bacterial load in the respiratory tract

    c. Soothing irritated pharyngeal mucosa

    d. Thinning pharyngeal mucus

20. _____, a mast cell stabilizer given orally or by intranasal inhalation, seems effective in reducing the symptoms and duration of the common cold but it is not FDA approved for this purpose.

CHAPTER 47

Physiology of the Cardiovascular System

■ Section I: Learning Objectives

1. Recognize the functions of the heart, blood vessels, and blood in supplying oxygen and nutrients to body tissues.
2. Describe the role of vascular endothelium in maintaining homeostasis.
3. Discuss atherosclerosis as the basic disorder causing many cardiovascular disorders for which drug therapy is required.
4. Manage the care of individuals with cardiovascular disorders for which drug therapy is a major treatment modality.

■ Section II: Assessing Your Understanding

ACTIVITY A

Fill in the Blanks

1. The cardiovascular or circulatory system is composed of the heart, blood vessels, and _____.
2. The general functions of the cardiovascular and circulatory systems are to carry oxygen, nutrients, hormones, _____, and other substances to all body cells and to remove waste products of cell metabolism (carbon dioxide and others).
3. The efficiency of the cardiovascular and circulatory systems depends on the heart's ability to pump blood, the _____ and functions of blood vessels, and the quality and quantity of blood.
4. The heart is a hollow, muscular organ that functions as a _____-_____ pump to circulate five to six liters of blood through the body every minute.
5. The heart has four chambers: two atria and two ventricles. The _____ are receiving chambers.

ACTIVITY B

Matching

Match the term in Column A with the definition in Column B.

COLUMN A

1. _____ Platelets
2. _____ Leukocytes
3. _____ Erythrocytes
4. _____ Solid particles or cells
5. _____ Plasma

COLUMN B

A. Function primarily to transport oxygen
B. Fragments of large cells, called *megakaryocytes*, found in the bone marrow
C. Comprises approximately 55% of the total blood volume and is more than 90% water
D. Function primarily as a defense mechanism against microorganisms
E. Comprise approximately 45% of total blood volume

ACTIVITY C

Short Answers

Briefly answer the following questions.

1. Describe the role of the atria as it relates to circulation.
2. Describe the role of the ventricles as it relates to circulation.
3. Identify the muscular wall that separates the right and left sides of the heart.
4. What is the role of the myocardium as it relates to circulation?
5. Define and locate the epicardium and the pericardium of the heart.

■ Section III: Applying Your Knowledge

ACTIVITY D
Case Study

Consider the scenario and answer the questions.

You are part of a group of student nurses studying the structure and function of the heart. Your contribution to the group is the conduction system.

1. What are the components of the conduction system.
2. What is the normal pacemaker of the heart? How does electrical current flow over the heart? What is a unique characteristic of the heart's conduction?
3. What happens if the SA node fails to fire?
4. How do the sympathetic nerves of the autonomic nervous system influence the heart rate?

■ Section IV: Practicing for NCLEX

Answer the following questions.

1. Which of the following is the goal of drug therapy in cardiovascular disorders?
   a. To restore homeostasis
   b. To heal physiologic deficits
   c. To heal disorders
   d. To increase the ability to conduct activities of daily living

2. Cardiovascular drugs may be given to achieve which of the following effects? (Select all that apply.)
   a. Increase or decrease cardiac output
   b. Alter heart rhythm
   c. Increase or decrease blood clotting
   d. Foster healing of damaged cardiac muscle

3. Which of the following disorders are usually treated with surgery rather than drug therapy? (Select all that apply.)
   a. Atherosclerosis
   b. Cardiac dysrhythmias
   c. Peripheral vascular disease
   d. Valvular disease

4. Because the _____ system is a closed system, a disorder in one part of the system eventually disturbs the function of all other parts.

5. Most vascular diseases result from the malfunction of _____ _____ or smooth muscle cells.

6. Which of the following is a major factor in atherosclerosis, acute coronary syndromes, hypertension, and thromboembolic disorders?
   a. Myocardial ischemia
   b. Dysfunctional endothelium
   c. Valvular incompetency
   d. Conduction disturbance

7. Pathologic changes in the structure of the capillary and venular endothelium also results in which of the following conditions?
   a. Edema
   b. Dysrhythmia
   c. Myocardial ischemia
   d. Valvular incompetence

8. Platelets are essential for which of the following processes?
   a. Cellular reproduction
   b. Blood coagulation
   c. Cirrhosis
   d. Prevention of infection

9. Platelets have no _____ and cannot replicate.

10. What is the main cause of endothelial dysfunction?
    a. Ischemia
    b. Hyponatremia
    c. Leukocytosis
    d. Injury to the blood vessel wall

11. Almost all oxygen (95% to 97%) is transported in combination with _____; very little is dissolved in blood.

12. What is the role of serum albumin in body system homeostasis?
    a. Tissue reproduction
    b. To maintain intracellular fluid volume by exerting colloid osmotic pressure
    c. To maintain blood volume by exerting colloid osmotic pressure
    d. Reproduction of red blood cells to maintain oxygen transport

13. What are the functions of blood? (Select all that apply.)
    a. To foster gastrointestinal homeostasis
    b. To nourish and oxygenate body cells
    c. To protect the body from invading microorganisms
    d. To initiate leukocytosis when a blood vessel is injured

14. Which of the following is included in the role of blood within the gastrointestinal tract?
    a. Transport of waste to the duodenum
    b. Transport metabolic wastes from tissues to the kidneys
    c. Transport of waste to the colon
    d. Transport of oxygen to the lungs

15. When injury occurs, the blood transfers which of the following components of blood to the site of the injury?
    a. Hemoglobin   c. Albumin
    b. Platelets   d. Leukocytes

16. Blood vessel walls are composed of two types of cells, smooth muscle cells and which other type?
    a. Epithelial cells   c. Glucothelial cells
    b. Endothelial cells   d. Exothelial cells

17. What is the inner lining of the blood vessel called?
    a. Intima   c. Exothelium
    b. Endothelium   d. Epithelium

18. Coronary arteries originate at the base of the aorta in the aortic cusps and fill during which stage of the cardiac cycle?
    a. Systole   c. Tricuspid contraction
    b. Diastole   d. Mitral contraction

19. The _____ valve separates the right ventricle and pulmonary artery.

20. The _____ valve separates the left ventricle and aorta.

CHAPTER 48

Drug Therapy for Heart Failure

■ Section I: Learning Objectives

1. Recognize major manifestations of heart failure (HF).
2. Discuss the role of endothelial dysfunction in HF.
3. Differentiate the types of drugs used to treat HF.
4. Identify the role of digoxin in the management of HF and atrial fibrillation.
5. List characteristics of digoxin in terms of effects on myocardial contractility and cardiac conduction, indications for use, principles of therapy, and nursing process implications.
6. Differentiate digitalizing doses and maintenance doses of digoxin.
7. Explain the roles of potassium chloride, lidocaine, atropine, and digoxin immune Fab in the management of digoxin toxicity.

■ Section II: Assessing Your Understanding

ACTIVITY A

Fill in the Blanks

1. _____ _____ is a complex clinical condition that occurs when the heart cannot pump enough blood to meet tissue needs for oxygen and nutrients.
2. Impaired myocardial contraction during systole is called _____ _____.
3. Impaired relaxation and filling of ventricles during diastole is called _____ _____.
4. HF has also been referred to as congestive heart failure (CHF), because frequently there are congestion and _____ _____ in the lungs and peripheral tissues.

5. At the cellular level, _____ _____ stems from dysfunction of contractile myocardial cells and the endothelial cells that line the heart and blood vessels.

ACTIVITY B

Matching

Match the term in Column A with the definition in Column B.

COLUMN A

1. _____ Digoxin (Lanoxin)

2. _____ Milrinone IV (Primacor)

3. _____ Nesiritide (Natrecor)

4. _____ Digoxin immune Fab (Digibind)

5. _____ Lidocaine

COLUMN B

A. Most commonly used cardiotonic–inotropic agents for short-term management of acute, severe HF that is not controlled by digoxin, diuretics, and vasodilators

B. First in its class of drugs to be used in the management of acute HF

C. Antidysrhythmic local anesthetic agent used to decrease myocardial irritability

D. The only commonly used digitalis glycoside

E. Digoxin-binding antidote derived from antidigoxin antibodies produced in sheep

ACTIVITY C

Short Answers

Briefly answer the following questions.

1. Discuss the primary causes of heart failure.
2. Discuss a compensatory mechanism of heart failure involving neurohormones.
3. What are the symptoms of heart failure?
4. What impact does the renin–angiotensin–aldosterone system have on congestive heart failure?
5. Define cardiac or ventricular remodeling.

■ Section III: Applying Your Knowledge

ACTIVITY D

Case Study

Consider the scenario and answer the questions.

Mrs. White is diagnosed with atrial fibrillation. Her physician orders digoxin 0.125 mg daily. You are responsible for her education plan.

1. Mrs. White asks if she should administer the medication on an empty or a full stomach. How would you respond?
2. Mrs. White is stabilized on a tablet formation of digoxin. She asks if the physician can change the formulation to Lanoxicaps, which may be easier to swallow. The physician changes the formulation but orders digoxin levels to be drawn at routine intervals. Why did the physician make this order?
3. Mrs. White develops chronic renal failure. She returns to the physician's office for a routine visit. The morning before the visit, she presents to the laboratory for assessment of her digoxin level. The level is 3. Based on this laboratory result, what would you expect the physician to do?
4. Discuss the teaching you would give Mrs. White concerning her digoxin prescription, including the reason that she is taking digoxin, the onset of action and peak effect of the drug, and the difference between IV and oral digoxin.

■ Section IV: Practicing for NCLEX

Answer the following questions.

1. Mrs. Pease's digoxin level is 0.125. You understand that this level is which of the following?
   a. Normal   c. Toxic
   b. Elevated   d. Low

2. _____ toxicity is one of the most commonly encountered drug-related reasons for hospitalization, because the drug has a narrow therapeutic index, and the endpoint of effective therapy is often difficult to define and measure.

3. Mr. Zander presents to your emergency department with signs and symptoms of acute congestive heart failure. Assessment findings and tests confirm the diagnosis. Which type of diuretic would be the drug of choice to treat the client?
   a. Thiazide   c. Potassium-sparing
   b. Loop   d. Calcium-wasting

4. Mr. Donati is admitted to the hospital secondary to hypoxia and acute congestive heart failure. At discharge, the client notes that the physician discontinued his beta-blockers. You explain that beta-blockers may do which of the following?
   a. Cause increased shortness of breath
   b. Cause anginal episodes
   c. Decrease myocardial contractility
   d. Increase atrioventricular conductivity

5. Mr. Roberts, age 65, presents to the physician's office with complaints of shortness of breath on exertion, edema in his ankles, and waking up in the middle of the night unable to breathe. You suspect that his symptoms are indicative of which of the following?

   a. Asthmatic bronchitis
   c. Heart failure
   b. Pulmonary edema
   d. Myocardial infarction

6. The most common conditions leading to HF are coronary artery disease and _____.

7. Heart failure may result from which of the following? (Select all that apply.)

   a. Impaired myocardial contraction during systole

   b. Impaired relaxation and filling of ventricles during diastole

   c. A combination of systolic and diastolic dysfunction

   d. Impaired conduction from the SA node

8. Mr. Harbor takes natural licorice for his arthritis. He complains that he is more short of breath. You understand that licorice blocks the effects of spironolactone by causing which of the following?

   a. Sodium retention and potassium loss

   b. Increased cardiac afterload

   c. Renal insufficiency

   d. Potassium retention and dysrhythmia

9. Mrs. Beattie's drugs include a furosemide, digoxin, and hydralazine. She is unable to afford all of her medications, so she takes them intermittently to make them last longer. As her home care nurse, in addition to making a referral to social service, you tell the client which of the following?

   a. Different types of drugs have different actions and produce different responses.

   b. Over-the-counter drugs may be viable substitutes for the more expensive medications.

   c. Her plan is acceptable if the physician is aware and laboratory studies are done more frequently.

   d. Changes in doses may be better than alternating medications.

10. Mr. King is diagnosed with cirrhosis of the liver. He also takes digoxin for a diagnosis of atrial fibrillation. You would expect the physician to do which of the following?

   a. Lower the digoxin dose

   b. Increase the digoxin dose

   c. Check the client's digoxin level

   d. Maintain the current digoxin dose

11. Mr. Billings is diagnosed with renal failure secondary to diabetes mellitus. Based on the new diagnosis, the physician may safely reduce the client's digoxin dose to which of the following?

   a. 0.25 mg every other day

   b. 0.125 mg every day

   c. 0.125 mg three times a week

   d. 0.25 mg five times a week

12. The pediatric cardiologist orders digoxin for your patient. You understand that, during the initial doses, which of the following may occur?

   a. The patient may experience an increased heart rate initially, then a decreased rate.

   b. The patient may be monitored by ECG.

   c. The patient may experience a hypertensive crisis.

   d. The patient may experience an exacerbation of congestive heart failure.

13. _____ _____ _____ is a digoxin-binding antidote derived from antidigoxin antibodies produced in sheep.

14. Mrs. Farrell presents to the emergency department with nausea, vomiting, and a heart rate of 45 beats per minute. Her husband states that she takes digoxin, Lasix, and nitroglycerin for chest pain. Laboratory results confirm digoxin toxicity. You would expect the physician to order which of the following medications to treat the bradycardia?

   a. Atropine
   c. Nitroglycerin
   b. Nifedipine
   d. Nesiritide

15. Mr. Sweet is diagnosed with heart failure. The physician orders a loading dose of digoxin. Loading doses are necessary for which of the following reasons?

    a. Digoxin's short half-life increases the risk for toxicity.

    b. The client is at risk for dysthymia with titrated doses.

    c. Digoxin's long half-life makes therapeutic serum levels difficult to obtain without loading.

    d. Oral digoxin is ineffective for the treatment of heart failure.

16. Mr. Ames is diagnosed with chronic heart failure. He is hospitalized for the second time this year for symptoms of hypokalemia. The physician changes his diuretic to one that is which of the following types?

    a. Potassium-wasting   c. Sodium-sparing

    b. Potassium-sparing   d. Sodium-wasting

17. For chronic heart failure, an ACE inhibitor or ARB and a _____ are the basic standards of care.

18. For acute HF, the first drugs of choice may include an IV loop diuretic, a cardiotonic–inotropic agent, and _____.

19. Mr. Levinson is diagnosed with heart failure. He is 6 feet tall and weight 275 pounds. By losing weight, he will do which of the following?

    a. Increase his cardiac contractility and myocardial oxygen demand

    b. Decrease his systemic vascular resistance and myocardial oxygen demand

    c. Decrease his cardiac output

    d. Reduce his risk for hypotensive crisis

20. Administering oxygen to a patient in heart failure will do which of the following? (Select all that apply.)

    a. Relieve dyspnea

    b. Decrease pulmonary oxygenation

    c. Reduce the work of breathing

    d. Decrease constriction of pulmonary blood vessels

CHAPTER 49

Antidysrhythmic Drugs

■ Section I: Learning Objectives

1. Provide an overview of the cardiac electrophysiology and specific cardiac dysrhythmias affecting rhythm.
2. Discuss the roles of sodium channel, beta-adrenergic, potassium channel, and calcium channel blockers along with two unclassified drugs in the management of dysrhythmias.
3. Describe the nursing process implications and actions related to caring for patients using selected antidysrhythmic drugs.
4. Describe the principles of therapy, including nonpharmacologic and pharmacologic measures to manage tachydysrhythmias.
5. Differentiate between supraventricular and ventricular dysrhythmias in terms of etiology and hemodynamic effects on the patient.
6. Discuss the effects of dysrhythmias in special populations.

■ Section II: Assessing Your Understanding

ACTIVITY A

Fill in the Blanks

1. _____, sometimes called arrhythmias, are abnormalities in heart rate or rhythm.
2. The mechanical or "pump" activity of the heart resides in _____ tissue.
3. _____ is the heart's ability to generate an electrical impulse.
4. Initiation of an electrical impulse depends predominately on the movement of sodium and _____ ions into a myocardial cell and movement of potassium ions out of the cell.
5. The ability of a cardiac muscle cell to respond to an electrical stimulus is called _____.

ACTIVITY B

Matching

Match the term in Column A with the definition in Column B.

COLUMN A

1. _____ Procainamide
2. _____ Disopyramide
3. _____ Lidocaine
4. _____ Dofetilide
5. _____ Diltiazem and verapamil

COLUMN B

A. Similar to quinidine in pharmacologic actions and may be given orally to adults with ventricular tachydysrhythmias
B. Indicated for the maintenance of NSR in symptomatic patients who are in A-Fib of more than 1 week's duration
C. The only calcium channel blockers approved for management of dysrhythmias
D. Related to the local anesthetic procaine and is similar to quinidine in actions and uses
E. An antidysrhythmic for treating serious ventricular dysrhythmias associated with acute myocardial infarction, cardiac catheterization, cardiac surgery, and digitalis-induced ventricular dysrhythmias

ACTIVITY C

Short Answers

Briefly answer the following questions.

1. Describe how the electrophysiology of the heart causes it to beat.
2. What is automaticity, and how does it affect the heart beat?
3. What is excitability, and how does it affect the heart beat?
4. Define absolute refractory period as it relates to the electrophysiology of the heart.
5. Define conductivity as it relates to the electrophysiology of the heart.

■ Section III: Applying Your Knowledge

ACTIVITY D

Case Study

Consider the scenario and answer the questions.

Mr. Bennet presents to the emergency department with palpitations, dizziness, shortness of breath, and crushing chest pain. The physician diagnoses serious ventricular dysrhythmias related to myocardial infarction and begins treatment. He orders the administration of lidocaine via an intravenous route.

1. What is the mechanism of action of lidocaine? If Mr. Bennet were to develop an atrial dysrhythmia, what would you expect the physician to do with his lidocaine prescription?
2. Initially the physician orders a bolus dose of lidocaine to treat Mr. Bennet. What effect does a bolus dose have?
3. Mr. Bennet's wife arrives and informs you that her husband is an alcoholic and is diagnosed with cirrhosis of the liver. How would treatment of this patient change based on this new information? If the patient's history revealed that he broke out in hives after receiving procaine, how would this information change the treatment approach?
4. The physician orders measurement of Mr. Bennet's lidocaine serum levels, and the laboratory indicates that the level is 0.75 mcg/mL. What does this result tell you?

■ Section IV: Practicing for NCLEX

Answer the following questions.

1. Which of the following is a life-threatening risk associated with the use of amiodarone?
   a. Decreased myocardial contractility
   b. Mitral atresia
   c. Ventricular irritability
   d. Pulmonary toxicity

2. Amiodarone is a potassium channel blocker that prolongs conduction in all cardiac tissues. Which of the following is another effect of amiodarone? (Select all that apply.)
   a. It decreases heart rate.
   b. It diminishes bradydysrhythmias.
   c. It increases contractility of the left ventricle.
   d. It decreases contractility of the left ventricle.

3. The FDA has issued a black box warning for disopyramide because of its known _____ properties.

4. Which two class IV drugs are the only calcium channel blockers approved for the management of dysrhythmias?
   a. Diltiazem   c. Amlodipine
   b. Nifedipine   d. Verapamil

5. Mr. King is released from the hospital after a myocardial infarction. The physician prescribes a class II beta-adrenergic blocker drug. Why does the physician choose this drug?
   a. It is effective in reducing mortality after myocardial infarction.
   b. It is the drug of choice for clients who experience myocardial infarction.
   c. It is the drug of choice for clients with pulmonary edema.
   d. It is the drug of choice for the treatment of pneumonia.

6. Flecainide, propafenone, and moricizine are unique in that they have no effect on the repolarization phase but do have which of the following effects?

   a. They increase conduction in the ventricles.

   b. They decrease conduction in the atria.

   c. They increase conduction in the atria.

   d. They decrease conduction in the ventricles.

7. Lidocaine is the prototype of class IB antidysrhythmics used for treating serious ventricular dysrhythmias associated with which of the following conditions? (Select all that apply.)

   a. Cardiac catheterization

   b. Cardiac surgery

   c. Digitalis-induced ventricular dysrhythmias

   d. Digitalis-induced atrial dysrhythmias

8. Which of the following is an effect of quinidine, the prototype of class IA antidysrhythmics? (Select all that apply.)

   a. It reduces automaticity.

   b. It speeds conduction.

   c. It prolongs the refractory period.

   d. It slows the refractory period.

9. Initiation of an electrical impulse depends predominately on the movement of _____ and _____ ions into a myocardial cell and movement of potassium ions out of the cell.

10. _____ _____ is the most common dysrhythmia.

11. You are visiting the home of a client who is prescribed antidysrhythmic medication. Part of your teaching will include the reporting of which of the following?

   a. Increased energy

   b. Improved functional status

   c. Dizziness

   d. Improved mentation

12. Mr. Garnet is admitted to the critical care unit after experiencing a myocardial infarction and subsequent serious dysrhythmias. He is treated successfully for ventricular dysrhythmia, and the physician orders continuous IV therapy. Which of the following may cause further development of dysrhythmias?

   a. Elevated LFTs   c. Electrolyte imbalances

   b. Hypotension   d. Elevated blood glucose

13. Mrs. Bertram is prescribed digoxin. Six months later, she is diagnosed with impaired liver function. As her long-term care nurse, which of the following would you expect the physician to do?

   a. Increase the dose of digoxin

   b. Continue to monitor the client

   c. Decrease the dosage of the digoxin

   d. Discontinue the digoxin

14. Mrs. Gainer is diagnosed with a ventricular dysrhythmia. The physician orders antidysrhythmic drug therapy. Three months later, she is diagnosed with chronic renal insufficiency. Which of the following would be ordered? (Select all that apply.)

   a. Plasma drug levels

   b. Routine ECG

   c. Monitor for symptoms of drug toxicity

   d. Routine CBC

15. Mr. Carter, age 75, presents to his physician with a cardiac dysrhythmia. The physician chooses to treat the dysrhythmia because of which of the following types of symptoms?

   a. Symptoms related to circulatory impairment

   b. Symptoms related to diabetic neuropathy

   c. Symptoms related to Meniere's disease

   d. Symptoms related to cardiomyopathy

16. _____ is more common in children with structural heart disease or significant dysrhythmias.

17. _____ is the beta-blocker most commonly used in children.

18. Michael S. is treated in the pediatric unit with adenosine. He weighs less than 50 kg. How would you expect the intravenous dose to be administered?
    a. Initially, a 0.2 mg/kg IV push is given, with a maximum dose administration of 6 mg
    b. Initially, a 0.2 mg/kg IV push is given, with a maximum dose administration of 10 mg
    c. Initially, a 0.1 mg/kg IV push is given, with a maximum dose administration of 8 mg
    d. Initially, a 0.1 mg/kg IV push is given, with a maximum dose administration of 6 mg

19. Mrs. Benz presents to the emergency department with dizziness, shortness of breath, and palpitations. This is the third episode of A-Fib for this client in 1 month. A low dose of which of the following drugs is the pharmacologic choice for preventing recurrent A-Fib after electrical or pharmacologic conversion?
    a. Diltiazem   c. Amiodarone
    b. Nifedipine   d. Amlodipine

20. Nonpharmacologic management for PSVT with mild or moderate symptoms includes which of the following techniques? (Select all that apply.)
    a. Valsalva's maneuver   c. Warm baths
    b. Carotid sinus massage   d. Brisk exercise

CHAPTER 50

Antianginal Drugs

■ Section I: Learning Objectives

1. Describe the types, causes, and effects of angina pectoris.
2. Describe general characteristics and types of antianginal drugs.
3. Discuss nitrate antianginals in terms of indications for use, routes of administration, adverse effects, nursing process implications, and drug tolerance.
4. Differentiate between short-acting and long-acting dosage forms of nitrate antianginal drugs.
5. Teach patients ways to prevent, minimize, or manage acute anginal attacks.
6. Use the nursing process in the care of individuals on antianginal and adjunctive therapy for treatment of myocardial ischemia.

■ Section II: Assessing Your Understanding

ACTIVITY A

Fill in the Blanks

1. _____ _____ is a clinical syndrome characterized by episodes of chest pain.
2. Angina pectoris occurs when there is a deficit in _____ oxygen supply in relation to myocardial oxygen demand.
3. Angina is most often caused by atherosclerotic plaque in the coronary arteries but may also be caused by coronary _____.
4. The development and progression of atherosclerotic plaque is called _____ _____ _____.
5. There are three main types of angina: classic angina, _____ angina, and unstable angina.

ACTIVITY B

Matching

Match the term in Column A with the definition in Column B.

COLUMN A

1. _____ Nitroglycerin (e.g., Nitro-Bid)
2. _____ Isosorbide dinitrate (Isordil)
3. _____ Propranolol
4. _____ Ranolazine (Ranexa)
5. _____ Calcium channel blockers

COLUMN B

A. Used to reduce the frequency and severity of acute anginal episodes
B. Represents a new classification of antianginal medication, metabolic modulators, used in individuals with chronic angina
C. Prototype drug, used to relieve acute angina pectoris, prevent exercise-induced angina, and decrease the frequency and severity of acute anginal episodes
D. Act on contractile and conductive tissues of the heart and on vascular smooth muscle
E. Used to reduce the frequency and severity of acute attacks of angina

ACTIVITY C

Short Answers

Briefly answer the following questions.

1. Describe typical anginal symptoms for the male.
2. Describe typical anginal symptoms for the female.
3. Describe how the elderly experience anginal symptoms.
4. Define atherosclerosis.
5. What are the causes myocardial ischemia?

■ Section III: Applying Your Knowledge

ACTIVITY D

Case Studies

Consider the scenarios and answer the questions.

Case Study 1

Mrs. Smith, age 45, is diagnosed with coronary artery disease. She self-administers a calcium channel blocker, an antilipidemic, and an antianginal medication. You are responsible for an education plan using nonpharmacologic methods for management of her disease process.

1. Mrs. Smith has these risk factors: obesity, elevated triglycerides, reduced HDL, hypertension, and elevated fasting glucose. What are these factors indicative of?
2. Mrs. Smith asks you what nonpharmacologic management can do to improve her health and cardiac status. How would you respond?

Case Study 2

Mr. Newsome is diagnosed with coronary artery disease and angina. The physician orders nitrates. You are responsible for the client's education plan.

1. Mr. Newsome is fearful that the nitrates will not control his chest pain. He asks you how they will help him when he is in pain. How would you explain the action of nitrates?
2. The physician orders sublingual nitroglycerin. What can you tell Mr. Newsome about this drug? What are some contraindications to the use of sublingual nitroglycerin?

3. During an education session, Mr. Newsome confides that he self-administers sildenafil (Viagra) periodically. What further teaching regarding nitrates is required for this patient?

■ Section IV: Practicing for NCLEX

Answer the following questions.

1. The physician prescribes a small dose of antianginal medication to a client newly diagnosed with coronary artery disease. Which of the following is the reason for starting with a small dose?
   a. Small doses minimize angina.
   b. Small doses minimize adverse effects.
   c. Small doses minimize myocardial enervation.
   d. Small doses minimize oxygenation to the myocardium.

2. Mr. Anspar asks you why the doctor has added combined aspirin, antilipemics, and antihypertensives to his medication regimen when he feels fine and hasn't experienced an anginal episode in a year. Which of the following does this combination of drugs do?
   a. Prevents episodic hypertensive crisis and subsequent CVA
   b. Prevents cerebral edema and subsequent CVA
   c. Prevents progression of myocardial ischemia to MI
   d. Reduces afterload that fosters an MI

3. The physician prescribes calcium channel blockers for Mr. Smith, who is diagnosed with angina pectoris. Which of the following do calcium channel blockers do?
   a. Induce coronary artery vasospasm
   b. Increase blood pressure to increase oxygenation to the myocardium
   c. Improve blood supply to the myocardium
   d. Prevent anginal episodes

4. Mr. Moore presents to the physician's office for a regular visit. He takes nitrates on a regular schedule for his anginal episodes and has done so for 3 years. Which of the following statements would you expect from the patient about the action of the nitrates?

    a. "They eliminate my chest pain as they always have."

    b. "They do not work as well to manage my chest pain as they used to."

    c. "They're causing dizziness, which I haven't experienced in the past."

    d. "They're causing increased chest pain and discomfort."

5. Mr. Aaron, age 75, is being treated for diabetes type 2, hypertension, gout, angina, coronary artery disease, and peptic ulcer disease. You are concerned because he is taking a traditional antianginal drug in combination with seven other medications. Which of the following could be the consequence?

    a. A greater incidence of adverse drug effects

    b. Decreased effectiveness of the antianginal drug

    c. Decreased effectiveness of the antihypertensive

    d. A greater incidence of hyperglycemic episodes

6. Mr. Kovak is at risk for silent ischemia after experiencing a transmural MI. Which of the following would you expect the physician to order?

    a. Nitrates

    b. Calcium channel blockers

    c. Antilipidemics

    d. Beta-blockers

7. Common drugs used for myocardial ischemia are the organic _____, the beta-adrenergic blocking agents, and the calcium channel blocking agents.

8. Which of the following are routes of choice for nitroglycerin? (Select all that apply.)

    a. Oral   c. Transmucosal

    b. IV   d. Transdermal

9. Which of the following are the goals of antianginal drug therapy? (Select all that apply.)

    a. To relieve acute anginal pain

    b. To prevent anginal episodes

    c. To improve exercise tolerance and quality of life

    d. To prevent MI and sudden cardiac death.

10. Mr. Conner is diagnosed with atherosclerosis. In your explanation to the patient, what would you say is the most likely cause of his angina?

    a. Decreased oxygenation to the myocardium

    b. A reduction in plaque secondary to arthrosclerosis

    c. Hypertension of the myocardium

    d. Decreased musculature of the myocardium related to plaque

11. Which of the following do the home care nurse's responsibilities include? (Select all that apply.)

    a. Monitoring the patient's response to antianginal medications

    b. Teaching patients and caregivers how to use, store, and replace medications to ensure a constant supply

    c. Discussing the benefits of exercise to decrease the oxygen demands of the heart

    d. Discussing circumstances for which the patient should seek emergency care

12. You visit your client in the home care setting. On assessment, you find that he has gained 6 pounds in 2 days, has 4+ pitting edema from his ankles to his patella bilaterally, and has course crackles throughout his lung fields. In the middle of the examination, he states that he is experiencing an anginal episode. In this case, you expect which of the following when the patient uses his nitroglycerin?

    a. Its effect will be impaired.

    b. It will be effective.

    c. It will cause hypertensive crisis.

    d. It will exacerbate his congestive heart failure.

13. Antianginal drugs are most often used to manage which of the following? (Select all that apply.)
    a. Severe angina
    b. Severe postural hypotension
    c. Severe hypertension
    d. Serious cardiac dysrhythmias

14. A metabolic modulator is _____ in patients with hepatic impairment.

15. During surgery, a child develops hypertension. The physician orders nitroglycerin IV. The initial dose will be adjusted for weight, and later doses will be adjusted to which factor?
    a. Response   c. Age
    b. Weight   d. Relief of chest pain

16. For relief of acute angina and for prophylaxis before events that cause acute angina, which of the following is the primary drug of choice?
    a. Nitroglycerin   c. Nifedipine
    b. Diltiazem   d. Furosemide

17. Mr. Quint does not respond to traditional treatment for his chronic angina. The physician orders ranolazine (Ranexa) and orders a baseline ECG prior to medication administration. Three months later, the physician orders a repeat ECG. For which of the following is the physician monitoring the client?
    a. Dose-dependent QT prolongation
    b. Dose-dependent ST elevation
    c. Dose-dependent ectopic beats
    d. Dose-dependent premature ventricular beats

18. Mr. Randolph presents to the physician's office for the results of his exercise-tolerance test and for modification of his medication regimen. The physician informs Mr. Randolph that he experiences tachycardia which, based on his history, may precipitate anginal episodes. Based on this information, which of the following would you expect the physician to order?
    a. Nifedipine   c. Propranolol
    b. Isosorbide   d. Nitroglycerin

19. Isosorbide mononitrate (Ismo, Imdur) is the metabolite and active component of
    _____ _____.

20. The physician determines the maximum tolerable of isosorbide dinitrate (Isordil) by increasing the dose until which of the following happens?
    a. A headache occurs.
    b. Hypertension is managed.
    c. Postural hypotension occurs.
    d. Anginal symptoms dissipate.

CHAPTER 51

Drugs Used in Hypotension and Shock

■ Section I: Learning Objectives

1. Identify patients at risk for development of hypovolemia and shock.
2. Identify common causes of hypotension and shock.
3. Discuss the assessment of a patient in shock.
4. Describe therapeutic and adverse effects of vasopressor drugs used in the management of hypotension and shock.

■ Section II: Assessing Your Understanding

ACTIVITY A

Fill in the Blanks

1. _____ is a clinical condition of insufficient perfusion of cells and vital organs causing tissue hypoxia.
2. _____ shock involves a loss of intravascular fluid volume that may be due to actual blood loss or relative loss from fluid shifts within the body.
3. _____ shock occurs when the myocardium has lost its ability to contract efficiently and maintain an adequate cardiac output.
4. _____ or vasogenic shock is characterized by massive vasodilation, which results in a relative hypovolemia.
5. Distributive shock is further divided into anaphylactic, _____, and septic shock.

ACTIVITY B

Matching

Match the term in Column A with the definition in Column B.

COLUMN A

1. _____ Dobutamine
2. _____ Dopamine
3. _____ Epinephrine
4. _____ Metaraminol
5. _____ Phenylephrine (Neo-Synephrine)

COLUMN B

A. A naturally occurring catecholamine produced by the adrenal glands
B. Used mainly for hypotension associated with spinal anesthesia; acts indirectly by releasing norepinephrine from sympathetic nerve endings
C. Useful in hypovolemic and cardiogenic shock
D. An adrenergic drug that stimulates alpha-adrenergic receptors
E. A synthetic catecholamine developed to provide less vascular activity than dopamine

ACTIVITY C

Short Answers

Briefly answer the following questions.

1. Discuss the signs and symptoms related to the clinical condition of shock.
2. What is the impact of anaerobic metabolism on the human body?
3. What causes anaphylactic shock?
4. What causes septic shock to occur in the body?
5. What causes neurogenic shock in the human body?

■ Section III: Applying Your Knowledge

ACTIVITY D

Case Study

Consider the scenario and answer the questions.

Mrs. Jenks, age 45, presents to the emergency department with symptoms of anaphylactic shock. The patient presents with minor respiratory distress and swelling of her face and tongue. Mrs. Jenks' husband states that she is allergic to bees and that approximately 15 minutes ago she was stung by several bees while gardening.

1. The physician orders epinephrine. Explain what you know about low doses of epinephrine. What would you expect the epinephrine to do in Mrs. Jenks' case?
2. Why is epinephrine the drug of choice for management of anaphylactic shock? Why is it administered by subcutaneous injection to treat anaphylactic shock?
3. If Mrs. Jenks experienced cardiac arrest secondary to anaphylactic shock, how would the epinephrine be administered?
4. What adverse effects of epinephrine should you be monitoring Mrs. Jenks for?

■ Section IV: Practicing for NCLEX

Answer the following questions.

1. Mr. Smith is admitted to the critical care unit in your facility after a motor vehicle accident and subsequent hypovolemic shock. Despite fluid replacement therapy and stabilization of the patient's electrolyte imbalance, his cardiac output remains low. Which of the following are the treatments of choice? (Select all that apply.)
   a. Dobutamine   c. Epinephrine
   b. Dopamine   d. Phenylephrine

2. In hypotension and shock, drugs with alpha-adrenergic activity (e.g., norepinephrine, phenylephrine) are used for which of the following purposes?
   a. To increase peripheral vascular resistance
   b. To decrease peripheral vascular resistance
   c. To resolve hypertensive crisis
   d. To correct fluid volume deficit

3. Mr. Vento presents to the emergency department in hypovolemic shock secondary to a traumatic amputation of his left hand. The physician orders alpha-adrenergic medication to be administered. During the infusion of the medication, it is important to monitor which of the following values?
   a. Electrolytes   c. Albumin level
   b. Blood pressure   d. Temperature

4. Mr. Goldman is treated for hypotension and shock in your emergency department. Which of the following is an overall goal in the treatment of hypotension and shock? (Select all that apply.)
   a. To decrease vascular volume
   b. To maintain vascular volume
   c. To maximize oxygen delivery to the tissues
   d. To maintain serum albumin levels

5. Mrs. Peters is diagnosed with hypovolemic shock secondary to injuries incurred in a motor vehicle accident. You understand that Mrs. Peters is at risk for which of the following conditions?

   a. Hypertensive crisis
   b. Tissue hypoxia
   c. Hyperkalemia
   d. Pleural effusion

6. Mr. Smith, who was brought in after a construction accident, is experiencing multiple organ hypoxia precipitated by hypovolemic shock. To adequately monitor his condition, which of the following assessment methods should you be using?

   a. Intermittent noninvasive hemodynamic monitoring
   b. Vital signs every 10 minutes
   c. Hemoglobin and hematocrit every 30 minutes
   d. Continuous invasive hemodynamic monitoring

7. Ms. Dolinger's diagnoses include diabetes mellitus type 2, hypertension, and mild cirrhosis of the liver. She is prescribed adrenergic medication. Based on her impaired liver function, which of the following would you expect the physician to do?

   a. Increase the dose of the adrenergic medication gradually over 2 weeks
   b. Maintain the dose of the adrenergic medication
   c. Monitor liver function and adjust the medication as needed
   d. Reduce the dose of the adrenergic medication

8. Which of the following is a risk in older patients with diagnoses such as atherosclerosis, peripheral vascular disease, and diabetes mellitus who are prescribed anticholinergics?

   a. Fluid volume depletion
   b. Fluid volume excess
   c. Alteration in blood volume
   d. Hypoglycemia

9. You are caring for Lily, age 4. Treatment for hypovolemic shock in a child of Lily's age may include anticholinergic medications. The physician will base the dosage of the medication on which of the following factors?

   a. Height
   b. Hemoglobin and hematocrit
   c. Blood pressure
   d. Weight

10. Anaphylactic shock is often managed by _____ drugs as well as epinephrine.

11. Cardiogenic shock may be complicated by pulmonary congestion. For pulmonary congestion, which of the following is true? (Select all that apply.)

    a. Antiarrhythmic drugs are indicated.
    b. Diuretic drugs are indicated.
    c. 0.9 normal saline, 40 to 60 mL/hour, is indicated.
    d. IV fluids are contraindicated (except to maintain a patent IV line).

12. Clients diagnosed with hypovolemic shock may require volume replacement to optimize the SVO_2 (saturation of venous oxygen) and, thus, mixed venous oxygen consumption. As the nurse caring for this client, you are careful to avoid which of the following conditions?

    a. Hyperthermia
    b. Hypothermia
    c. Diathermia
    d. Bacteremia

13. For distributive shock characterized by severe vasodilation and decreased peripheral vascular resistance, a _____ drug, such as norepinephrine, is the first drug of choice.

14. The choice of drug depends primarily on the pathophysiology involved. For cardiogenic shock and decreased cardiac output, which of the following is the drug of choice?

    a. Dobutamine   c. Epinephrine

    b. Dopamine   d. Norepinephrine

15. With severe heart failure characterized by decreased cardiac output and high peripheral vascular resistance, which of the following drugs may be given in addition to the cardiotonic drugs?

    a. Nitroprusside   c. Lisinopril

    b. Digoxin   d. Lopressor

16. Norepinephrine (Levophed) stimulates alpha-adrenergic receptors and increases blood pressure primarily by which of the following mechanisms?

    a. Vasodilation

    b. Increasing cardiac contractility

    c. Vasoconstriction

    d. Reducing edema related to congestive heart failure

17. Milrinone, a treatment for heart failure, is also used to manage _____ shock in combination with other inotropic agents or vasopressors.

18. Dobutamine is a synthetic catecholamine developed to provide less vascular activity than dopamine. It acts mainly on beta$_1$ receptors in the heart to do which of the following?

    a. Decrease the force of myocardial contraction

    b. Increase heart rate

    c. Decrease blood pressure

    d. Increase the force of myocardial contraction

19. Dobutamine may _____ blood pressure with large doses.

20. Dobutamine must be administered by which of the following routes?

    a. Subcutaneous   c. Intravenous

    b. Intramuscular   d. Via a central line

CHAPTER 52

Antihypertensive Drugs

■ Section I: Learning Objectives

1. Describe factors that control blood pressure.
2. Define and describe hypertension.
3. Identify patients at risk for development of hypertension and its sequelae.
4. Discuss nonpharmacologic measures to control hypertension.
5. Review the effects of alpha-adrenergic blockers, beta-adrenergic blockers, calcium channel blockers, and diuretics in hypertension.
6. Discuss angiotensin-converting enzyme inhibitors and angiotensin II receptor blockers in terms of mechanisms of action, indications for use, adverse effects, and nursing process implications.
7. Describe the rationale for using combination drugs in the management of hypertension.
8. Discuss interventions to increase therapeutic effects and minimize adverse effects of antihypertensive drugs.
9. Discuss the use of antihypertensive drugs in special populations.

■ Section II: Assessing Your Understanding

ACTIVITY A

Fill in the Blanks

1. _____ blood pressure reflects the force exerted on arterial walls by blood flow.
2. Blood pressure normally remains constant because of _____ mechanisms that adjust blood flow to meet tissue needs.
3. The two major determinants of arterial blood pressure are _____ _____ (systolic pressure) and peripheral vascular resistance (diastolic pressure).

4. _____ _____ equals the product of the heart rate and stroke volume.
5. _____ _____ is the amount of blood ejected with each heartbeat (approximately 60 to 90 mL).

ACTIVITY B

Matching

Match the term in Column A with the definition in Column B.

COLUMN A

1. _____ ARBs
2. _____ Antiadrenergic (sympatholytic) drugs
3. _____ Beta-adrenergic blocking agents
4. _____ Calcium channel blockers
5. _____ Diuretics

COLUMN B

A. Inhibit activity of the SNS

B. Dilate peripheral arteries and decrease peripheral vascular resistance by relaxing vascular smooth muscle

C. Cause antihypertensive effects usually attributed to sodium and water depletion

D. Developed to block the strong blood pressure–raising effects of angiotensin II

E. Decrease heart rate, force of myocardial contraction, cardiac output, and renin release from the kidneys

ACTIVITY C

Short Answers

Briefly answer the following questions.

1. Define and discuss autoregulation.
2. Define and discuss the action of histamines.
3. What is the role of kinins as they relate to the vascular system?
4. What is the role of serotonin as it relates to the vascular system?
5. What is the role of prostaglandins as they relate to the vascular system?

■ Section III: Applying Your Knowledge

ACTIVITY D

Case Studies

Consider the scenarios and answer the questions.

Case Study 1

Mrs. Bartley has her blood pressure taken at the local elder health clinic. Her blood pressure at that time is 145/90. She is concerned because she never had an elevated blood pressure before. She calls her physician's office and asks for medication to treat her hypertension.

1. What is the definition of hypertension?
2. Mrs. Bartley is diagnosed with secondary hypertension. What are some causes of secondary hypertension?

Case Study 2

Mrs. Goodman, age 70, is diagnosed with isolated systolic hypertension.

1. What would you expect her blood pressure to be?
2. You understand that hypertension alters cardiovascular function by increasing the workload of the heart. What does this cause?

■ Section IV: Practicing for NCLEX

Answer the following questions.

1. Mr. Magahi is diagnosed with severe hypertension. The physician prescribes minoxidil. Three months later, Mr. Magahi presents to the emergency department with angina. You are concerned because minoxidil can have which of the following effects?

   a. Exacerbate angina and precipitate effusion

   b. Cause rebound hypertension when a dose is missed

   c. Precipitate cardiovascular accidents

   d. Exacerbate pancreatitis

2. Mrs. Grogan, age 35, controls the symptoms of her cardiovascular disease with ACE inhibitors. She discovers that she is pregnant and contacts her primary physician regarding her medication regimen. Which of the following would you expect the physician to do?

   a. Discontinue the drug

   b. Increase the dosage of the drug

   c. Decrease the dosage of the drug

   d. Maintain the current dosage of the drug

3. Mr. Frank's friend tells him to stop taking his metoprolol because he read that it causes cancer. You encourage the client to consult his physician, because abrupt withdrawal from the drug may cause which of the following effects?

   a. Postural hypotension and falls

   b. Bradycardia

   c. Exacerbation of his angina

   d. Atrial dysrhythmias

4. African Americans are more likely to have severe hypertension and to require multiple drugs, for which of the following reasons? (Select all that apply.)

   a. Low circulating renin

   b. Increased salt sensitivity

   c. A higher incidence of obesity

   d. Increased potassium sensitivity

204 CHAPTER 52 ■ Antihypertensive Drugs

5. Mr. Yu, an Asian executive visiting the United States, presents to the emergency department with a severe headache and an elevated blood pressure. He is admitted to the hospital for treatment and regulation of his medication regimen. The client is concerned because the dosage prescribed for his antihypertensive medication is lower than what he researched on the Internet. Which of the following is an accurate response for you to make?

a. "There is an error on the prescription."

b. "I will contact the physician immediately."

c. "People of Asian descent excrete the drugs more rapidly, so the doses prescribed are smaller."

d. "People of Asian descent excrete the drugs more slowly, so the doses prescribed are smaller."

6. Mr. Jones, age 45, is diagnosed with high-renin hypertension. Which of the following types of drugs would you expect the physician to order?

a. Ace inhibitors

b. Beta blockers

c. Diuretics

d. Calcium channel blockers

7. ACE inhibitors and _____ are equally effective at controlling blood pressure.

8. You instruct Mr. Montgomery to administer his alpha$_1$-adrenergic receptor blocking agent at night. Which of the following does this practice help to minimize?

a. Postural hypertension

b. First-dose phenomenon

c. Hypoglycemic reaction

d. Hyperglycemic reaction

9. Key behavioral determinants of blood pressure are related to which of the following factors?

a. Minimal body mass

b. Dietary consumption of calories and salt

c. Dietary consumption of sugars and fat

d. Comorbidities

10. Mr. Solomon, age 57, presents to the physician's office for the second consecutive month with an elevated blood pressure. His hypertension has been successfully managed with his current drug regimen for 2 years. When asked about his drug history, he states that the only new drug is the herb, yohimbe. What is yohimbe?

a. An over-the-counter antihyperglycemic

b. A central nervous system stimulant

c. An autonomic nervous system stimulant

d. A diuretic

11. Whether the patient or another member of the household is taking antihypertensive medications, the home care nurse may be helpful in which of the following tasks? (Select all that apply.)

a. Modification of drug dosage

b. Monitoring for drug effects

c. Promoting compliance with the prescribed pharmacologic modifications

d. Promoting compliance with the prescribed lifestyle modifications

12. A client presents to the emergency department in hypertensive crisis. You anticipate that the physician will order medication that will lower the blood pressure yet prevent stroke, MI, and acute renal failure, within what period of time?

a. Immediately

b. Within 5 minutes

c. Within 7 minutes

d. Over several minutes to several hours

13. Mr. Grant is admitted to your critical care unit with severe hypertension and myocardial ischemia. The physician orders nitroglycerin titrated according to which of the following factors?

a. Amount of chest pain or pressure

b. Weight

c. Blood pressure response

d. Renal function

Copyright © 2009. Wolters Kluwer Health I Lippincott Williams & Wilkins. *Study Guide for Abrams'*
Clinical Drug Therapy: Rationales for Nursing Practice, 9th ed.

14. Mr. Brands presents to the emergency room with a significantly elevated blood pressure. The physician chooses oral captopril for treatment and prescribes which of the following dosages every 1 to 2 hours?
    a. 25 to 50 mg
    b. 10 to 20 mg
    c. 5 to 10 mg
    d. 50 to 75 mg

15. Mr. Bacon presents to the physician's office for his annual visit. His prescription regimen includes ACE inhibitors. You find that his liver enzymes are elevated. Which of the following would you expect the physician to do?
    a. Increase the dosage of the drug
    b. Decrease the dosage of the drug
    c. Discontinue the drug
    d. Identify a source for the elevation other than the ACE inhibitors

16. Mrs. Stanley successfully treats her heart failure with an ACE inhibitor. She does not have evidence of severe or preexisting renal impairment. Her most recent laboratory results indicate increased BUN and serum creatinine levels. Which of the following would you expect the physician to do?
    a. Increase the dosage of the drug
    b. Decrease the dosage of the drug
    c. Discontinue the drug
    d. Maintain the dosage of the drug

17. In systolic hypertension, the systolic blood pressure is greater than _____ mm Hg, but diastolic pressure is lower than 90 mm Hg.

18. Nonpharmacologic management should be tried alone or with drug therapy. Which of the following are methods of nonpharmacologic management of hypertension? (Select all that apply.)
    a. Weight reduction
    b. Limited alcohol intake
    c. Moderate sodium restriction
    d. Diet including no concentrated sweets

19. The National High Blood Pressure Education Program Working Group on High Blood Pressure in Children and Adolescents states that prehypertension in children is defined as an average of systolic or diastolic pressures within which of the following ranges?
    a. 85th to 90th percentiles
    b. 90th to 95th percentiles
    c. 80th to 90th percentiles
    d. 80th to 85th percentiles

20. Beta blockers are used in children of all ages and are the preferential drug for children with hypertension and migraine headache; they should probably be avoided in children with resting pulse rates lower than _____ beats per minute.

CHAPTER 53

Diuretics

■ Section I: Learning Objectives

1. List characteristics of diuretics in terms of mechanism of action, indications for use, principles of therapy, and nursing process implications.
2. Discuss major adverse effects of thiazide, loop, and potassium-sparing diuretics.
3. Identify patients at risk for developing adverse reactions to diuretic administration.
4. Recognize commonly used potassium-losing and potassium-sparing diuretics.
5. Discuss the rationale for using combination products containing a potassium-losing and a potassium-sparing diuretic.
6. Discuss the rationale for concomitant use of a loop diuretic and a thiazide or related diuretic.
7. Teach patients to manage diuretic therapy effectively.
8. Discuss important elements of diuretic therapy in special populations.

■ Section II: Assessing Your Understanding

ACTIVITY A

Fill in the Blanks

1. Diuretics are drugs that increase renal excretion of water, sodium, and other electrolytes, thereby increasing urine formation and _____.
2. The primary function of the kidneys is to regulate the volume, _____, and pH of body fluids.
3. Each nephron is composed of a _____ and a tubule.
4. The glomerulus is a network of _____ that receives blood from the renal artery.
5. _____ _____ is a thin-walled structure that surrounds the glomerulus, then narrows and continues as the tubule.

ACTIVITY B

Matching

Match the term in Column A with the definition in Column B.

COLUMN A

1. _____ Thiazide diuretics
2. _____ Loop diuretics
3. _____ Potassium-sparing diuretics
4. _____ Osmotic agents
5. _____ Diuretic combinations

COLUMN B

A. Act at the distal tubule to decrease sodium reabsorption and potassium excretion
B. Produce rapid diuresis by increasing the solute load (osmotic pressure) of the glomerular filtrate
C. Synthetic drugs that are chemically related to the sulfonamides
D. Used to prevent potassium imbalances
E. Diuretics that inhibit sodium and chloride reabsorption in the ascending limb of the loop of Henle

ACTIVITY C

Short Answers

Briefly answer the following questions.

1. Explain how convoluted tubules enhance renal function.
2. Describe the three processes by which the nephron functions.
3. Describe the process of glomerular filtration.
4. What happens to the fluid processed during glomerular filtration?
5. What happens to blood that does not become part of the glomerular filtrate?

■ Section III: Applying Your Knowledge

ACTIVITY D
Case Study
Consider the scenario and answer the questions.

You are part of a group of nursing students studying the structure and function of the renal system. Your section is the renal tubules.

1. Define *reabsorption* as it relates to renal function. Where does reabsorption occur, and what substances are primarily reabsorbed?
2. Discuss what happens in the loop of Henle.
3. Explain the hormonal contribution to reabsorption.
4. Define *secretion* as it relates to renal function. Where does it occur, and what substances are secreted?

■ Section IV: Practicing for NCLEX

Answer the following questions.

1. Mrs. Watson, age 75, is diagnosed with atrial fibrillation and chronic congestive heart failure. The physician orders a combination of digoxin and diuretics to treat her diseases. Recent laboratory results indicate that the client's potassium level is 2 mEq/L. This patient is at risk for which of the following?
   a. Exacerbation of the atrial fibrillation
   b. Subtherapeutic levels of serum digoxin
   c. Digoxin toxicity
   d. Congestive heart failure

2. Mr. Bingham presents to the emergency room with shortness of breath, dizziness, and confusion. He is diagnosed with severe congestive heart failure. The physician orders high-dose furosemide continuous IV infusions. You would expect that the rate of dosage would be which of the following to decrease adverse effect?
   a. 4 mg/minute or less   c. 6 mg/minute or less
   b. 5 mg/minute or less   d. 8 mg/minute or less

3. Mrs. Carter is diagnosed with chronic congestive heart failure and hypertension. You would expect the physician to order which of the following types of diuretics?
   a. Loop   c. Thiazide
   b. Osmotic   d. Potassium-wasting

4. There is a known cross-sensitivity of some sulfonamide-allergic patients to which of the following sulfonamide nonantibiotics?
   a. Hydrochlorothiazide   c. Bumetanide
   b. Furosemide   d. Torsemide

5. Mr. Hackmore is prescribed potassium-sparing diuretics to treat his disease process. During his annual visit to the physician, he complains that he is experiencing muscle weakness and tingling in his fingers. Which of the following conditions do you suspect?
   a. Hypokalemia   c. Hypocalcemia
   b. Hyperkalemia   d. Hypercalcemia

6. Mrs. Kingman is diagnosed with hyponatremia. Which of the following diuretics would most likely promote this symptom?
   a. Osmotic   c. Potassium-sparing
   b. Thiazide   d. Loop

7. Mr. Tabor is excited because it is football season. He has season tickets and attends most games with his friends. At his latest appointment, Mr. Tabor's blood pressure is elevated. Which of the following do you suspect is the cause?
   a. He is anxious about his team.
   b. He is consuming excessive salty foods at the games.
   c. He is developing comorbidities.
   d. He has become a vegetarian until his team wins the championship.

8. A body weight change of _____ lb may indicate a gain or loss of 1000 mL of fluid.

9. Diuretic drugs act on the kidneys to decrease _____ of sodium, chloride, water, and other substances.

10. Diuretics are often taken in the home setting. The home care nurse may need to assist patients and caregivers by doing which of the following tasks? (Select all that apply.)

    a. Monitoring patient responses

    b. Assessing use of over-the-counter medications that may aggravate the patient's condition

    c. Weighing the patient daily

    d. Appropriating all sodium-rich foods in the home

11. Mr. Gardner is critically ill with a diagnosis of congestive heart failure exacerbated by a myocardial infarction. Which of the following fast-acting diuretics would be appropriate for the physician to order? (Select all that apply.)

    a. Furosemide   c. Hydrochlorothiazide

    b. Diazide   d. Bumetanide

12. Which of the following methods of administration of fast-acting diuretics would be most effective and least likely to produce adverse effects in a critically ill client with pulmonary edema?

    a. Intravenous bolus doses

    b. Continuous intravenous infusion

    c. Subcutaneous doses

    d. Intramuscular doses

13. Although they are needed to reduce ascites in clients with hepatic impairment, diuretics may precipitate which of the following conditions?

    a. Ammonia absorption

    b. Subtherapeutic drug levels

    c. Hepatic encephalopathy

    d. Hepatomegaly

14. To prevent metabolic alkalosis or hypokalemia, which of the following drugs may be administered to patients with cirrhosis in addition to diuretic therapy?

    a. Spironolactone   c. Hydrochlorothiazide

    b. Diazide   d. Bumetanide

15. Potassium-sparing diuretics are contraindicated in patients with renal impairment because of the high risk of hyperkalemia. If they are used at all, which of the following would be a priority?

    a. Administration of concurrent potassium

    b. Monitoring of serum electrolytes, creatinine, and BUN

    c. Administration of a thiazide diuretic

    d. Monitoring of CBC and serum albumin

16. To prevent accelerated degradation of furosemide, which of the following IV solutions should be used to mix the drug?

    a. D5W

    b. D51/2 NS

    c. Lactated Ringer's solution

    d. D51/4 NS

17. Mr. Andrews, age 71, is hospitalized with pulmonary edema; he is discharged with a prescription for a loop diuretic. He presents to the physician's office 1 week later with symptoms indicating excessive diuresis. This patient is also at risk for which of the following?

    a. Rebound hypertension

    b. Hypervolemia

    c. Embolism

    d. Gastric ulcer disease

18. The physician orders hydrochlorothiazide for Mr. Bunting. He has multiple comorbidities, and the physician chooses the smallest effective dose of the drug. You expect the physician to order a daily dose in which of the following ranges?

    a. 0.25 to 0.50 milligrams

    b. 0.50 to 0.75 milligrams

    c. 8 to 12 milligrams

    d. 12.5 to 25 milligrams

19. Thiazide drugs become ineffective when the GFR is less than which of the following levels?

    a. 30 mL/minute c. 50 mL/minute

    b. 40 mL/minute d. 60 mL/minute

20. The physician orders furosemide for your pediatric client. The established dose of the drug should not exceed how many milligrams per kilogram of body weight per day?

    a. 4 c. 8

    b. 6 d. 10

CHAPTER 54

Drugs That Affect Blood Coagulation

■ Section I: Learning Objectives

1. Describe important elements in the physiology of hemostasis and thrombosis.
2. Discuss potential consequences of blood clotting disorders.
3. Compare and contrast heparin and warfarin in terms of indications for use, onset and duration of action, routes of administration, blood tests used to monitor effects, and nursing process implications.
4. Discuss antiplatelet agents in terms of indications for use and effects on blood coagulation.
5. Describe thrombolytic agents in terms of indications and contraindications for use, routes of administration, and major adverse effects.
6. Describe systemic hemostatic agents for treating overdoses of anticoagulant and thrombolytic drugs.
7. Use the nursing process in the care of patients taking anticoagulant, antiplatelet, and thrombolytic agents.

■ Section II: Assessing Your Understanding

ACTIVITY A

Fill in the Blanks

1. Thrombosis involves the formation (*thrombogenesis*) or presence of a _____ in the vascular system.
2. _____ _____ is a normal body defense mechanism to prevent blood loss.
3. When part of a thrombus breaks off and travels to another part of the body, it is called a/an _____.
4. Atherosclerosis begins with accumulation of lipid-filled _____ on the inner lining of arteries.

5. In atherosclerosis, _____ _____ develop in response to elevated blood lipid levels and eventually become fibrous plaques (i.e., foam cells covered by smooth muscle cells and connective tissue).

ACTIVITY B

Matching

Match the term in Column A with the definition in Column B.

COLUMN A

1. _____ Heparin
2. _____ Low-molecular-weight heparins (LMWHs)
3. _____ Warfarin
4. _____ Aspirin
5. _____ Fondaparinux

COLUMN B

A. The most commonly used oral anticoagulant; acts in the liver to prevent synthesis of vitamin K–dependent clotting factors
B. Analgesic–antipyretic–anti-inflammatory drug with potent antiplatelet effects
C. The first of a new class of pentasaccharide antithrombotic agents that produces anticoagulant effects by directly binding to circulating and clot-bound factor Xa, accelerating the activity of antithrombin and inhibiting thrombin production
D. A pharmaceutical preparation of the natural anticoagulant produced primarily by mast cells in pericapillary connective tissue.
E. Contain the low-molecular-weight fraction and are as effective as IV heparin in treating thrombotic disorders

ACTIVITY C

Short Answers

Briefly answer the following questions.

1. Define hemostasis.
2. Explain the process of clot lysis.
3. Discuss the predisposing factors for arterial thrombosis.
4. Discuss the predisposing factors for venous thrombosis.
5. Discuss the two mechanisms by which venous thrombi cause disease.

■ Section III: Applying Your Knowledge

ACTIVITY D

Case Study

Consider the scenario and answer the questions.

Mrs. Adams is hospitalized in her fourth month of pregnancy with a pulmonary embolism. The physician prescribes heparin to be administered in the home daily until she returns to his office in 2 weeks. He also asks the nurse to schedule blood to be drawn for laboratory analysis by the home care nurse on a daily basis, with reports to him each day by 2 PM. You are the home care nurse in charge of Mrs. Adams' education and care.

1. Mrs. Adams asks you how the heparin will help to prevent a recurrence of the pulmonary embolism. What is your understanding of how heparin works?
2. The client is concerned because she received intravenous heparin during most of her stay in the hospital. She asks if the subcutaneous drug will be just as effective. What is the difference between the intravenous and the subcutaneous administration?
3. Mrs. Adams is concerned that the drug will cause her fetus to bleed internally. What do you know about the effect of injected heparin on a fetus?
4. Mrs. Adams' condition resolves. However, she is placed on bedrest for the duration of her pregnancy. Based on Mrs. Adams' history, what would you expect the physician to order while Mrs. Adams is on bedrest?

5. After delivery of a healthy baby girl, Mrs. Adams develops DIC. What is DIC? What is the goal of treatment? What would you expect the physician to prescribe as part of the treatment?

■ Section IV: Practicing for NCLEX

Answer the following questions.

1. The physician orders thrombolytic agents when treating a client diagnosed with acute myocardial infarction. Which of the following drugs should you keep readily available when blood flow is re-established?
   a. Anticoagulants
   b. Antidysrhythmics
   c. Antihypertensives
   d. Antianginals

2. The FDA has issued a black box warning for the use of protamine sulfate due to the risk of which of the following conditions? (Select all that apply.)
   a. Severe hypotension
   b. Cardiovascular collapse
   c. Cardiogenic pulmonary edema
   d. Pulmonary hypertension

3. _____ _____ is the antidote for standard heparin and LMWHs.

4. You are concerned that the physician does not order routine aPTTs when your client is receiving LMWH for thromboembolism prophylaxis. When you call the physician with your concern, which of the following will be his response?
   a. aPTTs should be drawn daily.
   b. aPTTs should be drawn weekly.
   c. aPTTs are not needed.
   d. INRs should be drawn weekly.

5. The physician reorders dalteparin for your client. The pharmacy informs you that the drug is not available. You call the physician and ask if you can replace the dalteparin with another LMWH. You expect that the physician's response will be which of the following?

   a. "I'll change the order to enoxaparin."

   b. "I'll change the drug to Lovenox."

   c. "The drugs are not interchangeable; have the pharmacy obtain the drug ordered."

   d. "The drugs are interchangeable; the pharmacy can substitute another LMWH."

6. The black box warning associated with warfarin concerns its risk of causing which of the following conditions?

   a. DIC

   b. Severe coagulopathy

   c. Hypotension

   d. Major or fatal bleeding

7. _____ _____ (Mephyton) is the antidote for warfarin.

8. Mr. Bannister presents to the physician's office because the physician is unable to regulate his Coumadin dosage. During the interview, you find that the client began taking which of the following substances, which might increase the effects of the warfarin?

   a. Ginseng to improve his energy

   b. Red meat to increase his protein intake

   c. Milk to increase his calcium level and prevent cramps

   d. Chamomile tea to help him sleep

9. Mr. Benewah is prescribed warfarin. His INR is 5.2. At what level is this dose?

   a. Subtherapeutic

   b. Therapeutic

   c. Elevated

   d. Within prescribed limits

10. Ms. Baxter is admitted to the hospital after a suicide attempt. You discover that she overdosed on aspirin. Which of the following do you expect the physician to do?

    a. Prescribe the antidote

    b. Prescribe a transfusion of platelets

    c. Prescribe a transfusion of whole blood

    d. Order an IV infusion of Ringer's lactate at 100 mL/hour

11. Mrs. Anderson is prescribed a thrombolytic agent. You understand that the purpose of this order may be to achieve which of the following effects? (Select all that apply.)

    a. Dissolve thrombi

    b. Limit tissue damage

    c. Prevent tissue damage from thrombi

    d. Increase coagulation

12. Antiplatelet drugs are used to prevent _____ thrombosis.

13. The physician discovers a clot in Mr. Proffit's left lower leg. He prescribes anticoagulant drugs to prevent formation of new clots and to achieve which other effect?

    a. Increase coagulation

    b. Regulate PTT

    c. Regulate PT, INR

    d. Prevent extension of clots already present

14. Mr. Norton takes warfarin daily for DVT prevention. He also takes a multivitamin with minerals. Which of the following instructions should you give him?

    a. Discontinue the multivitamin with minerals

    b. Increase the dose of the multivitamin with minerals

    c. Change his vitamins to ones that do not contain minerals

    d. Take his vitamins with minerals consistently

15. You are the home care nurse caring for Mr. Brown. He is learning to self-administer his heparin daily. You also draw blood every 2 to 3 days to monitor his platelet levels. Which of the following platelet counts would you report to the physician as a critical laboratory result?

    a. 150,000   c. 90,000

    b. 160,000   d. 400,000

16. Mr. Wilson is diagnosed with hepatitis A, diabetes type 1, and portal hypertension. He develops a DVT, and the physician prescribes warfarin. You are concerned, for which of the following reasons?

    a. The client is more likely to experience bleeding.

    b. The client is less likely to achieve a therapeutic dose.

    c. The client is at risk for further liver impairment.

    d. The client is at risk for hyperglycemic episodes.

17. Mrs. Farquhar is diagnosed with chronic renal insufficiency. Her vascular access site becomes incompetent, and the physician orders urokinase to dissolve the clot. Which of the following should you do?

    a. Administer the drug as ordered

    b. Hold the drug until you can contact the physician to verify the order

    c. Refuse to administer the drug

    d. Ask the physician to administer the drug

18. Mr. Sheffield, age 75, presents to the physician's office with complaints of bleeding gums and multiple bruises. When you review his drug history, you understand that he is prescribed aspirin 81 mg/day. Which of the following drugs may cause increased bleeding when used in conjunction with the aspirin?

    a. Antibiotics

    b. Antihypertensives

    c. NSAIDs

    d. Antidysrhythmics

19. Heparin solutions containing _____ _____ as a preservative should not be given to premature infants, because fatal reactions have been reported.

20. A stable daily dose of warfarin is reached when which of the following parameters is achieved?

    a. The PTT is within the therapeutic range.

    b. The PT and INR are within their therapeutic ranges and the dose does not cause bleeding.

    c. The INR is between 4 and 5.

    d. The INR is between 1 and 2 and the dose does not cause bleeding.

CHAPTER 55

Drugs for Dyslipidemia

■ Section I: Learning Objectives

1. Recognize the role of dyslipidemia in the metabolic syndrome.
2. Identify sources and functions of cholesterol and triglycerides.
3. Describe dyslipidemic drugs in terms of mechanism of action, indications for use, major adverse effects, and nursing process implications.
4. Educate patients in pharmacologic and nonpharmacologic measures to prevent or reduce dyslipidemia.
5. Use the nursing process in the care of patients with dyslipidemia.

■ Section II: Assessing Your Understanding

ACTIVITY A

Fill in the Blanks

1. _____ drugs are used in the management of elevated blood lipids, a major risk factor for atherosclerosis and vascular disorders such as coronary artery disease, strokes, and peripheral arterial insufficiency
2. Blood lipids, which include cholesterol, phospholipids, and triglycerides, are derived from the diet or synthesized by the liver and _____.
3. Most cholesterol is found in body cells, where it is a component of _____ _____ and performs other essential functions.
4. In cells of the adrenal glands, ovaries, and testes, cholesterol is required for the synthesis of _____ hormones.
5. In liver cells, cholesterol is used to form _____ _____, which is conjugated with other substances to form bile salts; bile salts promote absorption and digestion of fats.

ACTIVITY B

Matching

Match the term in Column A with the definition in Column B.

COLUMN A

1. _____ Atorvastatin
2. _____ Cholestyramine
3. _____ Gemfibrozil, fenofibrate
4. _____ Niacin (nicotinic acid)
5. _____ Ezetimibe

COLUMN B

A. Similar to endogenous fatty acids
B. Binds bile acids in the intestinal lumen
C. Decreases both cholesterol and triglycerides
D. Acts in the small intestine to inhibit absorption of cholesterol and decrease the delivery of intestinal cholesterol to the liver
E. Most widely used statin and one of the most widely used drugs in the United States

ACTIVITY C

Short Answers

Briefly answer the following questions.

1. Discuss the process by which blood lipids are transported.
2. Describe how lipoprotein density is determined.
3. Identify the risk factors associated with the metabolic syndrome.
4. How do these risk factors affect the cardiovascular, cerebrovascular, and peripheral vascular systems?
5. Discuss the first line of treatment for metabolic syndrome.

■ Section III: Applying Your Knowledge

ACTIVITY D
Case Study
Consider the scenario and answer the questions.

Mr. Best, age 45, presents to the physician's office for an employment-related physical examination. His last physical was 7 years ago. He leads a sedentary lifestyle and works in a high-stress environment. He is approximately 35 pounds overweight. His medication history includes ibuprofen periodically for headaches. He does not take vitamins or herbal supplements. Before the examination, the physician ordered the following laboratory studies: CBC, electrolyte panel, lipid panel, and electrocardiogram. The physician diagnoses Mr. Best with dyslipidemia.

1. Mr. Best asks you if the doctor is sure that he has dyslipidemia; he noticed that his HDL was low, and asks, "Isn't that good?" What do you know about the major risk factors for coronary artery disease?
2. Three months later, the physician orders a lipid profile and triglycerides. What instructions should you give Mr. Best about preparing for the tests?
3. What are some recommendations for reducing Mr. Best's risk factors for cardiovascular disease?

■ Section IV: Practicing for NCLEX

Answer the following questions.

1. Mr. Vandever's triglycerides are still elevated despite lifestyle changes. You expect the physician to order which of the following?
   a. Fenofibrate
   b. Cholestyramine
   c. Niacin
   d. Atorvastatin

2. Mrs. Custer presents to the physician's office with complaints of a recurrence of her "hot flashes." You understand that she is taking which of the following drugs to treat her dyslipidemia?
   a. Fenofibrate
   b. Cholestyramine
   c. Niacin
   d. Atorvastatin

3. You instruct your client to take his lovastatin in which of the following ways?
   a. In the morning 1 hour before breakfast
   b. At night 2 hours after a meal
   c. With food
   d. Without regard to food or time of the day

4. When your client asks what she can do to improve her cholesterol levels, you suggest which of the following?
   a. Smoking cessation
   b. Diet high in polysaturated fats
   C. Limit exercise to the weekends
   d. Weight lifting

5. Which of the following cardiac risk factors are related to metabolic syndrome? (Select all that apply.)
   a. Central adiposity
   b. Elevated triglycerides
   c. Reduced high-density lipoprotein cholesterol
   d. Postural hypotension

6. The physician orders a lipid profile without triglycerides for his client. When you phone the client with his appointment, you tell him which of the following?
   a. Fast for 12 hours before the test.
   b. Fast for 6 hours before the test.
   c. Fast for 4 hours before the test.
   d. Fasting is not needed.

7. Mr. Clark does not have a genetic disorder of lipid metabolism. You suspect that his elevated cholesterol is directly related to which of the following?

    a. His dietary intake of saturated fat

    b. His sedentary lifestyle

    c. His waist size

    d. His alcohol intake

8. Mr. Finnegan presents to the physician's office with symptoms of hyperglycemia. He is taking his oral antidiabetic mediation and has not modified his diet or exercise program in any way. When you interview the client, he states that he now takes flax seed to reduce his cholesterol level. You understand that flax seed may do which of the following?

    a. Increase absorption of his drugs

    b. Decrease absorption of his drugs

    c. Increase liver metabolism

    d. Decrease excretion of the drug through the kidneys

9. The physician prescribes fibrate for his client with elevated triglycerides. The client begins to self-administer niacin approximately 3 mg daily. Which of the following would you expect the physician to order?

    a. LFTs   c. Electrolyte panel

    b. CBC   d. Fibrate level

10. Mr. Jacobson takes cholesterol absorption inhibitors as a monotherapy without statins. He develops mild hepatic insufficiency. Which of the following would you expect the physician to do?

    a. Increase the dosage of his medication

    b. Decrease the dosage of his mediation

    c. Maintain the current dosage of his medication

    d. Discontinue his medication

11. Mr. Costa presents to the physician's office for his annual visit. He takes statins to control his hyperlipidemia. When he reviews the client's laboratory results, the physician notes that there is an unexplained elevation in the serum aspartate. Which of the following would you expect the physician to do?

    a. Increase the dose of the statin

    b. Discontinue the statin

    c. Decrease the dose of the statin

    d. Maintain the current dose of the statin

12. The physician is caring for a client who is a 2-year kidney transplant survivor. You would expect him to order which of the following drugs for the client's hyperlipidemia?

    a. Atorvastatin   c. Lovastatin

    b. Fluvastatin   d. Pravastatin

13. Mrs. Dina, age 57, is postmenopausal. Lifestyle changes have not made a significant impact on her lipids. Which of the following would you expect the physician to suggest?

    a. Fenofibrate

    b. Cholestyramine

    c. Niacin

    d. Estrogen replacement therapy

14. Randy H., age 8, requires treatment for dyslipidemia. Which of the following would you expect the physician to order?

    a. Pravastatin   c. Cholestyramine

    b. Fenofibrate   d. Niacin

15. Patients of which ethnic group may find diet and exercise more useful than lipid-lowering drugs?

    a. African Americans   c. Native Americans

    b. Asian Americans   d. Italian Americans

16. Mr. Griffin's laboratory results indicate that both cholesterol and triglycerides are elevated. Which of the following medications may be ordered? (Select all that apply.)

    a. Statin

    b. Cholesterol absorption inhibitor

    c. Gemfibrozil

    d. Bile acid sequestrant

17. A fibrate–statin combination should be avoided because of increased risks of which of the following conditions?

    a. Severe myopathy

    b. Rebound dyslipidemia

    c. Cardiac dysrhythmia

    d. Postural hypotension

18. Which of the following drugs or drug classes decreases the delivery of intestinal cholesterol to the liver?

    a. Statin

    b. Fibrate

    c. Cholesterol absorption inhibitor

    d. Bile acid sequestrant

19. Which of the following drugs or drug classes inhibits mobilization of free fatty acids from peripheral tissues?

    a. Statin   c. Cholesterol absorption inhibitor

    b. Fibrate   d. Niacin

20. Bile acid sequestrants bind bile acids in the _____ lumen.

CHAPTER 56

Physiology of the Digestive System

■ Section I: Learning Objectives

1. Review the roles of the main digestive tract structures.
2. List common signs and symptoms affecting gastrointestinal functions.
3. Identify general categories of drugs used to treat gastrointestinal disorders.
4. Discuss the effects of nongastrointestinal drugs on gastrointestinal functioning.

■ Section II: Assessing Your Understanding

ACTIVITY A

Fill in the Blanks

1. The digestive system comprises the alimentary canal, a tube extending from the oral cavity to the _____.
2. The digestive system also comprises accessory organs including the salivary glands, gallbladder, _____, and pancreas.
3. The main function of the system is to provide the body with fluids, nutrients, and electrolytes in a form that can be used at the _____ level.
4. The system also disposes of waste products that result from the digestive process; this is called _____.
5. The _____ canal has the same basic structure throughout.

ACTIVITY B

Matching

Match the term in Column A with the definition in Column B.

COLUMN A

1. _____ oral cavity

2. _____ esophagus

3. _____ stomach

4. _____ small intestine

5. _____ large intestine

COLUMN B

A. Where chewing mechanically breaks food into smaller particles, which can be swallowed more easily and provide a larger surface area for enzyme action

B. Consists of the duodenum, jejunum, and ileum and is approximately 20 feet (6 m) long

C. A musculofibrous tube about 10 inches (25 cm) long; its main function is to convey food from the pharynx to the stomach

D. Consists of the cecum, colon, rectum, and anus

E. A dilated area that serves as a reservoir

ACTIVITY C

Short Answers

Briefly answer the following questions.

1. What is the function of the pancreas in the gastrointestinal system?
2. What is the function of the gallbladder in the gastrointestinal system?
3. What is the function of mucus in the gastrointestinal system?
4. What is the function of saliva in the gastrointestinal system?
5. What is the role of hydrochloric acid in the gastrointestinal system?

■ Section III: Applying Your Knowledge

ACTIVITY D

Case Study

Consider the scenario and answer the questions.

You are participating in a study group of student nurses. Your assignment is to outline and define the structure and function of the liver.

1. Describe the circulation of blood as it relates to the liver. What is the liver's role in the case of hypovolemic shock?
2. Discuss the function of the Kupffer cells in the liver.
3. What is the role of the liver in metabolizing drugs? What methods does the liver use to detoxify substances?

■ Section IV: Practicing for NCLEX

Answer the following questions.

1. The liver plays numerous roles in digestion, including which of the following? (Select all that apply.)
   a. Metabolism of carbohydrates, fats, and proteins
   b. Storage of fat-soluble vitamins
   c. Storage of vitamin B_{12}
   d. Storage of carbohydrates

2. The gallbladder stores and releases bile into the small intestine when _____ are present in the duodenum.

3. Pancreatic juices are rich in bicarbonate and which other substance?
   a. Digestive enzymes   c. Insulin
   b. Hydrochloric acid   d. Carbonic acid

4. Most nutrients and drugs are absorbed in which organ?
   a. Large intestine   c. Esophagus
   b. Stomach   d. Small intestine

5. Mucus and _____ protect the stomach from the acidic pH of the gastric secretions.

6. Gastrin, _____, and histamine stimulate secretion of gastric acid.

7. To effectively digest proteins, which of the following does pepsin require?
   a. Basic pH   c. Acidic pH
   b. Histamine   d. Hydrocarbons

8. Food is mixed with gastric juices, which contain mucus and digestive enzymes such as which of the following? (Select all that apply.)
   a. Pepsin   c. Histamine
   b. Hydrochloric acid   d. Carbonic acid

9. Which of the following is the result of failure of the lower esophageal sphincter?
   a. Reflux of gastric contents into the stomach
   b. Reflux of gastric contents into the small intestine
   c. Reflux of gastric contents into the large intestine
   d. Reflux of gastric contents into the esophagus

10. The esophagus is bordered by _____ at each end and serves to convey food to the stomach.

11. Digestion begins in the oral cavity with mastication and digestion of which of the following components of food?
    a. Starches   c. Carbohydrates
    b. Proteins   d. Fats

12. _____ stimulation promotes sphincter function and inhibits motility.

13. Peristalsis propels food through the digestive tract and mixes the food bolus with which of the following substances?
    a. Insulin   c. Pepsin
    b. Digestive juices   d. Histamine

14. Which of the following are the main functions of the digestive system? (Select all that apply.)
    a. Provide the body with useable nutrition
    b. Dispose of waste products
    c. Create protein for brain metabolism
    d. Create carbohydrates for cardiac function

15. The digestive system and drug therapy have a reciprocal relationship. As a result, which of the following symptoms may be related to drug therapy?

    a. Dizziness
    b. Somnolence
    c. Tachycardia
    d. Nausea

16. The hormone _____ causes the gallbladder to contract and release bile into the small intestine when fats are present in intestinal contents.

17. The major digestive enzyme in gastric juice is pepsin, a proteolytic enzyme. However, the names of most digestive enzymes have which of the following endings?

    a. -ace
    b. -ase
    c. -ese
    d. -ece

18. Which of the following tasks is a function of the liver?

    a. Metabolism of insulin
    b. Creation of phagocytes
    c. Production of body heat
    d. Functioning as the body's "cooling system"

19. Formation of urea removes _____ from body fluids.

20. Excess glucose that cannot be converted to _____ is converted to fat.

CHAPTER 57

Nutritional Support Products, Vitamins, and Mineral–Electrolytes

■ Section I: Learning Objectives

1. Assess patients for risk factors and manifestations of protein-calorie undernutrition.
2. Identify patients at risk for development of vitamin and/or mineral–electrolyte deficiency or excess.
3. Describe adverse effects associated with overdoses of vitamins.
4. Discuss the rationale for administering vitamin K to newborns.
5. Describe signs, symptoms, and treatment of sodium, potassium, magnesium, and chloride imbalances.
6. Describe signs, symptoms, and treatment of iron deficiency anemia.
7. Discuss the chelating agents used to remove excessive copper, iron, and lead from body tissues.
8. Apply nursing process skills to prevent, recognize, or treat nutritional imbalances.
9. Monitor laboratory reports that indicate nutritional status.

■ Section II: Assessing Your Understanding

ACTIVITY A

Fill in the Blanks

1. _____ are structural and functional components of all body tissues; the recommended amount for adults is 50 to 60 grams daily.
2. _____ and fats mainly provide energy for cellular metabolism.
3. Energy is measured in _____ per gram of food oxidized in the body.
4. Carbohydrates and _____ supply 4 kcal per gram; fats supply 9 kcal per gram.
5. _____ are required for normal body metabolism, growth, and development.

ACTIVITY B

Matching

Match the term in Column A with the definition in Column B.

COLUMN A

1. _____ Sodium polystyrene sulfonate (Kayexalate)
2. _____ Desferasirox (Exjade)
3. _____ Deferoxamine (Desferal)
4. _____ Penicillamine (Cuprimine)
5. _____ Succimer (Chemet)

COLUMN B

A. A parenteral drug used to remove excess iron from storage sites (e.g., ferritin, hemosiderin) in the body
B. Chelates copper, zinc, mercury, and lead to form soluble complexes that are excreted in the urine
C. Chelates lead to form water-soluble complexes that are excreted in the urine
D. Used to treat hyperkalemia
E. An oral iron-chelating agent used to treat chronic iron overload

ACTIVITY C

Short Answers

Briefly answer the following questions.

1. Discuss how nutritional deficiency states may occur.
2. What are liquid enteral products and why are they administered?
3. When are IV fluids used instead of liquid enteral products? What types of solutions are used?
4. Under what circumstances are pancreatic enzymes used, and what is their purpose to maintain a client's health and well-being?
5. What is considered the best source of vitamins to maintain health? Why do clients take commercially prepared vitamins?

■ Section III: Applying Your Knowledge

ACTIVITY D

Case Study

Consider the scenario and answer the questions.

Mrs. Angelis presents to the physician's office with symptoms of fatigue, listlessness, and dyspnea on exertion. She is diagnosed with iron deficiency anemia. The physician orders ferrous sulfate. You are responsible for Mrs. Angelis' education care plan.

1. In addition to treating iron deficiency anemia, how are iron preparations used to prevent iron deficiency anemia?
2. Mrs. Angelis asks you how long the iron will take to work. What can you tell her about how the iron preparation works? How would you respond if she asks for an enteric-coated preparation?
3. What are some adverse effects of this drug? What adjustments to the treatment might be made in reaction to some of these effects?

■ Section IV: Practicing for NCLEX

Answer the following questions.

1. Mrs. Ridley presents to the physician's office for her yearly physical examination. When you ask about her current drug regimen, she states that she self-administers megadoses of vitamin C to prevent cancer. Which of the following statements is an appropriate response?
   a. "You require large doses of multiple vitamins to prevent cancer."
   b. "Large doses of single vitamins do not prevent cancer."
   c. "Large doses of vitamin C will also prevent cardiovascular disease."
   d. "Large doses of vitamin C will also prevent HIV."

2. Mr. Theodore tells you that he obtains all of his nutrients from vitamins. Which of the following is the correct explanation to give this patient?
   a. "The effectiveness of the vitamins depends on the brand."
   b. "You cannot obtain enough vitamin B_6 from vitamins."
   c. "You should consult your physician for the correct strength of the vitamins."
   d. "Nutrients are best obtained from foods."

3. Which of the following are fat-soluble vitamins? (Select all that apply.)
   a. A   c. K
   b. D   d. B

4. Which of the following are water-soluble vitamins? (Select all that apply.)
   a. B complex   c. C
   b. K   d. A

5. As the home care nurse visiting a patient, which of the following is included in your responsibilities?

   a. Providing care to the client with physician's orders

   b. Assessing the nutritional status of the client you have physician's orders to visit

   c. Assessing the nutritional status of all members of the household

   d. Providing nutrition counseling to the person who is the primary cook within the family

6. For patients receiving tube feedings at home, which of the following may be a subject of teaching by the home care nurse? (Select all that apply.)

   a. The goals of treatment and techniques of administration

   b. Preparation or storage of solutions

   c. Adjustment of the nutrition formula

   d. Monitoring of responses (e.g., weight, urine output)

7. You are caring for a critically ill patient in the unit. An IV is dedicated to fluid and electrolyte replacement. To prevent imbalances and adverse reactions, which of the following should you closely monitor?

   a. Hemoglobin and hematocrit levels

   b. Serum electrolyte levels

   c. Serum albumin levels

   d. BUN and creatine levels

8. You are responsible for the administration of total parental nutrition for a client. The physician orders a fat emulsion. How should the fat emulsion be administered?

   a. Rapidly over 30 minutes

   b. Over 1 to 2 hours

   c. Slowly over an 8-hour period

   d. Slowly over 24 hours

9. You are comparing the recipe for a TPN with the physician's orders for an adult male, age 35. How will vitamin K be administered?

   a. Separately by injection

   b. Separately orally

   c. Included in the TPN order

   d. Monthly subcutaneously

10. Mr. Springer is diagnosed with COPD. His enteral feeding formula will be individualized and will contain which of the following combinations of nutrients?

    a. More carbohydrates and less protein

    b. Less carbohydrate and more fat

    c. Less carbohydrate and more protein

    d. Less fat and more protein

11. Patients with cardiac or renal impairment who require fluid restriction may benefit from a more _____ enteral formula (e.g., 1.5 kcal/mL).

12. Mr. Powers is admitted to your unit for treatment of pneumonia. His diagnoses include cirrhosis of the liver. You would expect his diet to include restriction of which of the following elements?

    a. Carbohydrate   c. Calcium

    b. Fat   d. Protein

13. With enteral nutrition, _____- _____ may be given to provide amino acids, carbohydrates, and a few electrolytes for patients with renal failure.

14. IV fat emulsions should not be given to patients with ARF if serum triglyceride levels exceed which of the following levels?

    a. 400 mg/dL   c. 200 mg/dL

    b. 300 mg/dL   d. 100 mg/dL

15. Mr. Smith, age 75, is admitted to your unit. His diagnoses include diabetes mellitus type 2, arthrosclerosis, and a PMH of MI in 1989. You should be concerned if his enteral feeding contains which of the following elements?

    a. Animal fats

    b. Low amounts of glucose

    c. Potassium

    d. Calcium

16. To prevent accidental ingestion of iron-containing medications by children, products with 30 mg or more of iron must be provided in which of the following ways?

    a. They must have childproof caps.

    b. They must be packaged as individual doses.

    c. They must be supplied by prescription only.

    d. They must be prescribed only for adults.

17. All such drugs should be kept out of reach of young children and should never be referred to as "_____."

18. Preterm infants need proportionately more vitamins than term infants, for which of the following reasons?

    a. They often experience electrolyte imbalances.

    b. Their growth rate is faster.

    c. Their metabolism is slower.

    d. Their growth rate is slower.

19. Mrs. Pearson is diagnosed with a seizure disorder, and the physician prescribes phenytoin. She is preparing to conceive her second child and begins to self-administer folic acid. The concurrent use of these medications places the client at risk for which of the following adverse effects?

    a. Phenytoin toxicity

    b. Seizures

    c. Folic acid toxicity

    d. Subtherapeutic levels of folic acid

20. Niacin may increase the risk of _____ with statin cholesterol-lowering drugs (e.g., atorvastatin [Lipitor]).

CHAPTER 58

Drugs Used to Aid Weight Management

■ Section I: Learning Objectives

1. Promote healthful lifestyle measures to maintain body weight within a desirable range and avoid obesity.
2. Assess patients for risk factors and manifestations of obesity.
3. Calculate body mass index (BMI).
4. Counsel patients about the health consequences of obesity.
5. Assist overweight patients to develop and maintain a safe and realistic weight-loss program.
6. Identify reliable sources for information about nutrition, weight loss, and weight maintenance.
7. Assist patients with effective use of approved weight-loss drugs, when indicated.

■ Section II: Assessing Your Understanding

ACTIVITY A

Fill in the Blanks

1. _____ is defined as a *body mass index* (BMI) of 25 to 29.9.
2. _____ is defined as a BMI of 30 or more.
3. The _____ reflects weight in relation to height and is a better indicator than weight alone.
4. The desirable range for _____ is 18.5 to 24.9.
5. A large waist circumference (greater than 35 inches for women or 40 inches for men) is another risk factor for overweight and _____.

ACTIVITY B

Matching

Match the term in Column A with the definition in Column B.

COLUMN A

1. _____ Phentermine (Adipex-P)
2. _____ Sibutramine (Meridia)
3. _____ Orlistat (Xenical, Alli)
4. _____ Glucomannan
5. _____ Guarana

COLUMN B

A. Schedule IV drug and most commonly prescribed anti-obesity drug
B. Most frequently prescribed adrenergic anorexiant
C. Decreases absorption of dietary fat from the intestine
D. Major source of commercial caffeine; found in weight-loss products and many other supplements and other food products
E. Expands on contact with body fluids

ACTIVITY C

Short Answers

Briefly answer the following questions.

1. What is the primary cause of obesity?
2. What is central or visceral obesity?
3. What is the prevalence of obesity in the United States?
4. What is the etiology of excessive weight gain?
5. Explain how energy expenditure influences weight control.

■ Section III: Applying Your Knowledge

ACTIVITY D

Case Study

Consider the scenario and answer the questions.

During a routine physician's appointment, Mrs. Romano requests more information about orlistat. She is concerned about her obesity and does not want to take a prescription medication. You are responsible for her education plan.

1. Mrs. Romano asks how orlistat works. How would you respond?
2. Mrs. Romano wants to know whether the drug will lower her cholesterol. What is your understanding of the relationship between weight loss and effects on cholesterol with this drug?
3. Explain the absorption of the drug. Does it cause any adverse effects? What are the disadvantages of taking orlistat?
4. Mrs. Romano asks if there are any other medications or supplements that she should take with the orlistat to remain healthy. What can you suggest?

■ Section IV: Practicing for NCLEX

Answer the following questions.

1. Mr. Gibson presents to the physician's office 1 year after losing 50 pounds. He complains that he is rapidly regaining his weight and doesn't know what to do about it. Which of the following should you review? (Select all that apply.)
   a. His lifestyle habits
   b. His exercise habits
   c. His work habits
   d. His eating habits

2. Mrs. Salas presents to the physician's office for a routine physical examination. She is 10 pounds overweight and asks the physician for a prescription for a weight-loss drug. She is healthy and her laboratory values are within normal limits. The physician does which of the following?
   a. Orders the medication with a short-term prescription
   b. Encourages the client to increase her exercise and eat a healthy diet
   c. Refuses to order the weight-loss drugs because her HMO will not pay for them
   d. Orders an open prescription of a weight-loss drug.

3. Reducing _____ _____ and increasing caloric expenditure are part of any successful weight-loss program.

4. Mr. Gonzales asks the physician how to lose weight without drugs. The physician suggests decreasing his intake by 500 calories per day to lose which of the following?
   a. 2 pounds per week
   b. 4 pounds per week
   c. 3 pounds per week
   d. 1 pound per week

5. Overweight and obesity are major concerns because of their association with numerous health problems, including which of the following? (Select all that apply.)
   a. Diabetes   c. Hypoglycemia
   b. Hypertension   d. Hypokalemia

6. You are the home care nurse for Mr. and Mrs. Stanley. Mrs. Stanley states that she found a weight-loss program on the Internet for $200.00 that will help her to lose 50 pounds safely in 30 days. She asks you about the program. You do which of the following?
   a. Encourage the client to purchase the program, because it will improve her blood glucose.
   b. Encourage the client to purchase the program, because she will eventually decrease her dependence on prescription medications
   c. Discourage the purchase, because the diet promises unrealistic weight loss expectations
   d. Discourage the purchase, because the cost of the diet is prohibitive.

7. Mr. Wilson is diagnosed with diabetes mellitus, hyperlipidemia, obesity, and cirrhosis of the liver. He asks the physician to prescribe sibutramine for weight loss. You would expect the physician to do which of the following?

   a. Order the prescription, because weight loss will improve the client's overall health

   b. Order the prescription, because administration of the medication will decrease the client's lipids

   c. Refuse to order the medication, because the drug is excreted in the kidneys

   d. Refuse to order the medication, because the drug is metabolized in the liver

8. Mrs. Fleming is diagnosed with end-stage renal disease. She asks the physician to prescribe sibutramine to help her to lose weight. She states that she has friends with renal disease who take the drug and assumes that it is safe. The physician does which of the following?

   a. Orders the drug

   b. Orders the drug with an increased dosage

   c. Orders the drug with a decreased dosage

   d. Does not order the drug

9. With orlistat, the manufacturer recommends conservative use and dosage, because in older adults which of the following is often decreased? (Select all that apply.)

   a. Renal function   c. Pancreatic function

   b. Cardiac function   d. Hepatic function

10. Mrs. Goodrich brings her overweight child to the pediatrician's office. She requests medication to help her child lose weight. The physician does not order medication. You are responsible for the family education plan and focus your teaching on which of the following?

    a. Decreasing physical activity

    b. Putting the child on a diet

    c. Increasing physical activity

    d. Decreasing the child's BMI

11. Mrs. Goodrich's child exceeds optimal adult weight. The goal of the treatment plan established with Mrs. Goodrich and her child is a weight loss of how many pounds per year until the optimal adult weight is reached?

    a. 10 to 12 pounds   c. 12 to 15 pounds

    b. 6 to 8 pounds   d. 25 to 30 pounds

12. Mrs. Lang brings her 16-year-old daughter to the physician's office for a weight-loss program. The patient is 100 pounds overweight, and diets have been unsuccessful in the past. The physician orders which of the following?

    a. Phentermine   c. Glucomannan

    b. Orlistat   d. Sibutramine

13. Mrs. Inserra asks you which commercial program will offer her psychological support and positive reinforcement for weight loss. She knows what is available in her community but is concerned about the success rates of the programs. You state that reviews suggest that which of the following programs has the best success rates?

    a. OPTIFAST   c. Weight Watchers

    b. Jenny Craig   d. L.A. Weight Loss

14. Mrs. Rose takes orlistat for weight loss. The weight loss is not progressing as quickly as she would like, and she asks her physician to order sibutramine for her. She hopes that the combination will decrease her appetite and foster quicker weight loss. The physician does which of the following?

    a. Orders the medication combination

    b. Orders a low dose of sibutramine to use with the orlistat

    c. Does not order the combination due to possible adverse reactions

    d. Does not order the combination because it does not improve weight loss

15. Mr. Devens is diagnosed with diabetes type 2. He presents to the physician's office after a weight loss of 25 pounds. You would expect the physician to do which of the following?

    a. Tell the client that his diabetes is cured

    b. Decrease his diabetic medications

    c. Increase his diabetic medications

    d. Diagnose the client with hypoglycemia

16. For a client with cardiovascular disease, the benefits of weight loss include which of the following? (Select all that apply.)

    a. Lower blood pressure

    b. Decreased HDL cholesterol

    c. Increased HDL cholesterol

    d. Lower serum triglycerides

17. Ms. Adler is 35 pounds overweight. She asks the physician for a referral to a surgeon for bariatric surgery. You would expect the physician to do which of the following?

    a. Make the referral

    b. Decline to make the referral

    c. Refer the client to a psychologist

    d. Refer the client to a pharmacologist for an OTC diet supplement

18. Ms. Kay presents to the physician's office with complaints of weakness, dizziness, and heart palpitations. She takes over-the-counter Super Dieter's Tea. You expect the physician to order which of the following?

    a. Serum electrolytes

    b. Hemoglobin and hematocrit

    c. Serum albumin

    d. CO_2

19. Ms. Kelly presents to the physician's office with complaints of abdominal pain. During the interview, you discover that the client is using guar gum as a weight-loss product. In addition, she limits her fluid intake to reduce retention. Ms. Kelly is at risk for which of the following?

    a. Pancreatitis

    b. Peptic ulcer disease

    c. Intestinal obstruction

    d. Esophageal varices

20. Products containing glucomannan should not be used by people with _____.

CHAPTER 59

Drugs Used for Peptic Ulcer and Acid Reflux Disease

■ Section I: Learning Objectives

1. Describe the main elements of peptic ulcer disease and gastroesophageal reflux disease (GERD).
2. Differentiate the types of drugs used to treat peptic ulcers and acid reflux disorders.
3. Discuss the advantages and disadvantages of proton pump inhibitors.
4. Differentiate between prescription and over-the-counter uses of histamine$_2$ receptor–blocking agents.
5. Discuss significant drug–drug interactions with cimetidine.
6. Describe characteristics, uses, and effects of selected antacids.
7. Discuss the rationale for using combination antacid products.
8. Teach patients nonpharmacologic measures to manage peptic ulcers and GERD

■ Section II: Assessing Your Understanding

ACTIVITY A

Fill in the Blanks

1. _____ _____ _____ is characterized by ulcer formation in the esophagus, stomach, or duodenum, areas of the gastrointestinal (GI) mucosa that are exposed to gastric acid and pepsin.
2. Gastric and _____ ulcers are more common than esophageal ulcers.
3. Peptic ulcers are attributed to an imbalance between cell-destructive and cell-_____ effects.
4. Cell-destructive effects include those of gastric acid (hydrochloric acid), _____, *Helicobacter pylori* infection, and ingestion of nonsteroidal anti-inflammatory drugs (NSAIDs).

5. _____ _____, a strong acid that can digest the stomach wall, is secreted by parietal cells in the mucosa of the stomach antrum, near the pylorus.

ACTIVITY B

Matching

Match the term in Column A with the definition in Column B.

COLUMN A

1. _____ Antacids
2. _____ H2RAs
3. _____ PPIs
4. _____ Naturally occurring prostaglandin E
5. _____ Sucralfate

COLUMN B

A. Produced in mucosal cells of the stomach and duodenum, inhibits gastric acid secretion and increases mucus and bicarbonate secretion, mucosal blood flow, and perhaps mucosal repair
B. A preparation of sulfated sucrose and aluminum hydroxide that binds to normal and ulcerated mucosa; used to prevent and treat peptic ulcer disease
C. Inhibits both basal secretion of gastric acid and the secretion stimulated by histamine, acetylcholine, and gastrin
D. Strong inhibitors of gastric acid secretion
E. Alkaline substances that neutralize acids

ACTIVITY C

Short Answers

Briefly answer the following questions.

1. Explain the mechanism of action of antacids.
2. Explain the effect that histamines have on the gastrointestinal system.
3. What are proton pump inhibitors, and how do they affect the gastrointestinal system?
4. What effect does naturally occurring prostaglandin E have on the gastrointestinal system?
5. What disease process is sucralfate used for, and what is its mechanism of action?

■ Section III: Applying Your Knowledge

ACTIVITY D

Case Study

Consider the scenario and answer the questions.

Mr. Dinwiddie, a construction worker, self-administers ibuprofen 800 mg four times a day for pain related to arthritis and his work. He presents to the physician's office with stomach pain that has become chronic within the past 2 weeks. The physician orders misoprostol.

1. Why did the physician order misoprostol? What is misoprostol? How will this drug help with the stomach pain?
2. Mr. Dinwiddie asks if misoprostol is safe for his wife. She has chronic back pain and also self-administers NSAIDs prescribed by her physician. Would you refer Mrs. Dinwiddie to her physician for the same treatment?
3. What is the most common adverse reaction related to misoprostol use? What is the most common indication for misoprostol?

■ Section IV: Practicing for NCLEX

Answer the following questions.

1. For sucralfate to be effective, the drug must be given under which of the following conditions?
   a. In an acid pH   c. On an empty stomach
   b. In a basic pH   d. On a full stomach

2. The PPIs bind irreversibility to the gastric proton pump to prevent the release of gastric acid from _____ cells into the stomach lumen.

3. PPIs are considered drugs of choice for treatment of which of the following conditions? (Select all that apply.)
   a. Duodenal ulcers
   b. Esophageal varices
   c. Zollinger-Ellison syndrome
   d. Gastric ulcers

4. The H2RAs inhibit secretion of gastric acid, decreasing the acidity of _____ _____.

5. Mr. Maffi is diagnosed with *H. pylori* infection. The physician will order amoxicillin and which of the following?
   a. Proton pump inhibitors
   b. Sucralfate
   c. H2RAs
   d. Antacids

6. Mrs. Gallant presents to the physician's office with increasing stomach acidity. She self-administers calcium antacids, and the more acid her stomach, the more antacids she takes. You suspect which of the following as her diagnosis?
   a. Hypocalcemia
   b. Rebound acidity
   c. Gastric reflux
   d. Hyperactive gastric mucosa

7. Mrs. Schwartz self-administers magnesium antacids. The more her stomach bothers her, the more antacids she takes. She presents to the office with symptoms of dizziness and weakness. These symptoms are secondary to which common adverse effect of magnesium antacids?
   a. Hypercalcemia   c. Diarrhea
   b. Hypocalcemia   d. GERD

8. Aluminum antacids have low neutralizing capacity and often cause _____.

9. Mr. Kinsey is overweight and lives a sedentary lifestyle. He presents to the office with complaints of acid regurgitation, especially at night. You suspect the physician's diagnosis will be which of the following?
   a. Gastritis
   b. Peptic ulcer disease
   c. Duodenal ulcer disease
   d. Gastroesophageal reflux disease

10. Alkalinization of gastric secretion is an example of which of the following?
   a. Cell-regenerative properties
   b. Presumptive gastric ulcer disease
   c. Cell-protective effects
   d. Esophageal erosion

11. Gastric acid and pepsin are indicative of which of the following conditions?
   a. Cell-destructive effects
   b. Alkaline mucosa
   c. Ingestion of magnesium antacids
   d. Alkaline gastric contents

12. The most common location for a peptic ulcer is the _____, followed by the stomach and esophagus.

13. Mrs. Scott is self-administering cimetidine. As her home care nurse, it is important for you to assess her medication regimen to identify which of the following?
   a. Adverse reactions
   b. Potential drug–drug interactions
   c. Allergic reactions
   d. Toxicity

14. Mr. Jackson has liver disease and is diagnosed with esophageal reflux. He asks the physician to prescribe PPIs. The use of PPIs in conjunction with a diagnosis of liver disease may result in which of the following?
   a. Decreased absorption of the PPIs
   b. Transient elevations in liver function tests
   c. PPI toxicity
   d. Subtherapeutic levels of PPIs in the bloodstream

15. Mrs. Soledad's diagnoses include diabetes mellitus, gastric ulcer disease, and chronic renal disease. When you review her medications with her, you discover that she self-administers antacids containing magnesium. Which of the following statements is true about antacids containing magnesium?
   a. They are an acceptable treatment for gastric ulcer disease.
   b. They are contraindicated for clients with renal disease.
   c. They may cause an exacerbation of her hyperglycemia.
   d. They may cause hypoglycemia for clients with chronic renal disease and diabetes.

16. Mrs. Richards, age 75, is diagnosed with diabetes mellitus type 2, hypertension, osteoporosis, and gastric ulcer disease. She is prescribed PPIs. Long-term (greater than 1 year) administration of PPIs may lead to which of the following?
   a. Increased risk for gastric cancer
   b. Increased risk for peptic ulcer disease
   c. Increased risk for hip fractures
   d. Increased risk for hypercalcemia

17. With H2RAs, older adults are more likely to experience adverse effects such as which of the following?
   a. Agitation   c. Hyperplasia
   b. Lethargy   d. Hypertension

18. Mr. Stillson, age 75, is treating his ulcer with antacids. Based on Mr. Stillson's age, you expect the physician to prescribe a dose of antacid that compares with the average prescribed dose in which of the following ways?

    a. Smaller than the average prescribed dose

    b. Larger than the average prescribed dose

    c. The same as the average prescribed dose

    d. No antacids, because they are contraindicated in the elderly

19. You are caring for Mr. O'Malley in your medical unit. He is fed via a nasogastric tube. The dose of antacid is based on which of the following factors?

    a. Signs and symptoms

    b. The pH of the stomach contents

    c. Patient age

    d. Disease processes

20. Mr. Everson is diagnosed with a duodenal ulcer. The physician chooses to treat the ulcer with PPIs. Mr. Everson asks how long he will have to take the medication. You inform him that, although treatment may be extended, most duodenal ulcers heal in about how long?

    a. 6 weeks   c. 4 weeks

    b. 8 weeks   d. 21 days

CHAPTER 60

Laxatives and Cathartics

■ Section I: Learning Objectives

1. Differentiate among the major types of laxatives according to effects on the gastrointestinal tract.
2. Differentiate the consequences of occasional use from those of chronic use.
3. Discuss rational choices of laxatives for selected patient populations or purposes.
4. Discuss bulk-forming laxatives as the most physiologic agents.
5. Discuss possible reasons for and hazards of overuse and abuse of laxatives.

■ Section II: Assessing Your Understanding

ACTIVITY A

Fill in the Blanks

1. Laxatives and cathartics are drugs used to promote bowel _____.
2. The term *laxative* implies mild effects and elimination of _____, _____ stool.
3. The term _____ implies strong effects and elimination of liquid or semiliquid stool.
4. _____ is normally stimulated by movements and reflexes in the gastrointestinal (GI) tract.
5. When the stomach and duodenum are distended with food or fluids, gastrocolic and _____ reflexes cause propulsive movements in the colon, which move feces into the rectum and arouse the urge to defecate.

ACTIVITY B

Matching

Match the term in Column A with the definition in Column B.

COLUMN A

1. _____ Bulk-forming laxatives (e.g., polycarbophil, psyllium seed)

2. _____ Surfactant laxatives (e.g., docusate calcium, potassium, or sodium)

3. _____ Saline laxatives (e.g., magnesium citrate, milk of magnesia)

4. _____ The stimulant cathartics

5. _____ Mineral oil

COLUMN B

A. Substances that are largely unabsorbed from the intestine

B. The strongest and most abused laxative products

C. Decrease the surface tension of the fecal mass to allow water to penetrate into the stool

D. The only lubricant laxative used clinically

E. Not well absorbed from the intestine; increase osmotic pressure in the intestinal lumen and cause water to be retained

ACTIVITY C

Short Answers

Briefly answer the following questions.

1. Explain the process that causes defecation within the human body.
2. Define constipation.
3. Why may cathartics and laxatives be indicated when caring for the elderly?
4. Why may cathartics and laxatives be indicated when caring for the client with a diagnosis of hypertension or myocardial infarction?
5. Why are cathartics and laxatives indicated for clients with the diagnosis of hepatic encephalopathy?

■ Section III: Applying Your Knowledge

ACTIVITY D

Case Study

Consider the scenario and answer the questions.

Mrs. Lomonaco presents to the physician's office with complaints of hard stool and no bowel movement for 5 days. After conducting a client history and physical examination, the physician diagnoses Mrs. Lomonaco with short-term constipation related to change in dietary pattern. The physician orders a saline laxative to be used short term. You are responsible for the client's teaching plan.

1. What can you tell the patient about the absorption of saline laxative? What kind of stool can the patient anticipate after taking the saline laxative?
2. Mrs. Lomonaco asks how long it will take milk of magnesia to work. She does not wish to be embarrassed during her church services and wishes to administer the medication so that she will evacuate before the evening service. How fast does milk of magnesia work?
3. Six weeks later, Mrs. Lomonaco presents to the physician's office with complaints of dizziness. When you take a drug history, you discover that the client has continued the short-term order for milk of magnesia daily for the past 6 weeks. The client states that she fears constipation and the milk of magnesia prevents recurrence. Based on the information accumulated, what do you suspect the client is experiencing?

4. The physician orders a colonoscopy and polyethylene glycol–electrolyte solution for Mrs. Lomonaco. What kind of teaching should you give Mrs. Lomonaco in preparation for this test?
5. Mrs. Lomonaco is diagnosed with occasional constipation. The physician orders polyethylene glycol solution (MiraLax). You are responsible for patient education. What can you tell Mrs. Lomanaco about this treatment?

■ Section IV: Practicing for NCLEX

Answer the following questions.

1. Ms. Rice is diagnosed with chronic idiopathic constipation. What is the drug of choice to treat this condition?
   a. Lubiprostone   c. Mineral oil
   b. Polycarbophil   d. Magnesium citrate

2. Mr. Medina is under treatment for acute congestive heart failure. His current drug regimen includes the potassium-wasting diuretic furosemide and replacement therapy that includes potassium. His current laboratory report indicates that his potassium level is 6.4. The physician will order Kayexalate in conjunction with which of the following?
   a. Milk of magnesia   c. Sorbitol
   b. Mineral oil enema   d. Colace

3. Mr. Givens is diagnosed with hepatic encephalopathy. His ammonia level is 60. The physician orders which of the following medications to decrease the production of the waste product, ammonia?
   a. Milk of magnesia   c. Sorbitol
   b. Colace   d. Lactulose

4. Mr. Bluestone is on aspiration precautions secondary to a CVA. He is experiencing constipation and has not had a bowel movement for 5 days. Digital examination reveals hard stool in the rectal vault. The physician orders a lubricant laxative. Mr. Bluestone is at risk for which of the following?
   a. Hemorrhoids
   b. Lipid aspiration pneumonia
   c. Decreased peristalsis secondary to the CVA
   d. Bowel obstruction secondary to the CVA

5. Ms. Shaw presents to the emergency room with skeletal muscle weakness, dysrhythmias, and hypotension. While taking a drug history, you learn that the client is taking stimulant cathartics to lose weight. Which of the following diagnoses do you suspect?
   a. Alcohol abuse
   b. Hemorrhage
   c. Fluid and electrolyte imbalance
   d. Crohn's disease

6. Polyethylene glycol–electrolyte solution is a nonabsorbable oral solution that rapidly evacuates the bowel within _____ hours.

7. Ms. Cheshire uses saline laxatives as a method of weight control. As part of your education plan, you inform the client that she is at risk for which of the following conditions?
   a. Electrolyte imbalances
   b. Hemorrhage
   c. Anorexia
   d. Binging and purging

8. Mr. Briggs has hemorrhoids, and the physician orders a surfactant laxative. Which of the following effects will this laxative have on the stool?
   a. Make it liquid and easier to expel
   b. Make it semiliquid and easier to expel
   c. Make it softer and easier to expel
   d. Make it formed and easier to expel

9. Which of the following is the most desirable type of laxative for long-term use?
   a. Surfactant laxatives
   b. Stimulant cathartics
   c. Saline laxatives
   d. Bulk-forming laxatives

10. Mr. Koh presents to the emergency department with severe abdominal pain. He states that he hasn't moved his bowels in 5 days. His bowel sounds are absent. He states that he wants a laxative. Which of the following would you expect the physician to order?
    a. Further tests   c. Mineral oil enema
    b. Saline laxative   d. A sedative

11. Which of the following are common reasons for abuse of laxatives and cathartics? (Select all that apply.)
    a. Eating disorders
    b. Desire for strict weight control
    c. Belief that a daily bowel movement is necessary for health
    d. General health colonics

12. _____ and _____ are drugs to promote bowel elimination.

13. Mrs. Decker fears that she is becoming addicted to laxatives. She asks you what she can do to treat her constipation. Which of the following lifestyle modifications would you recommend?
    a. Fluid restrictions
    b. Milk of magnesia every third day
    c. Increase fluid and fiber intake
    d. Limit exercise

14. _____ is the infrequent and painful expulsion of hard, dry stools.

15. Mr. Knight is diagnosed with upper neuron injuries after a motor vehicle accident. Which of the following treatment options will help this patient to evacuate his bowels?
    a. Bowel program
    b. Bladder training program
    c. Regimen of daily saline enemas
    d. Regimen of laxatives every other day

16. Mrs. Keene is a hospice client and is dependent for pain management on opioid analgesics, which slow her gastric motility and cause chronic constipation. Which of the following do you expect the physician to order?
    a. Lifestyle changes
    b. Routine laxative administration
    c. Suppositories each evening
    d. Reduction in the opioid analgesic

17. Parents should be advised not to give children any laxative more than _____ per _____ without consulting a healthcare provider.

18. Mrs. Childs presents to the pediatrician's office with her daughter, who is 4 years old and suffers from constipation. The physician does not order a laxative. You are responsible for the client's education plan. Which of the following would you encourage Mrs. Smith to do?

    a. Increase her daughter's intake of fluids and high-fiber foods

    b. Encourage a sedentary lifestyle for her daughter

    c. Decrease her daughter's exercise, because it leads to dehydration and constipation

    d. Increase pectin in her daughter's diet

19. Mrs. Belt is diagnosed with congestive heart failure. She suffers from periodic constipation. You are responsible for her education plan. Which of the following substances should she avoid using?

    a. Suppositories   c. Milk of magnesia

    b. Saline cathartics d. Colace

20. Oral use of mineral oil may cause potentially serious adverse effects, such as which of the following? (Select all that apply.)

    a. Decreased absorption of fat-soluble vitamins

    b. Decreased absorption of some drugs

    c. Hypertensive crisis

    d. Lipid pneumonia if aspirated into the lungs

CHAPTER 61

Antidiarrheals

■ Section I: Learning Objectives

1. Identify clients who are at risk for development of diarrhea.
2. Discuss guidelines for assessing diarrhea.
3. Describe types of diarrhea for which antidiarrheal drug therapy may be indicated.
4. Differentiate the major types of antidiarrheal drugs.
5. Discuss characteristics, effects, and nursing process implications of commonly used antidiarrheal agents.

■ Section II: Assessing Your Understanding

ACTIVITY A

Fill in the Blanks

1. _____ is a symptom of numerous conditions that increase bowel motility, cause secretion or retention of fluids in the intestinal lumen, and cause inflammation or irritation of the gastrointestinal (GI) tract.
2. *Escherichia coli* O157:H7–related hemorrhagic colitis most commonly occurs with the ingestion of undercooked _____ _____.
3. A serious complication of *E. coli* O157:H7 colitis is _____ _____ syndrome (HUS), which is characterized by thrombocytopenia, microangiopathic hemolytic anemia, and renal failure.
4. So-called travelers' diarrhea is usually caused by an _____ strain of *E. coli* (ETEC).
5. Consumption of improperly prepared poultry may result in diarrhea due to infection with _____ _____.

ACTIVITY B

Matching

Match the term in Column A with the definition in Column B.

COLUMN A

1. _____ Loperamide (Imodium)
2. _____ Octreotide acetate
3. _____ Polycarbophil and psyllium
4. _____ Cholestyramine or colestipol (bile-binding drugs)
5. _____ Rifaximin (Xifaxan)

COLUMN B

A. Structural analog of the antimycobacterial drug, rifampin
B. Useful in treating diarrhea due to bile salt accumulation in conditions such as Crohn's disease or surgical excision of the ileum
C. Synthetic derivative of meperidine that decreases GI motility by its effect on intestinal muscles
D. Synthetic form of somatostatin, a hormone produced in the anterior pituitary gland and in the pancreas
E. Most often used as bulk-forming laxatives

ACTIVITY C

Short Answers

Briefly answer the following questions.

1. How do people contract *Salmonella*?
2. How do people contract *Shigella*?
3. How does a lack of digestive enzymes or a deficiency of pancreatic enzymes affect digestion?
4. What is the mechanism by which inflammatory bowel disorders cause diarrhea?
5. What are the symptoms of irritable bowel syndrome (IBS)?

▪ Section III: Applying Your Knowledge

ACTIVITY D

Case Study

Consider the scenario and answer the questions.

Mrs. North, age 75, was diagnosed 5 years ago with diarrhea-predominant irritable bowel syndrome. She has experienced an overall 40% weight loss since the initial diagnosis. Multiple conventional therapies have been attempted to control her symptoms without success. She states that she has used medications prescribed by three physicians in the past and hopes that she will meet with success this time. After taking a thorough drug history, the physician orders alosetron (Lotronex). You are responsible for the education plan for Mrs. North.

1. Mrs. North asks why this medication has not been available to her in the past. How would you respond? What kind of drug is alosetron?
2. Mrs. North is diagnosed with an obsessive–compulsive disorder and is prescribed fluvoxamine by her psychiatrist. What kind of drug interaction would you expect? What would you expect the physician to do? What are some other contraindications for the use of alosetron?
3. Is Mrs. North's age a factor in the dosing of this drug? What other factors influence the prescription of alosetron?

▪ Section IV: Practicing for NCLEX

Answer the following questions.

1. Mr. Adler is diagnosed with bacterial gastroenteritis. On which of the following factors will treatment be based?
   a. Symptomatology
   b. Causative agent and susceptibility tests
   c. Number of days with diarrhea
   d. The country in which the organism originates

2. Specific therapy for diarrhea is directed at the cause of the symptom. Which of the following treatments may be applied? (Select all that apply.)
   a. Enzymatic replacement therapy
   b. Bile salt–binding drugs
   c. Corticosteroids
   d. 5-HT3 receptor antagonists

3. Polycarbophil is used to treat diarrhea by adsorbing toxins and water, thereby _____ the fluidity of stools.

4. Mr. and Mrs. Anderson present to the physician's office with traveler's diarrhea. Which of the following would you expect the physician to order?
   a. Cholestyramine   c. Octreotide acetate
   b. Psyllium   d. Bismuth subsalicylate

5. Mr. Everley is diagnosed with carcinoid syndrome. Which of the following would you expect the physician to order?
   a. Cholestyramine   c. Bismuth subsalicylate
   b. Octreotide   d. Psyllium

6. The most effective nonspecific therapy for symptomatic treatment of diarrhea is _____ and opiate derivatives.

7. _____ is the frequent expulsion of liquid or semiliquid stools resulting from increased bowel motility, increased secretion or retention of fluids in the intestinal lumen, or inflammation and irritation of the GI tract.

8. Mrs. Edwards is diagnosed with temporary acute diarrhea. Her other diagnoses include diabetes mellitus, dysrhythmia, and hepatic impairment. The physician orders loperamide. Based on her diagnoses, which of the following signs would you observe for in this patient?
   a. Signs of electrolyte imbalance
   b. Signs of hemorrhage
   c. Signs of hypercalcemia
   d. Signs of CNS toxicity

9. A physician orders diphenoxylate to treat a client who has severe hepatorenal disease. On what basis should you question this order?

   a. It may precipitate hepatic coma.

   b. It may precipitate hyperkalemia.

   c. It may precipitate hypercalcemia.

   d. It may precipitate hyperglycemia.

10. When administering diphenoxylate to children, you should observe for signs of which of the following conditions?

    a. Atropine overdose

    b. Opioid overdose

    c. Fluid and electrolyte imbalance

    d. Hypotensive crisis

11. In diarrhea caused by enzyme deficiency, _____ _____ are given, rather than antidiarrheal drugs.

12. Which of the following doses of morphine is considered effective to treat diarrheal episodes?

    a. 2 mg   c. 6 mg

    b. 4 mg   d. 1.25 mg

13. In antibiotic-associated colitis, which of the following is the initial treatment?

    a. Imodium

    b. Stopping the causative drug

    c. Administering a medication that will slow peristalsis

    d. Administering a low-dose opioid

14. Mrs. Franklin develops antibiotic-induced colitis. The symptoms have worsened within the past 72 hours. Which of the following would you expect the physician to order as the initial drug of choice?

    a. Loperamide   c. Metronidazole

    b. Bismuth subsalicylate   d. Psyllium

15. In ulcerative colitis, which of the following is one of the drugs of choice?

    a. Loperamide   c. Metronidazole

    b. Psyllium   d. Sulfonamide

16. For symptomatic treatment of diarrhea, which *two* of the following drugs would be initial choices for treatment?

    a. Diphenoxylate with atropine

    b. Psyllium

    c. Metronidazole

    d. Loperamide

17. The choice of antidiarrheal agent depends largely on the cause, severity, and _____ of the diarrhea.

18. In most cases of acute, nonspecific diarrhea in adults, fluid losses are not severe and clients need only simple replacement of fluids and electrolytes lost in the stool. Which of the following is an acceptable replacement fluid during the first 24 hours?

    a. 2 to 3 liters of clear liquids

    b. 1 to 2 liters of clear liquids

    c. 0.5 to 1 liter of clear liquids

    d. 3 to 4 liters of clear liquids

19. Contraindications to the use of antidiarrheal drugs include diarrhea caused by which of the following? (Select all that apply.)

    a. Toxic materials

    b. Microorganisms that penetrate intestinal mucosa

    c. Unknown origin

    d. Antibiotic-associated colitis

20. _____ is an antiprotozoal agent used specifically for treating diarrhea resulting from infection with *Giardia lamblia* or *Cryptosporidium parvum.*

CHAPTER 62

Antiemetics

■ Section I: Learning Objectives

1. Identify patients who are at risk of developing nausea and vomiting.
2. Discuss guidelines for preventing, minimizing, or treating nausea and vomiting.
3. Differentiate the major types of antiemetic drugs.
4. Discuss characteristics, effects, and nursing process implications of selected antiemetic drugs.

■ Section II: Assessing Your Understanding

ACTIVITY A

Fill in the Blanks

1. _____ drugs are used to prevent or treat nausea and vomiting.
2. _____ is an unpleasant sensation of abdominal discomfort accompanied by a desire to vomit.
3. _____ is the expulsion of stomach contents through the mouth.
4. Nausea and vomiting are the most common _____ _____ of drug therapy.
5. Vomiting occurs when the _____ _____, a nucleus of cells in the medulla oblongata, is stimulated.

ACTIVITY B

Matching

Match the term in Column A with the definition in Column B.

COLUMN A

1. _____ Prochlorperazine (Compazine) phenothiazines

2. _____ Dexamethasone and methylprednisolone

3. _____ Lorazepam (Ativan)

4. _____ Metoclopramide (Reglan)

5. _____ Ondansetron (Zofran), granisetron (Kytril), dolasetron (Anzemet), and palonosetron (Aloxi)

COLUMN B

A. Prokinetic agent that increases GI motility and the rate of gastric emptying by peripheral cholinergic effects

B. Effective in preventing or treating nausea and vomiting induced by drugs, radiation therapy, surgery, and most other stimuli

C. Often prescribed for patients who experience anticipatory nausea and vomiting before administration of anticancer drugs

D. Commonly used in the management of chemotherapy-induced emesis and postoperative nausea and vomiting

E. Antagonize serotonin receptors, preventing their activation by the effects of emetogenic drugs and toxins

ACTIVITY C

Short Answers

Briefly answer the following questions.

1. Identify three drugs most commonly associated with the adverse effects of nausea and vomiting.
2. Identify three causes other than drugs that may produce nausea and vomiting.
3. List five of the receptors located in the vomiting center, CTZ, and GI tract, which are stimulated by emetogenic drugs and toxins.
4. Describe the physiologic processes that occur during vomiting, beginning with the stimulation of the vomiting center and ending with the stomach contents' arriving toward the mouth for ejection.
5. Define the term *anticipatory nausea.*

■ Section III: Applying Your Knowledge

ACTIVITY D

Case Study

Consider the scenario and answer the questions.

Mrs. Homan was diagnosed with cancer and subsequently treated with chemotherapeutic agents. She develops moderate nausea and vomiting after chemotherapy; she is losing weight and stamina and has a significant fluid and electrolyte imbalance. The physician prescribes metoclopramide (Reglan). You are responsible for the client's education plan.

1. How does metoclopramide decrease nausea and vomiting? How is metoclopramide typically used?
2. What can you tell Mrs. Homan about when the effect of the medication begins and how long it lasts?
3. Mrs. Homan wishes to return to work part-time, now that her nausea is managed. What adverse effect may impact her decision? Mrs. Homan asks if she may have a few drinks during the Christmas party for cancer survivors next week. What do you know about the combination of alcohol and metoclopramide?
4. Mrs. Homan remains on the metoclopramide after chemotherapy for residual symptoms related to gastroparesis. Two years later, she develops Parkinson's disease. What would you expect the physician to do with Mrs. Homan's metoclopramide prescription?

■ Section IV: Practicing for NCLEX

Answer the following questions.

1. Mrs. Jenks is going on a cruise to Nova Scotia with her husband to celebrate their 15th wedding anniversary. She is concerned because she has experienced severe, debilitating, sea sickness in the past. Which of the following would you expect the physician to order?
   a. Scopolamine
   b. Dexamethasone
   c. Metoclopramide
   d. Ondansetron

2. Mrs. Blanching is receiving chemotherapy to treat her cancer. Several antiemetics have been prescribed, and each has been unsuccessful in treating her nausea and vomiting. The physician chooses to prescribe which of the following cannabinoid drug to manage her symptoms?
   a. Scopolamine
   b. Metoclopramide
   c. Ondansetron
   d. Dronabinol

3. Which of the following drugs antagonizes the neurokinin 1 receptor, preventing activation by emetogenic chemotherapeutic drugs?
   a. Metoclopramide
   b. Aprepitant
   c. Ondansetron
   d. Dronabinol

4. Which of the following 5-HT3 serotonin receptor antagonists antagonize serotonin receptors, thereby preventing their activation by emetogenic drugs and toxins?
   a. Metoclopramide
   b. Aprepitant
   c. Ondansetron
   d. Dronabinol

5. Which of the following drugs is a prokinetic agent that functions by increasing the release of acetylcholine from nerve endings in the GI tract, thereby increasing GI motility and gastric emptying?
   a. Metoclopramide
   b. Aprepitant
   c. Ondansetron
   d. Dronabinol

6. Mrs. Gantry prepares to begin her second round of chemotherapy. She tells the physician that she knows that the nausea and vomiting will be worse this time around. The physician orders lorazepam because it has which of the following effects? (Select all that apply.)

    a. Producing relaxation

    b. Relieving anxiety

    c. Inhibiting cerebral cortex input to the vomiting center

    d. Creating a sense of euphoria

7. Which of the following medications may be used in combination with a 5-HT3 serotonin receptor antagonist to manage chemotherapy-induced emesis?

    a. Scopolamine   c. Metoclopramide

    b. Dexamethasone   d. Ondansetron

8. Antiemetic drugs are most effective when given _____ nausea and vomiting occurs.

9. What tasks are included in the role of the home care nurse visiting a client who is receiving antiemetics? (Select all that apply.)

    a. Assessing patients for possible causes of nausea and vomiting

    b. Assisting patients and caregivers with appropriate use of the drugs

    c. Providing interventions to prevent fluid and electrolyte depletion

    d. Administering all antiemetics to clients who experience nausea and vomiting

10. As a result of chemotherapy, Mr. Redford experiences hepatic dysfunction. Part of the client's medication regimen includes the use of phenothiazines. Which of the following would you expect the physician to do?

    a. Use an alternative medication

    b. Increase the dose of the medication

    c. Decrease the dose of the medication

    d. Maintain the current dose of the medication

11. Most antiemetic drugs are metabolized in the liver and should be used cautiously in patients with impaired hepatic function. For clients diagnosed with hepatic impairment, the dose of ondansetron should not exceed which of the following amounts?

    a. 8 mg   c. 10 mg

    b. 6 mg   d. 12 mg

12. As an adverse effect of her chemotherapy, Mrs. Pearson develops moderate to severe renal impairment. She routinely takes metoclopramide for chemotherapy-related nausea and vomiting with success and does not wish to change drugs. Which of the following would you expect the physician to do?

    a. Maintain the current dose of the metoclopramide

    b. Decrease the dosage of the metoclopramide

    c. Increase the dosage of the metoclopramide

    d. Discontinue the metoclopramide

13. Mr. Benjamin, age 75, develops nausea and vomiting secondary to administration of a new drug regimen to treat his Parkinson's disease. He is at risk for which of the following?

    a. Increased extrapyramidal effects

    b. Fluid and electrolyte imbalance

    c. Prostatitis

    d. Anxiety-induced vomiting

14. The American Society of Clinical Oncology recommends the use of which of the following drug combinations before administration of high-dose chemotherapy or chemotherapy with high to moderate emetic risk to pediatric oncology patients?

    a. An 5-HT3 receptor antagonist plus a phenothiazine

    b. An 5-HT3 receptor antagonist plus a antianxiety agent

    c. An 5-HT3 receptor antagonist plus a cannabinoid

    d. An 5-HT3 receptor antagonist plus a corticosteroid

15. A black box warning alerts nurses that promethazine is contraindicated in children younger than 2 years of age because of which of the following risks?

    a. Fatal hypovolemia secondary to hemorrhage

    b. Life-threatening cardiac dysrhythmias

    c. Fatal respiratory depression

    d. Fatal hypertension and subsequent cerebral vascular accident

16. The _____ _____ _____ are usually considered the most effective antiemetics. They may be given in a single daily dose.

17. If nausea and vomiting are likely to occur because of travel, administration of emetogenic anticancer drugs, diagnostic tests, or therapeutic procedures, an antiemetic drug should be given before the emetogenic event. Pretreatment has which of the following effects? (Select all that apply.)

    a. Increasing patient comfort

    b. Allowing use of lower drug doses

    c. Possibly preventing aspiration

    d. Possibly preventing extrapyramidal symptoms

18. A client is experiencing nausea and vomiting related to nonobstructive gastric retention after abdominal surgery. Which of the following would you expect the physician to order?

    a. Scopolamine   c. Metoclopramide

    b. Dexamethasone   d. Ondansetron

19. A client develops labyrinthitis. What would you expect the physician to order?

    a. Scopolamine   c. Metoclopramide

    b. Dexamethasone   d. Meclizine

20. Promethazine (Phenergan), a phenothiazine, is often used clinically for its _____, antiemetic, and sedative effects.

CHAPTER 63

Drugs Used in Ophthalmic Conditions

■ Section I: Learning Objectives

1. Review characteristics of ocular structures that influence drug therapy for eye disorders.
2. Discuss selected drugs in relation to their use in ocular disorders.
3. Use correct techniques to administer ophthalmic medications.
4. Assess for ocular effects of systemic drugs and systemic effects of ophthalmic drugs.
5. Teach patients, family members, or caregivers correct administration of eye medications.
6. For a patient with an eye disorder, teach about the importance of taking medications as prescribed to protect and preserve eyesight.

■ Section II: Assessing Your Understanding

ACTIVITY A

Fill in the Blanks

1. Refractive errors that cause nearsightedness are called _____.
2. Refractive errors that cause farsightedness are called _____.
3. Refractive errors include myopia, hyperopia, _____, and astigmatism.
4. Conditions that cause refractive errors impair vision by interfering with the eye's ability to focus light rays on the _____.
5. Ophthalmic drugs are used only in the _____ of the refractive error conditions; treatment involves prescription of eyeglasses or contact lenses.

ACTIVITY B

Matching

Match the term in Column A with the definition in Column B.

COLUMN A

1. _____ Conjunctivitis
2. _____ Blepharitis
3. _____ Keratitis (inflammation of the cornea)
4. _____ Fungal infections
5. _____ Bacterial corneal ulcers

COLUMN B

A. Common eye disorder that may be caused by allergens, bacterial or viral infections, or physical or chemical irritants
B. Commonly occur and may often be attributed to frequent use of ophthalmic antibiotics and corticosteroids
C. Chronic infection of glands and lash follicles on the margins of the eyelids, characterized by burning, redness, and itching
D. Most often caused by pneumococci and staphylococci
E. May be caused by microorganisms, trauma, allergy, ischemia, and drying of the cornea

ACTIVITY C

Short Answers

Briefly answer the following questions.

1. Explain how the eyelids and lacrimal system function to protect the eye.
2. Explain the difference between miosis and mydriasis.
3. Outline the structure of the eyeball.
4. Discuss the process that causes vision to occur.
5. Define refraction.

■ Section III: Applying Your Knowledge

ACTIVITY D
Case Study

Consider the scenario and answer the questions.

Mrs. Lincoln, a 75-year-old African-American woman, is diagnosed with primary open-angle glaucoma. She also has hypertension. You are responsible for her education plan.

1. Mrs. Lincoln asks you how glaucoma is diagnosed and how the physician is sure that she has this illness. What is your understanding of a diagnosis of glaucoma? What is the range of intraocular pressure that is characteristic of glaucoma?
2. What are Mrs. Lincoln's risk factors for glaucoma? For which condition is Mrs. Lincoln further at risk because of her glaucoma?
3. As part of your patient teaching, what can you tell Mrs. Lincoln about glaucoma? What type of disease is it? What characterizes the disease?
4. If Mrs. Lincoln were to present to the physician's office with nausea, blurred vision with halo, and, when assessed, increased intraocular pressure and report that she had taken a tricyclic antidepressant, what diagnosis is likely?

■ Section IV: Practicing for NCLEX

Answer the following questions.

1. Mrs. Young is diagnosed with cardiac disease. She is also prescribed local eye medications. You caution Mrs. Young that local eye medications may cause which of the following effects?
   a. Increased visual acuity
   b. Systemic effects
   c. Local effects
   d. Exacerbation of her glaucoma

2. Under which of the following conditions should eye medications be kept?
   a. Refrigerated
   b. Sterile
   c. Clean
   d. In a warm environment

3. Mrs. Hinton complains that she must administer her eye drops several times because she blinks. How might this influence the therapeutic effects of the drops?
   a. Therapeutic effects depend on administration of the medication on a routine basis.
   b. Therapeutic effects may vary due to blinking.
   c. Therapeutic effects may vary due to the medication schedule.
   d. Therapeutic effects depend on accurate administration.

4. Drug therapy of eye disorders is unique because of which of the following factors? (Select all that apply.)
   a. Location of the eye
   b. Structure of the eye
   c. Function of the eye
   d. Proximity of the eye to the brain

5. Which of the following tasks does the role of the home care nurse caring for clients with acute or chronic eye disorders include? (Select all that apply.)
   a. Teaching patients and caregivers reasons for use of drugs
   b. Teaching accurate administration technique of drugs
   c. Assessment of therapeutic and adverse drug reactions
   d. Diagnosis of eye disorders

6. To prevent exacerbation of cardiac symptoms, which of the following should the nurse do?
   a. Schedule eye drugs to coincide with cardiac drugs
   b. Schedule eye drugs 2 hours before cardiac drugs
   c. Occlude the nasolacrimal duct in the inner canthus of the eye
   d. Schedule eye drugs 1 hour before cardiac drugs

7. A major use of topical ophthalmic drugs in children is to dilate the pupil and _____ accommodation for ophthalmoscopic examination.

8. You would expect a pediatrician to order which of the following drugs as a general rule for children?
   a. Long-acting mydriatics
   b. Cyclopentolate
   c. Gentamicin
   d. Fluoroquinolone

9. For chronic glaucoma, the goal of drug therapy is to slow disease progression by reducing IOP. What are the first-line drugs used to treat glaucoma?
   a. Topical ACE inhibitors
   b. Topical beta blockers
   c. Antibacterials
   d. Mydriatics

10. Ms. Lawrence, a contact lens wearer, presents to the physician with a corneal abrasion. Which of the following would you expect the physician to order?
    a. Topical ace inhibitor
    b. Topical beta blocker
    c. Antipseudomonal antibiotic
    d. Antistaphylococcal antibiotic

11. Most corneal abrasions heal in _____ to _____ hours.

12. Mr. Cotter presents to the physician's office with symptoms of an eye infection. He is diagnosed with a fungal infection. Which of the following would you expect the physician to prescribe?
    a. Amoxicillin   c. Penicillin
    b. Natamycin   d. Nystatin

13. Mr. Smith gets dust in his eyes when he is cleaning his furnace. He flushes his eyes in the sink and 3 days later presents to the physician's office with symptoms of a severe infectious process. The physician orders both a topical and a systemic antibiotic. Which of the following systemic antibiotics is appropriate?
    a. Natamycin   c. Erythromycin
    b. Ampicillin   d. Vancomycin

14. Four days later, Mr. Smith again presents to the physician's office, with increased inflammation to his eye. Which of the following would you expect the physician to prescribe?
    a. Gentamicin   c. Natamycin
    b. Dicloxacillin   d. Vancomycin

15. Mr. Benson presents to the physician's office with drainage and inflammation in his right eye. Which of the following would you expect the physician to do?
    a. Order a topical antibiotic
    b. Refer the client to an optometrist
    c. Order a systemic antibiotic
    d. Order a culture and sensitivity of the drainage

16. Ms. Gonzalez wears soft contact lenses. She uses eye drops containing benzalkonium. You teach the client that the medication should be instilled under which of the following conditions?
    a. 15 minutes or longer before inserting soft contacts
    b. While wearing the soft contacts
    c. 15 minutes after application of the soft contacts
    d. 5 minutes before inserting soft contacts

17. To increase safety and accuracy of ophthalmic drug therapy, the labels and caps of eye medications are _____ _____.

18. Mr. Holtz is prescribed a topical ophthalmic medication. When should he discard the medication? (Select all that apply.)
    a. After the expiration date
    b. If it becomes cloudy
    c. If the color changes
    d. If his condition improves

19. The physician prescribes medication for a client's eye disorder. His concern is that the client requires high concentrations of the drug. Which of the following would you expect the physician to order?
    a. Ointment   c. Distilled formulation
    b. Drop   d. Suspension

20. Absorption of eye medications is increased in eye disorders associated with _____ and inflammation.

CHAPTER 64

Drugs Used in Dermatologic Conditions

■ Section I: Learning Objectives

1. Review characteristics of skin structures that influence drug therapy for dermatologic disorders.
2. Discuss antimicrobial, anti-inflammatory, and selected miscellaneous drugs in relation to their use in dermatologic disorders.
3. Use correct techniques to administer dermatologic medications.
4. Teach patients, family members, or caregivers correct administration of dermatologic medications.
5. For patients with "open lesion" skin disorders, teach about the importance and techniques of preventing infection.
6. Practice and teach measures to protect the skin from the damaging effects of sun exposure.

■ Section II: Assessing Your Understanding

ACTIVITY A

Fill in the Blanks

1. The skin is the largest body organ and the interface between the internal and external _____.
2. Epidermal or epithelial cells begin in the _____ layer of the epidermis and migrate outward, undergoing degenerative changes in each layer.
3. The outer layer of the skin is called the _____ _____ and is composed of dead cells and keratin.
4. _____ is a tough protein substance that is insoluble in water, weak acids, and weak bases.
5. _____ are pigment-producing cells located at the junction of the epidermis and the dermis.

ACTIVITY B

Matching

Match the term in Column A with the definition in Column B.

COLUMN A

1. _____ Aloe
2. _____ Azelaic acid (Azelex)
3. _____ Oral isotretinoin (Accutane)
4. _____ Coal-tar preparations
5. _____ Hydrocortisone

COLUMN B

A. Has antibacterial activity against *P. acnes*
B. Have anti-inflammatory and antipruritic actions and can be used alone or with topical corticosteroids
C. Is often used as a topical remedy for minor burns and wounds (e.g., sunburn, cuts, abrasions) to decrease pain, itching, and inflammation and to promote healing
D. Is the corticosteroid most often included in topical otic preparations
E. May be used for patients with severe acne not responsive to safer drugs

ACTIVITY C

Short Answers

Briefly answer the following questions.

1. Describe melanocytes and identify their function.
2. Identify three dermal structures.
3. Describe the composition of mucous membranes.
4. Discuss the difference between primary and secondary dermatologic disorders.
5. Describe how the skin regulates body temperature.

■ Section III: Applying Your Knowledge

ACTIVITY D

Case Study

Consider the scenario and answer the questions.

Ms. Benjamin presents to the physician's office with a red, patchy area on her right forearm that is draining pus. The physician diagnoses the area as atopic dermatitis and prescribes an antibiotic.

1. The client asks you if the antibiotic will cure the atopic dermatitis. How would you respond?
2. Ms. Benjamin asks you if she contracted the dermatitis from her brother; she cared for him when he had the chicken pox. What can you tell Ms. Benjamin about the cause of atopic dermatitis?
3. The physician stages the atopic dermatitis as acute. When you inspect the affected area, what would you expect to find? What other disease process may be evident based on Mrs. Benjamin's diagnosis of atopic dermatitis?
4. You instruct Mrs. Benjamin to avoid possible causes or exacerbating factors. She asks you if she has to give up her job as a financial consultant. What factor related to her profession may cause an exacerbation of her dermatitis?
5. Mrs. Benjamin is concerned and asks you if the red patches on her child's elbows and forearms may be indicative of atopic dermatitis. What should you suggest to her?

■ Section IV: Practicing for NCLEX

Answer the following questions.

1. Mr. Billings is prescribed a combination of topical drugs to treat his atopic dermatitis. Which of the following statements by Mr. Billings indicates that he requires further education regarding his medication regimen?
   a. "The drug therapy will reduce the inflammation caused by my disease."
   b. "The drug therapy may cause dryness of the skin."
   c. "Local drug therapy will not be absorbed systemically."
   d. "The drug therapy may cause adverse effects."

2. Special precautions are needed for safe use of oral retinoids in which of the following patient populations?
   a. Male patients with a history of prostate disease
   b. Children with a diagnosis of diabetes type 1
   c. Female clients with asthmatic bronchitis
   d. Female patients of childbearing potential

3. Special precautions are needed for safe use of topical corticosteroids, especially in which group of patients?
   a. Males
   b. Females
   c. Children
   d. Females with comorbidities

4. The physician orders daily topical drugs to treat Mr. Wong's dermatitis. Which of the following factors is important to teach the patient?
   a. Accurate application to maximize therapeutic effects
   b. PRN usage
   c. Rationale for an open prescription
   d. Alternative medications that are available

5. Mr. Bingley, age 75, develops a red patchy area on his shin. To assist in the diagnosis of the lesion, which of the following must the nurse report? (Select all that apply.)
   a. Type of lesions   c. Location of lesions
   b. Age of client   d. Sex of the client

6. Which of the following are the most common bacterial causes of skin infection? (Select all that apply.)
   a. Staphylococci   c. *Morganella morgani*
   b. Enterococci   d. Streptococci

7. When a patient is treated for skin disorders, which of the following tasks are included in the role of the home care nurse? (Select all that apply.)
   a. Assessing patients and other members of the household
   b. Assessing the home environment for risks of skin disorders
   c. Researching genetic or environmental factors contributing to the skin disorder
   d. Assessing response to treatment

8. The physician orders a topical corticosteroid for a rash on Mr. Golden's elbow. Mr. Golden, age 75, also has hypertension, chronic congestive heart failure, and diabetes type 2. Which of the following is a concern in this situation?

   a. Corticosteroids may be absorbed systemically and exacerbate congestive heart failure symptoms.

   b. Corticosteroids should be used with caution on thin or atrophic skin.

   c. Corticosteroids may diminish signs of infection on the elbow.

   d. Corticosteroids may exacerbate symptoms related to diabetes type 2.

9. What is one rationale for the cautious use of topical agents in infants?

   a. Diminished absorption of the drug

   b. Infant skin is more permeable

   c. Inconsistent use of the drugs in the health care environment

   d. Infant skin is significantly less permeable

10. Which of the following adverse effects are associated with the use of topical corticosteroids in children? (Select all that apply.)

    a. Febrile episodes

    b. Cushing's disease

    c. Intracranial hypertension

    d. Postural hypotension

11. The physician orders topical corticosteroids for Jayme V, age 2, a patient in your pediatric unit. When noting the physician's order, which of the following would cause you concern?

    a. The smallest effective dose is ordered.

    b. The open-ended order includes the use of an occlusive dressing.

    c. The order is for the shortest effective time.

    d. The drug is ordered in a topical form.

12. Mrs. Gonzales is diagnosed with chronic histamine-induced urticaria. As part of your education plan, when would you teach the client to administer the antihistamine?

    a. Only when the lesions appear

    b. Before the symptoms appear and PRN thereafter

    c. Before the symptoms appear and round the clock thereafter

    d. When the symptoms appear and round the clock thereafter

13. _____ is the oral retinoid of choice for treatment of severe psoriasis.

14. Methotrexate is an antineoplastic drug that has long been used to treat psoriasis because it suppresses inflammation and proliferation of which of the following?

    a. B lymphocytes   c. M lymphocytes

    b. NK lymphocytes   d. T lymphocytes

15. Mr. Preston presents to the physician's office complaining that he has difficulty sleeping because of the intense itching related to his dermatitis. To relieve the itching and promote sleep, which of the following would you expect the physician to order?

    a. Diphenhydramine

    b. Oral isotretinoin (Accutane)

    c. Corticosteroids

    d. Antibiotic therapy

16. The physician may prescribe which of the following drugs to a female with high levels of androgens and acne?

    a. Estrogen   c. Anhydrin

    b. Antiandrogens   d. Androgens

17. Ms. Batten is prescribed retinoids for her moderate acne. She returns to the office 1 week later, disappointed because she does not see improvement in her condition. You explain to the client that improvement may not be seen for up to how many weeks?

    a. 5   c. 10

    b. 7   d. 12

18. _____ _____ are first-line treatment for patients with moderate to severe inflammatory acne.

19. Which of the following treatment modalities are most effective in treating skin conditions?

    a. Clindamycin

    b. Benzoyl peroxide

    c. Topical erythromycin

    d. Topical antibiotic and benzoyl peroxide

20. When treating skin conditions, on which of the following does dosage depend? (Select all that apply.)

    a. Length of application

    b. Drug concentration

    c. Area of application

    d. Method of application

CHAPTER 65

Drug Use During Pregnancy and Lactation

■ Section I: Learning Objectives

1. Discuss reasons for minimizing drug use during pregnancy and lactation.
2. Describe selected fetotoxic and teratogenic drugs.
3. Discuss guidelines for drug therapy of pregnancy-associated signs and symptoms.
4. Discuss guidelines for drug therapy of selected chronic disorders during pregnancy and lactation.
5. Discuss which immunizations are considered safe for use during pregnancy and which are contraindicated.
6. Teach women of childbearing potential to avoid prescribed and over-the-counter drugs when possible and to inform all health care providers if there is a possibility of pregnancy.
7. Discuss the role of the home care nurse working with a pregnant woman.
8. Discuss drugs used during pregnancy complications and during normal labor and delivery in terms of their effects on the mother and newborn infant.
9. Describe abortifacients in terms of characteristics and nursing process implications.

■ Section II: Assessing Your Understanding

ACTIVITY A

Fill in the Blanks

1. Drugs that are potentially harmful to the fetus are _____.
2. _____ (formation of fetal organs) occurs during the first 2 to 8 weeks after conception.
3. On the maternal side, _____ _____ _____ carries blood and drugs to the placenta.
4. Drugs used to stop preterm labor are _____.

5. Drugs ingested by a pregnant woman reach the fetus through the maternal–placental–fetal circulation, which is completed by about the _____ _____ after conception.

ACTIVITY B

Matching

Match the term in Column A with the definition in Column B.

COLUMN A

1. _____ Magnesium sulfate
2. _____ Nifedipine
3. _____ NSAIDs, such as indomethacin
4. _____ Terbutaline
5. _____ Erythromycin ointment 0.5%

COLUMN B

A. Inhibit uterine prostaglandins that help to initiate the uterine contractions of normal labor
B. Long given IV as a first-line agent, but now considered ineffective as a tocolytic
C. Applied to each eye at delivery; effective against both chlamydial and gonococcal infections
D. Calcium channel blocking drug that decreases uterine contractions
E. Beta-adrenergic agent that inhibits uterine contractions by reducing intracellular calcium levels

ACTIVITY C

Short Answers

Briefly answer the following questions.

1. How do the physiologic changes during pregnancy influence drug effects on the mother and fetus?
2. Explain how the fetus metabolizes and excretes most drugs.
3. What impact does the fetal blood–brain barrier have on the absorption of drugs into the brain?
4. What role does the maternal circulation have in the metabolism and excretion of drugs?
5. What is the impact on the fetus of drugs taken on a regular schedule by the mother?

■ Section III: Applying Your Knowledge

ACTIVITY D

Case Study

Consider the scenario and answer the questions.

Mrs. Waddell, age 25, discovers that she is pregnant with her second child. She presents to the physician's office for her first prenatal visit. The physician orders laboratory testing before the visit.

1. Mrs. Waddell is diagnosed with folic acid deficiency anemia. She states that she is healthy and takes a multivitamin with minerals once a day. What would you expect the physician to do?
2. Mrs. Waddell states that she took extra iron supplements with her last pregnancy to prevent anemia. The physician did not order it this time, and she is concerned. She wants a healthy baby. What do you know about iron supplementation in pregnancy?
3. Mrs. Waddell develops GERD in her sixth month of pregnancy. She asks whether antacids are an acceptable treatment for her condition. What do you know about the use of antacids during pregnancy? What nonpharmacologic treatments could this patient use for her GERD?
4. When the patient is in her eight month, she experiences constipation related to her pregnancy. She informs you that she routinely takes mineral oil because it softens the stool and does not irritate her hemorrhoids. What alternate treatment can you suggest? Why shouldn't the patient use mineral oil as a laxative?

■ Section IV: Practicing for NCLEX

Answer the following questions.

1. Mrs. Allen develops a headache and asks you if it is safe to take aspirin 1 hour before breastfeeding. Which of the following is an appropriate response?
   a. "The aspirin will not be absorbed by the baby."
   b. "Aspirin should be avoided during lactation; consult your physician."
   c. "Your headache may interfere with letdown; take the aspirin."
   d. "Aspirin is the drug of choice for pain during the lactation period."

2. Mrs. Sikes' friend offers her an herbal tea that helps to prevent miscarriage and promote fetal health. She asks you if the drug is safe. Which of the following would be your response?
   a. "Herbal drugs are safe during pregnancy in moderation."
   b. "Teas in general are safe during pregnancy."
   c. "The tea should be administered in moderation."
   d. "Drugs should be avoided during pregnancy."

3. To prevent neural tube defects, a physician may prescribe which of the following drugs during pregnancy?
   a. Folic acid
   b. Vitamin C
   c. Iron
   d. Multivitamin with minerals

4. Mrs. Smith is considering pregnancy; she is healthy and does not take prescription medications. She asks you for advice. Which of the following should you suggest this patient do?
   a. Avoid over-the-counter medications before pregnancy
   b. Begin fertility drugs as soon as possible
   c. Avoid multivitamins with minerals before pregnancy
   d. Double the dose of her multivitamins with minerals before pregnancy

5. Major concerns with drug use during pregnancy are fetotoxicity and _____.

6. Ms. Bergman is diagnosed with hyperemesis, and the physician orders a home care nurse to assess her during her pregnancy. In order to care for the client, what qualifications should the nurse have?

   a. Experience in care of obstetric clients

   b. Obstetric specialty

   c. Maternal home care nursing specialty

   d. Scheduled next as the nurse to admit new clients

7. The physician orders short-term therapy for a disease process in a patient who is breastfeeding. The medication is transferred to the baby during lactation. Which of the following should the patient do?

   a. Pump and discard her milk

   b. Disregard the prescription

   c. Continue to breastfeed

   d. Stop breastfeeding until the medication regimen is complete

8. Ms. Corday delivers a healthy daughter. The patient, who is HIV positive, asks when she should begin breastfeeding. What is the appropriate response?

   a. "Breastfeeding is based on your T-cell level."

   b. "As soon as the breastfeeding coach arrives."

   c. "You should not breastfeed."

   d. "When the child is hungry."

9. Mrs. Herrera discovers she is pregnant. She asks the physician for a rubella vaccination. Which of the following do you anticipate the physician will do?

   a. Decline, because the rubella vaccine is a live-virus vaccine

   b. Decline, because a titer was not drawn

   c. Administer the vaccine, because the client is in her first trimester

   d. Administer the vaccine regardless of the trimester, because of the risk-versus-benefit ratio

10. Mrs. Dorland suffers from migraine headaches. Her friend tells her that acetaminophen is safe to take during pregnancy. She asks you if it is safe to take the drug for her migraines. Which of the following statements is true?

    a. Acetaminophen is safe in this circumstance.

    b. The patient requires a stronger medication.

    c. Acetaminophen is the drug of choice for migraines.

    d. The physician should be consulted regarding diagnosis and the medication prescribed.

11. One hour after delivery, Mrs. East is concerned that her child is listless. You would evaluate which of the following?

    a. The child's ability to breastfeed

    b. Antibiotic administration to the mother before delivery

    c. Drugs received by the mother during labor and delivery

    d. Maternal nutrition

12. A mother asks why the nurse administers phytonadione to her newborn after delivery. Which of the following does the drug prevent?

    a. Syphilis   c. Calcium deficiency

    b. Gonorrhea   d. Hemorrhagic disease

13. Drug therapy should be initiated with low doses, especially with drugs that are highly bound to plasma _____.

14. Ophthalmia neonatorum is a form of bacterial conjunctivitis that may cause ulceration and blindness. This is most commonly caused by which of the following?

    a. Gonorrhea

    b. *Chlamydia trachomatis*

    c. *Staphylococcus aureus*

    d. Methicillin-resistant *Staphylococcus aureus*

15. Which of the following is one of the benefits of using regional anesthesia during labor and delivery?

    a. The neonate is rarely depressed.

    b. The mother sleeps during labor and delivery.

    c. The mother is semiconscious during labor and delivery.

    d. The neonate is lethargic after delivery.

16. Ms. Penn receives Duramorph through her epidural catheter after undergoing a cesarean section. For which of the following should you observe the client?
    a. Hypertension   c. Diarrhea
    b. Urinary retention   d. Dysrhythmia

17. Ms. Harbor received parenteral opioid analgesics during labor and deliver of her first child. You observe that the neonate is experiencing respiratory depression. Which of the following is the drug of choice in this case?
    a. Magnesium sulfate   c. Morphine sulfate
    b. Terbutaline   d. Naloxone

18. Pitocin is given to prevent which of the following conditions?
    a. Letdown
    b. Postpartum bleeding
    c. Postpartum hypotension
    d. Eclampsia

19. Prostaglandins $F_{2\alpha}$ and E_2 stimulate uterine contractions by increasing intracellular calcium concentrations and activating the _____–_____ contractile units of uterine muscle.

20. Mrs. Olinger exhibits symptoms related to preterm labor. She is 37 weeks' pregnant. The physician orders magnesium sulfate. You note symptoms of hypermagnesemia and report this to the physician. Which of the following would you expect the physician to order?
    a. Calcium gluconate   c. Magnesium sulfate
    b. Calcium magnate   d. Narcan

Answers

Chapter 1: Introduction to Pharmacology

SECTION II: ASSESSING YOUR UNDERSTANDING

ACTIVITY A
FILL IN THE BLANKS
1. Pharmacology
2. Drug therapy
3. Medications
4. Prototypes
5. Pharmacoeconomics

ACTIVITY B
MATCHING
1. D   2. E   3. B   4. A   5. C

ACTIVITY C
SEQUENCING

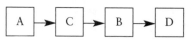

ACTIVITY D
SHORT ANSWERS
1. Drugs with local effects, such as sunscreen lotions and local anesthetics, act mainly at the site of application.
2. Drugs with systemic effects are taken into the body, circulated through the bloodstream to their sites of action in various body tissues, and eventually eliminated from the body.
3. Synthetic drugs are more standardized in their chemical characteristics, more consistent in their effects, and less likely to produce allergic reactions.
4. The process of biotechnology involves manipulating deoxyribonucleic acid (DNA) and ribonucleic acid (RNA) and recombining genes into hybrid molecules that can be inserted into living organisms (*Escherichia coli* bacteria are often used) and repeatedly reproduced. Each hybrid molecule produces a genetically identical molecule, called a clone.
5. Cloning makes it possible to identify the DNA sequence in a gene and to produce the protein product encoded by the gene, such as insulin. Cloning also allows production of adequate amounts of the drug for therapeutic or research purposes.

SECTION III: APPLYING YOUR KNOWLEDGE

ACTIVITY E
CASE STUDIES
1. Legally, American consumers have two routes of access to therapeutic drugs. One route is by *prescription* from a licensed health care provider, such as a physician, dentist, or nurse practitioner.
2. Over-the-counter (OTC) purchase of drugs that do not require a prescription. These routes are regulated by various drug laws.
3. Acquiring and using prescription drugs for nontherapeutic purposes, by persons who are not authorized to have the drugs or for whom they are not prescribed, is illegal.

SECTION IV: PRACTICING FOR NCLEX
1. a. *Rationale:* The FDA approves many new drugs annually. New drugs are categorized according to their review priority and therapeutic potential. A status of "1P" indicates a new drug reviewed on a priority (accelerated) basis and with some therapeutic advantages over drugs already available; a status of "1S" indicates standard review and drugs with few, if any, therapeutic advantages (i.e., the new drug is similar to one or more older drugs currently on the market). Most new drugs are "1S" prescription drugs.
2. b, c, and d. *Rationale:* The FDA also approves drugs for OTC availability, including the transfer of drugs from prescription to OTC status, and may require additional clinical trials to determine the safety and effectiveness of OTC use. For prescription drugs taken orally, transfer to OTC status may mean different indications for use and lower doses.
3. c. *Rationale:* Having drugs available OTC has potential advantages and disadvantages for consumers. Advantages include greater autonomy, faster and more convenient access to effective treatment, possibly earlier resumption of usual activities of daily living, fewer visits to a health care provider, and possibly increased efforts by consumers to learn about their symptoms or conditions and recommended treatments. Disadvantages include inaccurate self-diagnoses and potential risks of choosing a wrong or contraindicated drug, delayed treatment by a health care professional, and development of adverse drug reactions and interactions. When a drug is switched from prescription to OTC status, pharmaceutical companies' sales and profits increase and insurance companies' costs decrease. Costs to consumers increase because health insurance policies do not cover OTC drugs.
4. a and c. *Rationale:* When prevention or cure is not a reasonable goal, relief of symptoms can greatly improve a client's quality of life and ability to function in activities of daily living.
5. b. *Rationale:* Drugs are classified according to their effects on particular body systems, their therapeutic uses, and their chemical characteristics.
6. b. *Rationale:* The names of therapeutic classifications usually reflect the conditions for which the drugs are used (e.g., antidepressants, antihypertensives).
7. d. *Rationale:* Drugs may be prescribed and dispensed by generic name or by trade name.
8. c. *Rationale:* A new drug is protected by patent for several years, during which time only the pharmaceutical manufacturer that developed it can market it. This is seen as a return on the company's investment in developing a drug, which may require years of work and millions of dollars, and as an incentive for developing other drugs. Other pharmaceutical companies cannot manufacture and market the drug until the patent expires.
9. b. *Rationale:* Current drug laws and standards have evolved over many years. Their main goal is to protect the public by ensuring that drugs marketed for therapeutic purposes are safe and effective.

10. The Public Health Service regulates vaccines and other biologic products. The Federal Trade Commission can suppress misleading advertisements of nonprescription drugs.

11. c. *Rationale:* The Comprehensive Drug Abuse Prevention and Control Act was passed in 1970. Title II of this law, called the Controlled Substances Act, regulates the manufacture and distribution of narcotics, stimulants, depressants, hallucinogens, and anabolic steroids. These drugs are categorized according to therapeutic usefulness and potential for abuse and are labeled as controlled substances (e.g., morphine is a C-II or Schedule II drug).

12. a, c, and d. *Rationale:* Nurses are responsible for storing controlled substances in locked containers, administering them only to people, for whom they are prescribed, recording each dose given on agency narcotic sheets and on the client's medication administration record, maintaining an accurate inventory, and reporting discrepancies to the proper authorities.

13. a, b, and d. *Rationale:* The Drug Enforcement Administration (DEA) enforces the Controlled Substances Act. Individuals and companies that are legally empowered to handle controlled substances must be registered with the DEA, keep accurate records of all transactions, and provide for secure storage. Prescribers are assigned a number by the DEA and must include the number on all prescriptions they write for a controlled substance. Prescriptions for Schedule II drugs cannot be refilled; a new prescription is required.

14. b. *Rationale:* Historically, drug research was done mainly with young, white males as subjects. In 1993, Congress passed the National Institutes of Health (NIH) Revitalization Act, which formalized a policy of the NIH that women and minorities must be included in human subject research studies funded by the NIH and in clinical drug trials.

15. a. *Rationale:* Since 1962, newly developed drugs have been extensively tested before being marketed for general use. Initially, drugs are tested in animals, and the FDA reviews the test results. Next, clinical trials in humans are done, usually with a randomized, controlled experimental design that involves selection of subjects according to established criteria, random assignment of subjects to experimental groups, and administration of the test drug to one group and a control substance to another group.

16. b. *Rationale:* FDA approval of a drug for OTC availability involves evaluation of evidence that the consumer can use the drug safely, using information on the product label, and shifts primary responsibility for safe and effective drug therapy from health care professionals to consumers. With prescription drugs, a health care professional diagnoses the condition, often with the help of laboratory and other diagnostic tests, and determines a need for the drug.

17. b. *Rationale:* There are many sources of drug data, including pharmacology and other textbooks, drug reference books, journal articles, and Internet sites. For the beginning student of pharmacology, a textbook is the best source of information, because it describes groups of drugs in relation to therapeutic uses.

18. A placebo is an inactive substance similar in appearance to the actual drug.

19. c. *Rationale:* The Durham-Humphrey Amendment designates drugs that must be prescribed by a licensed physician or nurse practitioner and dispensed by a pharmacist.

20. The Food and Drug Administration (FDA) is charged with enforcing the law.

Chapter 2: Basic Concepts and Processes

SECTION II: ASSESSING YOUR UNDERSTANDING

ACTIVITY A
FILL IN THE BLANKS
1. Drugs
2. Cell membrane
3. Pharmacokinetics
4. Absorption
5. Faster
6. Additive effects
7. Synergism
8. Interference
9. Displacement
10. Antidote

ACTIVITY B
MATCHING
1. E   2. B   3. A   4. D   5. C

ACTIVITY C
SEQUENCING

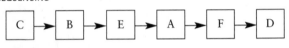

ACTIVITY D
SHORT ANSWERS
1. To act on body cells, drugs given for systemic effects must reach adequate concentrations in the blood and other tissue fluids surrounding the cells. Therefore, they must enter the body and be circulated to their sites of action (target cells). After they act on cells, they must be eliminated from the body.
2. Although cells differ from one tissue to another, their common characteristics include the ability to perform the following functions:
   - Exchange materials with their immediate environment
   - Obtain energy from nutrients
   - Synthesize hormones, neurotransmitters, enzymes, structural proteins, and other complex molecules
   - Duplicate themselves (reproduce)
   - Communicate with one another via various biologic chemicals, such as neurotransmitters and hormones.
3. Numerous factors affect the rate and extent of drug absorption, including dosage form, route of administration and blood flow to the site of administration, gastrointestinal function, the presence of food or other drugs, and other variables.
4. Rapid movement through the stomach and small intestine may increase drug absorption by promoting contact with absorptive mucous membrane; it also may decrease absorption, because some drugs may move through the small intestine too rapidly to be absorbed. For many drugs, the presence of food in the stomach slows the rate of absorption and may decrease the amount of drug absorbed.
5. Drug distribution into the CNS is limited because the blood–brain barrier, which is composed of capillaries with tight walls, limits movement of drug molecules into brain tissue. This barrier usually acts as a selectively permeable membrane to protect the CNS.

SECTION III: APPLYING YOUR KNOWLEDGE

ACTIVITY E

CASE STUDIES

1. A *serum drug level* is a laboratory measurement of the amount of a drug in the blood at a particular time; it reflects dosage, absorption, bioavailability, half-life, and the rates of metabolism and excretion. A minimum effective concentration (MEC) must be present before a drug exerts its pharmacologic action on body cells; this is largely determined by the drug dose and how well it is absorbed into the bloodstream.

2. A toxic concentration is an excessive level at which toxicity occurs. Toxic concentrations may stem from a single large dose, repeated small doses, or slow metabolism that allows the drug to accumulate in the body.

3. Between low and high concentrations is the therapeutic range, which is the goal of drug therapy—that is, enough drug to be beneficial, but not enough to be toxic.

SECTION IV: PRACTICING FOR NCLEX

1. d. *Rationale:* Bioavailability is the portion of a dose that reaches the systemic circulation and is available to act on body cells.

2. c. *Rationale:* An intravenous drug is virtually 100% bioavailable. An oral drug is almost always less than 100% bioavailable, because some of it is not absorbed from the gastrointestinal tract and some goes to the liver and is partially metabolized before reaching the systemic circulation.

3. c. *Rationale:* With chronic administration, some drugs stimulate liver cells to produce larger amounts of drug-metabolizing enzymes (called *enzyme induction*). Enzyme induction accelerates drug metabolism, because larger amounts of the enzymes (and more binding sites) allow larger amounts of a drug to be metabolized during a given time. As a result, larger doses of the rapidly metabolized drug may be required to produce or maintain therapeutic effects. Rapid metabolism may also increase the production of toxic metabolites with some drugs (e.g., acetaminophen). Drugs that induce enzyme production also may increase the rate of metabolism for endogenous steroidal hormones (e.g., cortisol, estrogens, testosterone, vitamin D). However, *enzyme induction does not occur for 1 to 3 weeks after an inducing agent is started*, because new enzyme proteins must be synthesized.

4. a and d. *Rationale:* Metabolism also may be decreased or delayed in a process called *enzyme inhibition*, which most often occurs with concurrent administration of two or more drugs that compete for the same metabolizing enzymes. In this case, smaller doses of the slowly metabolized drug may be needed to avoid adverse effects and toxicity from drug accumulation. *Enzyme inhibition occurs within hours or days of starting an inhibiting agent.* Cimetidine, a gastric acid suppressor, inhibits several CYP enzymes (e.g., CYP1A, CYP2C, CYP2D, CYP3A) and can greatly decrease drug metabolism.

5. a. *Rationale:* When drugs are given orally, they are absorbed from the gastrointestinal tract and carried to the liver through the portal circulation. Some drugs are extensively metabolized in the liver, with only part of a drug dose reaching the systemic circulation for distribution to sites of action. This is called the *first-pass effect* or presystemic metabolism.

6. a. *Rationale:* Some drugs or metabolites are excreted in bile and then eliminated in feces; others are excreted in bile, reabsorbed from the small intestine, and then returned to the liver in a process called *enterohepatic recirculation.*

7. c. *Rationale:* For most drugs, serum levels indicate the onset, peak, and duration of drug action. After a single dose of a drug is given, onset of action occurs when the drug level reaches the MEC.

8. a, c, e, and f. *Rationale:* In clinical practice, measurement of serum drug levels is useful in several circumstances:
   - When drugs with a narrow margin of safety are given, because their therapeutic doses are close to their toxic doses (e.g., digoxin, aminoglycoside antibiotics, lithium)
   - To document the serum drug levels associated with particular drug dosages, therapeutic effects, or possible adverse effects
   - To monitor unexpected responses to a drug dose, such as decreased therapeutic effects or increased adverse effects
   - When a drug overdose is suspected

9. *Serum half-life*, also called elimination half-life, is the time required for the serum concentration of a drug to decrease by 50%. It is determined primarily by the drug's rates of metabolism and excretion. A drug with a short half-life requires more frequent administration than one with a long half-life.

10. c. *Rationale:* When a drug is given at a stable dose, 4 to 5 half-lives are required to achieve steady-state concentrations and develop equilibrium between tissue and serum concentrations. Because maximal therapeutic effects do not occur until equilibrium is established, some drugs are not fully effective for days or weeks. To maintain steady-state conditions, the amount of drug given must equal the amount eliminated from the body. When a drug dose is changed, an additional 4 to 5 half-lives are required to re-establish equilibrium; when a drug is discontinued, it is eliminated gradually over several half-lives.

11. a. *Rationale:* Pharmacodynamics involves drug actions on target cells and the resulting alterations in cellular biochemical reactions and functions (i.e., "what the drug does to the body").

12. a, c, and d. *Rationale:* Relatively few drugs act by mechanisms other than combination with receptor sites on cells. Drugs that do not act on receptor sites include the following:
   - Antacids, which act chemically to neutralize the hydrochloric acid produced by gastric parietal cells and thereby raise the pH of gastric fluid
   - Osmotic diuretics (e.g., mannitol), which increase the osmolarity of plasma and pull water out of tissues into the bloodstream
   - Drugs that are structurally similar to nutrients required by body cells (e.g., purines, pyrimidines) and that can be incorporated into cellular constituents, such as nucleic acids. This interferes with normal cell functioning. Several anticancer drugs act by this mechanism.
   - Metal chelating agents, which combine with toxic metals to form a complex that can be more readily excreted

13. a. *Rationale:* Dosage refers to the frequency, size, and number of doses; it is a major determinant of drug actions and responses, both therapeutic and adverse. If the amount is too small or is administered infrequently, no pharmacologic action occurs, because the drug does not reach an adequate concentration at target cells. If the amount is too large or is administered too often, toxicity (poisoning) may occur. Overdosage may occur with a single large dose or with chronic ingestion of smaller doses.

14. b. *Rationale:* Most drug–diet interactions are undesirable because food often slows absorption of oral drugs by slowing gastric emptying time and altering gastrointestinal secretions and motility. Giving medications 1 hour before or 2 hours after a meal can minimize interactions that decrease drug absorption.

15. b. *Rationale:* An interaction occurs between tyramine-containing foods, and monoamine oxidase (MAO) inhibitor drugs. Tyramine causes the release of norepinephrine, a strong vasoconstrictive agent, from the adrenal medulla and sympathetic neurons. Normally, norepinephrine is quickly inactivated by MAO. However, because MAO inhibitor drugs prevent inactivation of norepinephrine, ingestion of tyramine-containing foods with an MAO inhibitor may produce severe hypertension or intracranial hemorrhage. MAO inhibitors include the antidepressants isocarboxazid and phenelzine and the antiparkinson drugs rasagiline and selegiline. Tyramine-rich foods to be avoided by patients taking MAO inhibitors include aged cheeses, sauerkraut, soy sauce, tap or draft beers, and red wines.

16. c. *Rationale:* An interaction may occur between warfarin (Coumadin), an oral anticoagulant, and foods containing vitamin K. Because vitamin K antagonizes the action of warfarin, large amounts of spinach and other green leafy vegetables may offset the anticoagulant effects and predispose the person to thromboembolic disorders.

17. a. *Rationale:* Grapefruit contains a substance that strongly inhibits the metabolism of drugs normally metabolized by the cytochrome P450 CYP3A4 enzyme. This effect greatly increases the blood levels of some drugs (e.g., the widely used "statin" group of cholesterol-lowering drugs) and the effect lasts for several days. Patients who take medications metabolized by the CYP3A4 enzyme should be advised against eating grapefruit or drinking grapefruit juice.

18. d. *Rationale:* In older adults (65 years and older), physiologic changes may alter all pharmacokinetic processes. Changes in the gastrointestinal tract include decreased gastric acidity, decreased blood flow, and decreased motility. Despite these changes, however, there is little difference in drug absorption. Changes in the cardiovascular system include decreased cardiac output and therefore slower distribution of drug molecules to their sites of action, metabolism, and excretion. In the liver, blood flow and metabolizing enzymes are decreased. Therefore, many drugs are metabolized more slowly, have a longer action, and are more likely to accumulate with chronic administration. In the kidneys, there is decreased blood flow, decreased glomerular filtration rate, and decreased tubular secretion of drugs; all of these changes tend to slow excretion and promote accumulation of drugs in the body. Impaired kidney and liver function greatly increases the risks of adverse drug effects. In addition, older adults are more likely to have acute and chronic illnesses that require the use of multiple drugs or long-term drug therapy. Therefore, possibilities for interactions among drugs and between drugs and diseased organs are greatly multiplied.

19. b. *Rationale:* Most drug information has been derived from clinical drug trials using white men. Interethnic variations became evident when drugs and dosages developed for Caucasians produced unexpected responses, including toxicity, when given to individuals from other ethnic groups. One common variation is that African Americans respond differently to some cardiovascular drugs. For example, for African Americans with hypertension, angiotensin-converting enzyme (ACE) inhibitors and beta-adrenergic blocking drugs are less effective, and diuretics and calcium channel blockers are more effective. Also, African Americans with heart failure seem to respond better to a combination of hydralazine and isosorbide than do Caucasian patients with heart failure.

20. b. *Rationale:* Drug *tolerance* occurs when the body becomes accustomed to a particular drug over time, so that larger doses must be given to produce the same effects. Tolerance may be acquired to the pharmacologic action of many drugs, especially opioid analgesics, alcohol, and other CNS depressants. Tolerance to pharmacologically related drugs is called *cross-tolerance*. For example, a person who regularly drinks large amounts of alcohol becomes able to ingest even larger amounts before becoming intoxicated—this is tolerance to alcohol. If the person is then given sedative-type drugs or a general anesthetic, larger-than-usual doses are required to produce a pharmacologic effect—this is cross-tolerance.

Chapter 3: Administering Medications

SECTION II: ASSESSING YOUR UNDERSTANDING

ACTIVITY A
FILL IN THE BLANKS
1. therapeutic purposes
2. Certified Medical Assistants (CMAs); Certified Medication Aides (nursing assistants with a short course of training, also called CMAs)
3. unit-dose
4. Controlled drugs
5. Medication Reconciliation

ACTIVITY B
MATCHING
1. C   2. D   3. E   4. A   5. B

ACTIVITY C
SEQUENCING

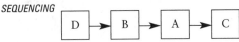

ACTIVITY D
SHORT ANSWERS
1. The five rights are as follows:
   - Right drug
   - Right dose
   - Right client
   - Right route
   - Right time
2. Medication errors commonly reported include giving an incorrect dose, not giving an ordered drug, and giving an unordered drug.

3. In the Computerized Provider Order Entry (CPOE) system, a prescriber types a medication order directly into a computer. This decreases errors associated with illegible handwriting and erroneous transcription or dispensing. CPOE, which is already used in many healthcare facilities, is widely recommended as the preferred alternative to error-prone handwritten orders.

4. The ISMP has long maintained a list of abbreviations that are often associated with medication errors, and the JCAHO now requires accredited organizations to maintain a "Do not use" list (e.g., u or U for units; IU for international units; qd for daily; qod for every other day; and others) that applies to all prescribers and transcribers of medication orders. Other abbreviations are not recommended, as well. In general, it is safer to write out drug names, routes of administration, and so forth and to minimize the use of abbreviations, symbols, and numbers that are often misinterpreted, especially when handwritten.

5. Medication orders should include the full name of the client; the name of the drug (preferably the generic name); the dose, route, and frequency of administration; and the date, time, and signature of the prescriber.

SECTION III: APPLYING YOUR KNOWLEDGE

ACTIVITY E
CASE STUDIES

1. Occasionally, verbal or telephone orders are acceptable. When taken, they should be written on the client's order sheet, signed by the person taking the order, and later countersigned by the prescriber.

2. Prescriptions for Schedule II controlled drugs cannot be refilled.

3. For discharge education, the following information should be part of the nurse's education plan: instructions for taking the drug (e.g., dose, frequency) and whether the prescription can be refilled.

SECTION IV: PRACTICING FOR NCLEX

1. c. *Rationale:* The sixth "right" is documentation.

2. c. *Rationale:* Learn essential information about each drug to be given (e.g., indications for use, contraindications, therapeutic effects, adverse effects, any specific instructions about administration).

3. a. *Rationale:* Interpret the prescriber's order accurately (i.e., drug name, dose, frequency of administration). Question the prescriber if any information is unclear or if the drug seems inappropriate for the client's condition.

4. b. *Rationale:* Read labels of drug containers for the drug name and concentration (usually in milligrams per tablet, capsule, or milliliter of solution). Many medications are available in different dosage forms and concentrations, and it is extremely important that the correct ones be used.

5. c. *Rationale:* Minimize the use of abbreviations for drug names, doses, routes of administration, and times of administration. This promotes safer administration and reduces errors. When abbreviations are used by prescribers or others, interpret them accurately or question the writer about the intended meaning.

6. c. *Rationale:* Measure doses accurately. Ask a colleague to double-check measurements of insulin and heparin, unusual doses (i.e., large or small), and any drugs to be given intravenously.

7. d. *Rationale:* Use the correct procedures and techniques for all routes of administration. For example, use appropriate anatomic landmarks to identify sites for intramuscular (IM) injections, follow the manufacturers' instructions for preparation and administration of intravenous (IV) medications, and use sterile materials and techniques for injectable and eye medications.

8. b. *Rationale:* Verify the identity of all clients before administering medications; check identification bands on clients who have them (e.g., in hospitals or long-term care facilities).

9. b. *Rationale:* The nurse may be held liable for not giving a drug or for giving a wrong drug or a wrong dose. In addition, the nurse is expected to have sufficient drug knowledge to recognize and question erroneous orders. If, after questioning the prescriber and seeking information from other authoritative sources, the nurse considers that giving a drug is unsafe, the nurse must refuse to give the drug. The fact that a physician wrote an erroneous order does not excuse the nurse from legal liability if he or she carries out that order.

10. a, c, and e. *Rationale:* Specific drugs often associated with errors and adverse drug events (ADEs) include insulin, heparin, and warfarin. The risk of ADEs increases with the number of drugs a patient uses.

11. c. *Rationale:* The bar code on the drug label contains the identification number, strength, and dosage form of the drug, and the bar code on the patient's identification band contains the MAR, which can be displayed when a nurse uses a hand-held scanning device. When administering medications, the nurse scans the bar code on the drug label, on the patient's identification band, and on the nurse's personal identification badge. A wireless computer network processes the scanned information; gives an error message on the scanner or sounds an alarm if the nurse is about to give the wrong drug or the right drug at the wrong time; and automatically records the time, drug, and dose given on the MAR.

12. d. *Rationale:* Drug preparations and dosage forms vary according to the drug's chemical characteristics, reason for use, and route of administration. Some drugs are available in only one dosage form, and others are available in several forms.

13. a. *Rationale:* Enteric-coated tablets and capsules are coated with a substance that is insoluble in stomach acid. This delays dissolution until the medication reaches the intestine, usually to avoid gastric irritation or to keep the drug from being destroyed by gastric acid.

14. c. *Rationale:* Several controlled-release dosage forms and drug delivery systems are available, and more continue to be developed. These formulations maintain more consistent serum drug levels and allow less frequent administration, which is more convenient for clients. Controlled-release oral tablets and capsules are called by a variety of names (e.g., timed release, sustained release, extended release), and their names usually include CR, SR, XL, or other indications that they are long-acting formulations.

15. b. *Rationale:* Because controlled-release tablets and capsules contain high amounts of drug intended to be absorbed slowly and act over a prolonged period of time, they should never be broken, opened, crushed, or chewed. Such an action allows the full dose to be absorbed immediately and constitutes an overdose, with potential organ damage or death.

16. The correct answer is two tablets. In this case, the answer can be readily calculated mentally. This is a simple example that also can be used to illustrate mathematical

calculations. This problem can be solved by several acceptable methods; the following formula is presented because of its relative simplicity for students lacking a more familiar method:

$$\frac{D}{H} = \frac{X}{V}$$

17. a, c, and d. *Rationale:* Common parenteral routes are subcutaneous (Sub-Q), intramuscular (IM) and intravenous (IV) injections. Injections require special drug preparations, equipment, and techniques.
18. c. *Rationale:* Use a filter needle to withdraw the medication from an ampule or vial, because broken glass or rubber fragments may need to be removed from the drug solution. Replace the filter needle with a regular needle before injecting the client.
19. b. *Rationale:* A 25-gauge needle is smaller than an 18-, 20-, or 22-gauge needle. Choice of needle gauge and length depends on the route of administration, the viscosity (thickness) of the solution to be given, and the size of the client. Usually, a 25-gauge, 5 ¼ 8-inch needle is used for Sub-Q injections, and a 22- or 20-gauge, 11 ¼ 2-inch needle is used for IM injections.
20. a, b, c, and d. *Rationale:* Sites for IM injections are the deltoid, dorsogluteal, ventrogluteal, and vastus lateralis muscles. These sites must be selected by first identifying anatomic landmarks.

Chapter 4: Nursing Process in Drug Therapy

SECTION II: ASSESSING YOUR UNDERSTANDING

ACTIVITY A
FILL IN THE BLANKS
1. nursing process
2. cognitive and psychomotor
3. Assessment
4. Nursing diagnoses
5. Interventions

ACTIVITY B
MATCHING
1. C   2. A   3. D   4. E   5. B

ACTIVITY C
SHORT ANSWERS
1. Assessment involves collecting data about client characteristics known to affect drug therapy. This includes observing and interviewing the client, interviewing family members or others involved in client care, completing a physical assessment, reviewing medical records for pertinent laboratory and diagnostic test reports, and other methods. Initially (before drug therapy is started or on first contact), assess age, weight, vital signs, health status, pathologic conditions, and ability to function in usual activities of daily living
2. Nursing diagnoses, as developed by the North American Nursing Diagnosis Association, describe client problems or needs and are based on assessment data. They should be individualized according to the client's condition and the drugs prescribed. The nursing diagnoses needed to adequately reflect a client's condition vary considerably. Because almost any nursing diagnosis may apply in specific circumstances, this text emphasizes those diagnoses that generally apply to drug therapy.

3. Planning/goals involves the expected outcomes of prescribed drug therapy. As a general rule, goals should be stated in terms of client behavior, not nurse behavior (e.g., "The client will. . . .")
4. Intervention involves implementing planned activities and includes any task performed directly with a client or indirectly on a client's behalf. Areas of intervention are broad and may include assessment, promoting compliance with prescribed drug therapy, and solving problems related to drug therapy, among others.
5. This step involves evaluating the client's status in relation to stated goals and expected outcomes. Some outcomes can be evaluated within a few minutes of drug administration (e.g., relief of acute pain after administration of an analgesic), but most require longer periods of time. Over time, the client is likely to experience brief contacts with many healthcare providers, which increases the difficulty of evaluating outcomes of drug therapy.

SECTION III: APPLYING YOUR KNOWLEDGE

ACTIVITY D
CASE STUDIES
CASE STUDY 1
1. b. *Rationale:* Assessment includes observing and interviewing the client, interviewing family members or others involved in client care, completing a physical assessment, reviewing medical records for pertinent laboratory and diagnostic test reports, and other methods. Initially (before drug therapy is started or on first contact), assess age, weight, vital signs, health status, pathologic conditions, and ability to function in usual activities of daily living.
2. a. *Rationale:* Subjective assessment includes the client's response to the interview. Subjective data is information that cannot be directly observed by the nurse.
3. b. *Rationale:* Objective data are directly observed by the nurse.

CASE STUDY 2
1. d. *Rationale:* All aspects of pediatric drug therapy must be guided by the child's age, weight, and level of growth and development.
2. a. *Rationale:* When pediatric dosage ranges are listed in drug literature, they should be used.
3. c. *Rationale:* Use the oral route of drug administration when possible. Try to obtain the child's cooperation; never force oral medications, because forcing may lead to aspiration.

SECTION IV: PRACTICING FOR NCLEX

1. c. *Rationale:* The American Society of Anesthesiologists recommends that all herbal products be discontinued 2 to 3 weeks before any surgical procedure. Some products (e.g., echinacea, feverfew, garlic, gingko biloba, ginseng, valerian, St. John's wort) can interfere with or increase the effects of some drugs, affect blood pressure or heart rhythm, or increase risks of bleeding; some have unknown effects when combined with anesthetics, other perioperative medications, and surgical procedures.
2. a. *Rationale:* Most herbal and dietary supplements should be avoided during pregnancy or lactation and in young children.
3. d. *Rationale:* Do not assume continued safety of an OTC medication you have taken for years. Older people are more likely to have adverse drug reactions and interactions because of changes in the heart, kidneys, and

other organs that occur with aging and various disease processes.

4. c. *Rationale:* Products are often advertised as "natural." Many people interpret this to mean that the products are safe and better than synthetic products. This is not true; "natural" does not mean safe, especially when taken concurrently with other herbals, dietary supplements, or drugs

5. b. *Rationale:* Read product labels carefully. The labels contain essential information about the name, ingredients, indications for use, usual dosage, when to stop using the medication or when to see a health care provider, possible adverse effects, and expiration date.

6. b. *Rationale:* Note that all OTC medications are not safe for everyone. Many OTC medications warn against use with certain illnesses (e.g., hypertension). Consult a healthcare provider before taking the product if you have a contraindicated condition. In addition, if taking any prescription medications, consult a healthcare provider before taking any OTC drugs to avoid undesirable drug interactions and adverse effects.

7. a. *Rationale:* Ask a healthcare provider before taking products containing aspirin if you are taking an anticoagulant (e.g., Coumadin).

8. d. *Rationale:* Do not take a laxative if you have stomach pain, nausea, or vomiting, to avoid worsening the problem.

9. c. *Rationale:* Ask a healthcare provider before taking other products containing aspirin if you are already taking a regular dose of aspirin to prevent blood clots, heart attack, or stroke. Aspirin is commonly used for this purpose, often in doses of 81 mg (a child's dose) or 325 mg.

10. a and b. *Rationale:* Avoid alcohol if taking sedating antihistamines, cough or cold remedies containing dextromethorphan, or sleeping pills. Because all of these drugs cause drowsiness when taken alone, combining any of them with alcohol may result in excessive and potentially dangerous sedation.

11. a, b, and d. *Rationale:* Store medications safely, in a cool, dry place. Do not store them in a bathroom; heat, light, and moisture may cause them to decompose. Do not store them near a dangerous substance, which could be taken by mistake. Keep medications in the container in which they were dispensed by the pharmacy, where the label identifies it and gives directions. Do not mix different medications in a single container.

12. b. *Rationale:* If a dose is missed, most authorities recommend taking the dose if remembered soon after the scheduled time, or omitting the dose if it is not remembered for several hours. If a dose is omitted, the next dose should be taken at the next scheduled time. Do not double the dose.

13. d. *Rationale:* If taking a liquid medication (or giving one to a child), measure with a calibrated medication cup or measuring spoon. A dose cannot be measured accurately with household teaspoons or tablespoons because they are different sizes and deliver varying amounts of medication. If the liquid medication is packaged with a measuring cup that shows teaspoons or tablespoons, that should be used to measure doses, for adults or children.

14. d. *Rationale:* Take most oral drugs at evenly spaced intervals around the clock. For example, if ordered once daily, a medication should be taken at about the same time every day. If ordered twice daily or morning and evening, doses should be taken about 12 hours apart.

15. b. *Rationale:* As a general rule, take oral medications with 6 to 8 oz of water, in a sitting or standing position. The water helps tablets and capsules dissolve in the stomach, "dilutes" the drug so that it is less likely to upset the stomach, and promotes absorption of the drug into the bloodstream.

16. a. *Rationale:* Get all prescriptions filled at the same pharmacy, if possible. This is an important safety factor in helping to avoid multiple prescriptions of the same or similar drugs and to minimize undesirable interactions of newly prescribed drugs with those already in use.

17. c. *Rationale:* Follow instructions for follow-up care (e.g., office visits, laboratory or other diagnostic tests that monitor therapeutic or adverse effects of drugs).

18. Meta-analysis involves a rigorous process of analyzing, comparing, and summarizing multiple studies.

19. When completing a drug history, the home care nurse should ask to see all prescribed and OTC medications that the client takes and should ask how and when the client takes each one.

20. Dosage requirements may vary among clients and within the same client at different times during an illness.

Chapter 5: Physiology of the Central Nervous System

SECTION II: ASSESSING YOUR UNDERSTANDING

ACTIVITY A
FILL IN THE BLANKS
1. brain and spinal cord
2. Afferent or sensory neurons
3. homeostasis
4. Electrical and chemical
5. neuron; glia

ACTIVITY B
MATCHING
1. B   2. D   3. A   4. C   5. E

ACTIVITY C
SEQUENCING

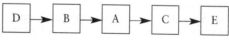

ACTIVITY D
SHORT ANSWERS
1. Characteristics that allow neurons to communicate with other body cells include excitability (the ability to produce an action potential or be stimulated) and conductivity (the ability to convey electrical impulses). Specific components of the communication network include neurotransmitters, synapses, and receptors.

2. Several factors affect the availability and function of neurotransmitters, including the following:
   - The availability of precursor proteins and enzymes required to synthesize particular neurotransmitters
   - The number and binding capacity of receptors in the cell membranes of presynaptic and postsynaptic nerve endings
   - Acid–base imbalances (acidosis decreases and alkalosis increases synaptic transmission)
   - Hypoxia, which causes CNS depression (coma occurs within seconds without oxygen)
   - Drugs, which may alter neurotransmitter synthesis, release, degradation, or binding to receptors to cause either CNS stimulation or depression

3. Norepinephrine is a catecholamine that is found in relatively large amounts in the hypothalamus and the limbic system and in smaller amounts in most areas of the brain, including the reticular formation.

4. CNS function in both health and disease is largely determined by interactions among neurotransmission systems. In health, complex mechanisms regulate the amounts and binding capacities of neurotransmitters and receptors, as well as the balance between excitatory and inhibitory forces.

5. When abnormalities occur in any of the elements listed for a healthy CNS, the resulting dysregulation and imbalances lead to signs and symptoms of CNS disorders. Overall, neurotransmission systems function interdependently; one system may increase, decrease, or otherwise modify the effects of another system.

SECTION III: APPLYING YOUR KNOWLEDGE

ACTIVITY E
CASE STUDIES

1. A prescription medication must be ordered by a physician or, in some states, a nurse practitioner. Prescriptions should not be shared.

2. CNS stimulants produce a variety of effects. Mild stimulation is characterized by wakefulness, mental alertness, and decreased fatigue. Increasing stimulation produces hyperactivity, excessive talking, nervousness, and insomnia. Excessive stimulation can cause convulsions, cardiac dysrhythmias, and death.

SECTION IV: PRACTICING FOR NCLEX

1. a, b, d, and e. *Rationale:* The cerebral cortex is involved in all conscious processes (e.g., learning, memory, reasoning, verbalization, and voluntary body movements).

2. a. *Rationale:* The thalamus receives impulses carrying sensations such as heat, cold, pain, and muscle position sense that produce a crude awareness in the thalamus. These sensations are relayed to the cerebral cortex, where they are interpreted regarding location, quality, intensity, and significance. The thalamus also relays motor impulses from the cortex to the spinal cord.

3. hypothalamus

4. c. *Rationale:* Oxytocin initiates uterine contractions to begin labor and delivery and helps release milk from breast glands during breastfeeding.

5. b. *Rationale:* When nerve impulses from the hypothalamus excite the vasomotor center, vasomotor tone is increased, and blood pressure is raised.

6. a. *Rationale:* The medulla contains groups of neurons that form the vital cardiac, respiratory, and vasomotor centers. For example, if the respiratory center is stimulated, respiratory rate and depth are increased. If the respiratory center is depressed, respiratory rate and depth are decreased. The medulla also contains reflex centers for coughing, vomiting, sneezing, swallowing, and salivating. The medulla and pons varolii also contain groups of neurons from which cranial nerves 5 through 12 originate.

7. c. *Rationale:* The reticular activating system is a network of neurons that extends from the spinal cord through the medulla and pons to the thalamus and hypothalamus. It receives impulses from all parts of the body, evaluates the significance of the impulses, and decides which impulses to transmit to the cerebral cortex. It also excites or inhibits motor nerves that control both reflex and voluntary movement. Stimulation of these neurons produces wakefulness and mental alertness, and depression causes sedation and loss of consciousness.

8. a. *Rationale:* Many nerve impulses from the limbic system are transmitted through the hypothalamus; this causes physiologic changes in blood pressure, heart rate, respiration, and hormone secretion to occur in response to emotions.

9. cerebellum

10. c. *Rationale:* The basal ganglia are concerned with skeletal muscle tone and orderly activity. Normal function is influenced by dopamine. Degenerative changes in one of these areas, the substantia nigra, cause dopamine to be released in decreased amounts. This process is a factor in the development of Parkinson's disease.

11. extrapyramidal

12. c. *Rationale:* Cerebral cortex cells are very sensitive to lack of oxygen (hypoxia), and interruption of blood supply causes immediate loss of consciousness. Brain stem cells are less sensitive to hypoxia.

13. a. *Rationale:* Thiamine deficiency can reduce the use of glucose by nerve cells and can cause degeneration of the myelin sheath. Such degeneration in central neurons leads to a form of brain damage known as Wernicke-Korsakoff encephalopathy.

14. peripheral nerves

15. b. *Rationale:* Reflexes are involuntary responses to certain nerve impulses received by the spinal cord (e.g., knee-jerk reflex, pupillary reflexes).

16. d. *Rationale:* When released from the synaptic vesicles, molecules of neurotransmitter cross the synapse, bind to receptors in the cell membrane of the postsynaptic neuron, and excite or inhibit postsynaptic neurons. Free neurotransmitter molecules (i.e., those not bound to receptors) are rapidly removed from the synapse by three mechanisms: transportation back into the presynaptic nerve terminal (reuptake) for reuse, diffusion into surrounding body fluids, or destruction by enzymes.

17. a. *Rationale:* A neurotransmitter–receptor complex may have an excitatory or inhibitory effect on the postsynaptic neuron.

18. cholinergic system

19. GABA

20. b. *Rationale:* Serotonin is synthesized from the amino acid tryptophan; the amount of tryptophan intake in the diet and the enzyme tryptophan hydroxylase control the rate of serotonin production.

Chapter 6: Opioid Analgesics and Pain Management

SECTION II: ASSESSING YOUR UNDERSTANDING

ACTIVITY A
FILL IN THE BLANKS

1. Pain
2. Opioid
3. Nociceptors
4. Nonopioid; nonopioids
5. black box warnings

ACTIVITY B
MATCHING

1. B   2. E   3. A   4. C   5. D

ACTIVITY C
SHORT ANSWERS

1. For a person to feel pain, the signal from the nociceptors in peripheral tissues must be transmitted to the spinal cord, then to the hypothalamus and cerebral cortex in the brain. The signal is carried to the spinal cord by two types of nerve cells, A-delta fibers and C fibers. A-delta fibers, which are myelinated and are found mainly in skin and muscle, transmit fast, sharp, well-localized pain signals. These fibers release glutamate and aspartate (excitatory amino acid neurotransmitters) at synapses in the spinal cord. C fibers, which are unmyelinated and are found in muscle, abdominal viscera, and periosteum, conduct the pain signal slowly and produce a poorly localized, dull or burning type of pain. Tissue damage resulting from an acute injury often produces an initial sharp pain transmitted by A-delta fibers, followed by a dull ache or burning sensation transmitted by C fibers. C fibers release somatostatin and substance P at synapses in the spinal cord. Glutamate, aspartate, substance P, and perhaps other chemical mediators enhance transmission of the pain signal.

2. Causes of tissue damage may be physical (e.g., heat, cold, pressure, stretch, spasm, ischemia) or chemical (e.g., pain-producing substances are released into the extracellular fluid surrounding the nerve fibers that carry the pain signal). These pain-producing substances activate pain receptors, increase the sensitivity of pain receptors, or stimulate the release of inflammatory substances.

3. Oral drugs undergo significant first-pass metabolism in the liver, which means that oral doses must be larger than injected doses to have equivalent therapeutic effects. The drugs are extensively metabolized in the liver, and metabolites are excreted in urine. Morphine and meperidine form pharmacologically active metabolites. Therefore, liver impairment can interfere with metabolism, and kidney impairment can interfere with excretion. Drug accumulation and increased adverse effects may occur if dosage is not reduced.

4. In the GI tract, opioids slow motility and may cause constipation and smooth muscle spasms in the bowel and biliary tract.

5. Capsaicin (Zostrix), a product derived from cayenne chili peppers, is applied topically to the skin to relieve pain associated with osteoarthritis, rheumatoid arthritis, postherpetic neuralgia after a herpes zoster infection (shingles), diabetic neuropathy, postsurgical pain (including pain after mastectomy or amputation), and other complex pain syndromes. It may be most effective in relieving arthritic pain in joints close to skin surfaces (e.g., fingers, elbows, knees). Its analgesic effects are attributed to depletion of substance P in nerve cells. Substance P enhances transmission of painful stimuli from peripheral tissues to the spinal cord. An additional analgesic effect may result from interference with production of prostaglandins and leukotrienes.

6. When opioids are used postoperatively, the goal is to relieve pain without excessive sedation, so that clients can do deep-breathing exercises, cough, ambulate, and participate in other activities to promote recovery. Strong opioids are usually given parenterally for a few days. Then, oral opioids or nonopioid analgesics are given.

SECTION III: APPLYING YOUR KNOWLEDGE
ACTIVITY D
CASE STUDIES

1. In severely burned clients, opioids should be used cautiously. A common cause of respiratory arrest in burned clients is excessive administration of analgesics. When opioids are necessary, they are usually given IV in small doses. Drugs given by other routes are absorbed erratically in the presence of shock and hypovolemia and may not relieve pain. In addition, unabsorbed drugs may be rapidly absorbed when circulation improves, with the potential for excessive dosage and toxic effects.

2. Agitation in a burned person may indicate hypoxia or hypovolemia rather than pain.

SECTION IV: PRACTICING FOR NCLEX

1. c. *Rationale:* Pain is a subjective experience. Stressors such as anxiety, depression, fatigue, anger, and fear tend to increase pain; rest, mood elevation, and diversionary activities tend to decrease pain. Pain is a complex physiologic, psychological, and sociocultural phenomenon that must be thoroughly assessed if it is to be managed effectively.

2. a. *Rationale:* With clients who are taking opioid analgesics for more than a few days, you should assess periodically for drug tolerance and the need for higher doses or more frequent administration. Do not assume that increased requests for pain medication indicate inappropriate drug-seeking behavior associated with drug dependence.

3. b. *Rationale:* Because pain is a subjective experience and cannot be objectively measured, assessment of intensity or severity is based on the client's description and the nurse's observations. Various scales have been developed to measure and quantify pain. These include verbal descriptor scales, in which the client is asked to rate pain as mild, moderate, or severe; numeric scales, with 0 representing no pain and 10 representing severe pain; and visual analog scales, in which the client chooses the location indicating the level of pain on a continuum.

4. b. *Rationale:* The term *referred pain* is used when pain arising from tissue damage in one area of the body is felt in another area. Patterns of referred pain may be helpful in diagnosis. For example, pain of cardiac origin may radiate to the neck, shoulders, chest muscles, and down the arms, often on the left side. This type of pain usually results from myocardial ischemia due to atherosclerotic plaque in coronary arteries.

5. d. *Rationale:* The nurse must assess every client in relation to pain, initially to determine appropriate interventions and later to determine whether the interventions were effective in preventing or relieving pain.

6. a. *Rationale:* Several lidocaine preparations are available to prevent or relieve pain. An oral preparation can be given to relieve mouth and throat pain, but it is not recommended for long-term use. A transdermal gel and patch (Lidoderm) may be used to relieve the pain of postherpetic neuralgia.

7. b. *Rationale:* Corticosteroids can reduce inflammation, irritability, and spontaneous discharge in injured nerves and other tissues. They are used to treat neuropathic, visceral, and bone pain.

8. c. *Rationale:* TCAs have long been used to relieve neuropathic pain. They inhibit the reuptake of norepinephrine and serotonin in nerve synapses, thereby making these neurotransmitters more available to inhibit pain signals. The drugs cause numerous adverse effects, especially in older adults, but their ability to promote sleep and relieve depression (which often accompanies chronic pain) may be beneficial enough to outweigh their disadvantages.

9. a. *Rationale:* Antiepileptic drugs (AEDs) are mainly used to treat neuropathic pain; they decrease the irritability of overexcited nerve cells that occurs in both epilepsy and neuropathic pain. Decreasing neuronal irritability means that the nerve cells carrying pain signals are less likely to discharge spontaneously or in response to stimuli. Gabapentin is commonly used for peripheral neuropathy.

10. a. *Rationale:* Acetaminophen acts on the parts of the brain that receive pain signals and is one of the safest analgesics for management of mild pain or as a supplement in management of more intense pain. It is especially useful in nonspecific musculoskeletal pain or pain associated with osteoarthritis. The maximum daily dose of acetaminophen is 4000 mg, and the drug should be avoided or the dosage reduced in clients with renal insufficiency or liver failure.

11. c. *Rationale:* NSAIDs (e.g., ibuprofen) reduce the production of prostaglandins, which in turn reduce inflammatory chemicals that cause, increase, or maintain pain signals. NSAIDs are useful in treating many pain conditions that are caused or aggravated by inflammation. They may be used for moderate to severe pain alone or with opioids. Adverse effects include GI bleeding.

12. Neuropathic

13. d. *Rationale:* Somatic pain results from stimulation of nociceptors in skin, bone, muscle, and soft tissue. It is usually well localized and described as sharp, burning, gnawing, throbbing, or cramping. It may be intermittent or constant, and acute or chronic. Sprains and other traumatic injuries are examples of acute somatic pain; the bone and joint pain of arthritis is an example of chronic somatic pain, although acute exacerbations may also occur. Somatic pain of low to moderate intensity may stimulate the sympathetic nervous system and produce increased blood pressure, pulse, and respiration; dilated pupils; and increased skeletal muscle tension, such as rigid posture or clenched fists.

14. a. *Rationale:* Chronic pain (i.e., pain lasting 3 months or longer) demands attention less urgently, may not be characterized by visible signs, and is often accompanied by emotional stress, increased irritability, depression, social withdrawal, financial distress, loss of libido, disturbed sleep patterns, diminished appetite, weight loss, and decreased ability to perform usual activities of daily living.

15. d. *Rationale:* Acute pain may be caused by injury, trauma, spasm, disease processes, and treatment or diagnostic procedures that damage body tissues. It is often described as sharp or cutting. The intensity of the pain is usually proportional to the amount of tissue damage, and the pain serves as a warning system by demanding the sufferer's attention and compelling behavior to withdraw from or avoid the pain-producing stimulus.

16. a. *Rationale:* Naloxone is the drug of choice for opioid overdose.

17. d. *Rationale:* When opioids are needed, use those with short half-lives (e.g., oxycodone, hydromorphone) are used because they are less likely to accumulate.

18. a. *Rationale:* Expressions of pain may differ according to age and developmental level. Infants may cry and have muscular rigidity and thrashing behavior. Preschoolers may behave aggressively or complain verbally of discomfort. Young school-aged children may express pain verbally or behaviorally, often with regression to behaviors used at younger ages. Adolescents may be reluctant to admit they are uncomfortable or need help. With chronic pain, children of all ages tend to withdraw and regress to an earlier stage of development.

19. c. *Rationale:* Opioids administered during labor and delivery may depress fetal and neonatal respiration. The drugs cross the blood–brain barrier of the infant more readily than that of the mother. Therefore, doses that do not depress maternal respiration may profoundly depress the infant's respiration. Respiration should be monitored closely in neonates, and the opioid antagonist naloxone should be readily available.

20. a. *Rationale:* Clonidine, an antihypertensive drug, is a nonopioid that may be used to treat opioid withdrawal. Clonidine reduces the release of norepinephrine in the brain and thus reduces symptoms associated with excessive stimulation of the sympathetic nervous system (e.g., anxiety, restlessness, insomnia). Blood pressure must be closely monitored during clonidine therapy.

Chapter 7: Analgesic–Antipyretic–Anti-inflammatory and Related Drugs

SECTION II: ASSESSING YOUR UNDERSTANDING

ACTIVITY A
FILL IN THE BLANKS
1. antiprostaglandin drugs
2. Prostaglandins
3. hypothalamus
4. Inflammation
5. –itis

ACTIVITY B
MATCHING
1. C   2. E   3. A   4. B   5. D

ACTIVITY C
SEQUENCING

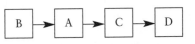

ACTIVITY D
SHORT ANSWERS
1. Prostaglandins are chemical mediators found in most body tissues; they help regulate many cell functions and participate in the inflammatory response. They are formed when cellular injury occurs and phospholipids in cell membranes release *arachidonic acid*. Arachidonic acid is metabolized by *cyclooxygenase (COX)* enzymes to produce prostaglandins, which act briefly in the area where they are produced and are then inactivated. Prostaglandins exert various and opposing effects in different body tissues.

2. Fever occurs when the set point of the hypothalamus is raised in response to the presence of *pyrogens* (fever-producing agents). Endogenous pyrogenes include cytokines such as interleukin-1, interleukin-6, and tumor necrosis factor. Exogenous pyrogens include bacteria and their toxins or other byproducts. The upward adjustment of the hypothalamic set point in response to the presence of a pyrogen is mediated by prostaglandin E_2. The body

responds to the higher hypothalamic set point by vasoconstriction of blood vessels and shivering, raising the core body temperature to the higher set point. Fever may accompany conditions such as dehydration, inflammation, infectious processes, some drugs, brain injury, or diseases involving the hypothalamus.

3. Systemic manifestations include leukocytosis, increased erythrocyte sedimentation rate, fever, headache, loss of appetite, lethargy or malaise, and weakness. Both local and systemic manifestations vary according to the cause and extent of tissue damage.

4. To relieve fever, aspirin and other NSAIDs act on the hypothalamus to decrease its response to pyrogens and reset the "thermostat" at a lower level. For inflammation, the drugs prevent prostaglandins from increasing the pain and edema produced by other substances released by damaged cells. Although these drugs relieve symptoms and contribute greatly to the client's comfort and quality of life, they do not cure the underlying disorders that cause the symptoms.

5. Aspirin and nonselective NSAIDs also have antiplatelet effects that differ in mechanism and extent. When aspirin is absorbed into the bloodstream, the acetyl portion dissociates and then binds irreversibly to platelet COX-1. This action prevents synthesis of thromboxane A_2, a prostaglandin derivative, thereby inhibiting platelet aggregation. A small, single dose (325 mg) of aspirin irreversibly acetylates circulating platelets within a few minutes, and effects last for the lifespan of the platelets (7 to 10 days). Most other NSAIDs bind reversibly with platelet COX-1, so that antiplatelet effects occur only while the drug is present in the blood. Therefore, aspirin has greater effects, but all of these drugs except acetaminophen and the COX-2 inhibitors inhibit platelet aggregation, interfere with blood coagulation, and increase the risk of bleeding.

SECTION III: APPLYING YOUR KNOWLEDGE

ACTIVITY E
CASE STUDIES

1. Degenerative joint disease (DJD), also known as osteoarthritis (OA), is a disease that affects the articular cartilage, subchondral bone, and synovium of weight-bearing joints. The joints of the fingers may also be affected by OA. Signs and symptoms of OA include pain, stiffness, and functional impairment. As joint cartilage deteriorates over time, there is less padding and lubricating fluid; underlying bone is exposed; and friction and abrasion lead to inflammation of the synovial membrane lining of the joint. Deformity of the joint occurs as the disease advances.

2. COX-2 is also normally present in several tissues (e.g., brain, bone, kidneys, GI tract, and female reproductive system). However, it is thought to occur in small amounts or to be inactive until stimulated by pain and inflammation. In inflamed tissues, COX-2 is induced by inflammatory chemical mediators such as interleukin-1 and tumor necrosis factor-alpha. In the GI tract, COX-2 is also induced by trauma and by *Helicobacter pylori* infection, a common cause of peptic ulcer disease. Overall, prostaglandins produced by COX-2 are associated with pain and other signs of inflammation. Inhibition of COX-2 results in the therapeutic effects of analgesia and anti-inflammatory activity. The COX-2 inhibitor drugs are NSAIDs designed to selectively inhibit COX-2 and relieve pain and inflammation with fewer adverse effects, especially stomach damage; however, with long-term use,

adverse effects still occur in the GI, renal, and cardiovascular systems.

SECTION IV: PRACTICING FOR NCLEX

1. b. *Rationale:* When colchicine is taken for acute gout, pain is usually relieved in 4 to 12 hours with IV administration or in 24 to 48 hours with oral administration. Inflammation and edema may not decrease for several days.

2. a. *Rationale:* With colchicine for chronic gout, carry the drug and take as directed when pain begins until relief is obtained or nausea, vomiting, and diarrhea occur.

3. d. *Rationale:* Drink 2 to 3 quarts of fluid daily with antigout drugs. An adequate fluid intake helps prevent formation of uric acid kidney stones. Fluid intake is especially important initially, when uric acid levels in the blood are high and large amounts of uric acid are being excreted in the urine.

4. c. *Rationale:* Acetaminophen is often the initial drug of choice for relieving mild to moderate pain and fever, because it does not cause gastric irritation or bleeding. It may be taken on an empty stomach.

5. a. *Rationale:* Acetaminophen is an effective aspirin substitute for pain or fever but not for inflammation or prevention of heart attack or stroke.

6. b. *Rationale:* Do not exceed recommended doses of acetaminophen due to risk of life-threatening liver damage. People with liver disorders such as hepatitis or those who ingest alcoholic beverages frequently should use extreme caution.

7. a. *Rationale:* If a client has a history of taking aspirin, including the low doses prescribed for antithrombotic effects, there is a risk of bleeding from common therapeutic procedures (e.g., intramuscular injections, venipuncture, insertion of urinary catheters or GI tubes) or diagnostic procedures (e.g., drawing blood, angiography).

8. c. *Rationale:* Older patients on long-term NSAIDs therapy should be evaluated for GI blood loss, renal dysfunction, edema, hypertension, and drug–drug or drug–disease interactions (Level A). Use of gastroprotective agents is recommended for individuals at risk of upper GI bleeding events (Level B). COX-2 inhibitors may be preferred in older adults, because they are less likely to cause gastric ulceration and bleeding; however this benefit must be weighed against the increased risk of cardiovascular events.

9. kidneys

10. b. *Rationale:* Ibuprofen also may be given for fever. Alternating acetaminophen and ibuprofen every 4 hours over a 3-day period to control fever in young children (ages 6 to 36 months) has been shown to be more effective than monotherapy with either agent.

11. d. *Rationale:* There is a risk of overdose and hepatotoxicity, because acetaminophen is a very common ingredient in OTC cold, flu, fever, and pain remedies. An overdose can occur with large doses of one product or smaller amounts of several different products. In addition, toxicity has occurred when parents or caregivers have given the liquid concentration intended for children to infants.

12. a. Cancer often produces chronic pain from tumor invasion of tissues or complications of treatment (chemotherapy, surgery, or radiation). As with acute pain, acetaminophen, aspirin, or other NSAIDs prevent

sensitization of peripheral pain receptors by inhibiting prostaglandin formation. NSAIDs are especially effective for pain associated with bone metastases.

13. b. Aspirin should generally be avoided for 1 to 2 weeks before and after surgery, because it increases the risk of bleeding. Most other NSAIDs should be discontinued approximately 3 days before surgery; nabumetone and piroxicam have long half-lives and must be discontinued approximately 1 week before surgery. NSAIDS, administered intraoperatively, have been shown to reduce postoperative pain and use of opioids after abdominal surgery.

14. overuse headaches, also called "rebound headaches"

15. c. *Rationale:* Both categories of migraine abortive drugs (e.g. ergot alkaloids and serotonin agonists) exert powerful vasoconstrictive effects and have the potential to raise blood pressure.

16. Reyes' syndrome

17. a. *Rationale:* If an ergot preparation is used, it should be given at the onset of headache, and the client should lie down in a quiet, darkened room.

18. c. *Rationale:* Preparations containing sedatives such as butalbital should be limited due to the possibility of overuse headaches and withdrawal issues (Level C).

19. Allopurinol, probenecid, or sulfinpyrazone may be given to reduce serum uric acid levels and prevent joint inflammation and renal calculi.

20. hyaluronic acid (Synvisc)

Chapter 8: Antianxiety and Sedative-Hypnotic Drugs

SECTION II: ASSESSING YOUR UNDERSTANDING

ACTIVITY A
FILL IN THE BLANKS
1. Antianxiety drugs, anxiolytics, sedatives
2. benzodiazepines, nonbenzodiazepine
3. Anxiety
4. Situational anxiety
5. gamma-aminobutyric acid (GABA)
6. Insomnia

ACTIVITY B
MATCHING
1. C   2. A   3. E   4. B   5. D

ACTIVITY C
SHORT ANSWERS
1. The pathophysiology of anxiety disorders is unknown, but there is evidence of a biologic basis and possible imbalances among several neurotransmission systems. A simplistic view involves an excess of excitatory neurotransmitters (e.g., norepinephrine) or a deficiency of inhibitory neurotransmitters (e.g., GABA).
2. The serotonin system, although not as well understood, is also thought to play a role in anxiety. Both selective serotonin reuptake inhibitors (SSRIs) and serotonin receptor agonists are now used to treat anxiety disorders. Research has suggested two possible roles for the serotonin receptor HT1A. During embryonic development, stimulation of HT1A receptors by serotonin is thought to play a role in development of normal brain circuitry necessary for normal anxiety responses. However, during adulthood, SSRIs act through HT1A receptors to reduce anxiety responses.
3. Activities that occur during the various sleep stages include increased tissue repair, synthesis of skeletal muscle protein, and secretion of growth hormone. At the same time, there are decreased body temperature, metabolic rate, glucose consumption, and production of catabolic hormones. Stage IV is followed by a period of 5 to 20 minutes of REM, dreaming, and increased physiologic activity.
4. Insomnia has many causes, including such stressors as pain, anxiety, illness, changes in lifestyle or environment, and various drugs. Occasional sleeplessness is a normal response to many stimuli and is not usually harmful. Insomnia is said to be chronic when it lasts longer than 1 month. As in anxiety, several neurotransmission systems are apparently involved in regulating sleep–wake cycles and producing insomnia.
5. The noradrenergic system is associated with the hyperarousal state experienced by clients with anxiety (i.e., feelings of panic, restlessness, tremulousness, palpitations, hyperventilation), which is attributed to excessive norepinephrine.

SECTION III: APPLYING YOUR KNOWLEDGE

ACTIVITY D
CASE STUDIES
CASE STUDY 1
1. Although some beneficial effects of buspirone may occur within 7 to 10 days, optimal effects may require 3 to 4 weeks. Because therapeutic effects may be delayed, buspirone is not considered beneficial for immediate effects or occasional (as-needed, or PRN) use.
2. Buspirone (BuSpar) differs chemically and pharmacologically from other antianxiety drugs. Its mechanism of action is unclear, but it apparently interacts with serotonin and dopamine receptors in the brain. Compared with the benzodiazepines, buspirone lacks muscle relaxant and anticonvulsant effects; does not cause sedation or physical or psychological dependence; does not increase the CNS depression of alcohol and other drugs; and is not a controlled substance.
3. Adverse effects of buspirone include nervousness and excitement. Therefore, clients who are wanting and accustomed to sedative effects may not like the drug or comply with instructions for its use.

CASE STUDY 2
1. Eszopiclone is rapidly absorbed after oral administration, reaching peak plasma levels 1 hour after administration. Onset of action may be delayed by approximately 1 hour if the drug is taken with a high-fat or heavy meal. Eszopiclone has a half-life of 6 hours.
2. Mr. Petski may be experiencing an adverse reaction to the medication. Adverse reactions include behavior changes such as reduced inhibition, aggression or bizarre behavior, worsening depression and suicidal ideation, hallucinations, and anterograde amnesia (short-term memory loss).
3. Review Mr. Petski's current drug regimen to determine whether he is taking any drugs that inhibit CYP3A4 enzymes (e.g., antidepressants, antifungals, erythromycin, grapefruit, protease inhibitors), which may require the physician to lower the dose of his medication to reduce adverse effects. Eszopiclone should not be taken with alcohol or other CNS depressants, to avoid additive effects.

SECTION IV: PRACTICING FOR NCLEX
1. b. *Rationale:* Eszopiclone (Lunesta) is the first oral nonbenzodiazepine hypnotic to be approved for long-term use (up to 12 months). During drug testing, tolerance to the hypnotic benefits of eszopiclone was not observed over a 6-month period.
2. c. *Rationale:* Eszopiclone is rapidly absorbed after oral administration, reaching peak plasma levels 1 hour after

administration. Onset of action may be delayed by approximately 1 hour if the drug is taken with a high-fat or heavy meal. Eszopiclone has a half life of 6 hours.

3. a. *Rationale:* Hydroxyzine (Vistaril) is an antihistamine with sedative and antiemetic properties. Clinical indications for use include anxiety, preoperative sedation, nausea and vomiting associated with surgery or motion sickness, and pruritus and urticaria associated with allergic dermatoses.

4. a. *Rationale:* Situational anxiety is a normal response to a stressful situation. It may be beneficial when it motivates the person toward constructive, problem-solving, coping activities. Symptoms may be quite severe, but they usually last only 2 to 3 weeks.

5. b. *Rationale:* Although there is no clear boundary between normal and abnormal anxiety, when anxiety is severe or prolonged and impairs the ability to function in usual activities of daily living, it is called an *anxiety disorder.*

6. d. *Rationale:* Benzodiazepines are widely used for anxiety and insomnia and are also used for several other indications. They have a wide margin of safety between therapeutic and toxic doses and are rarely fatal, even in overdose, unless combined with other CNS depressant drugs, such as alcohol. They are Schedule IV drugs under the Controlled Substances Act. They are drugs of abuse and may cause physiologic dependence; therefore, withdrawal symptoms occur if the drugs are stopped abruptly.

7. b. *Rationale:* Diazepam (Valium) is the prototype benzodiazepine. High-potency benzodiazepines such as alprazolam (Xanax), lorazepam (Ativan), and clonazepam (Klonopin) may be more commonly prescribed due to their greater therapeutic effects and rapid onset of action.

8. c. *Rationale:* Eszopiclone (Lunesta): Adverse reactions include behavior changes such as reduced inhibition, aggression or bizarre behavior, worsening depression and suicidal ideation, hallucinations, and anterograde amnesia (short-term memory loss).

9. d. *Rationale:* Ramelton does not cause physical dependence.

10. b. *Rationale:* Ramelton is rapidly absorbed orally, reaching peak plasma levels in about 45 minutes.

11. a. *Rationale:* Zaleplon is well absorbed, but bioavailability is only about 30% because of extensive presystemic or "first-pass" hepatic metabolism. Action onset is rapid and peaks in 1 hour. A high-fat, heavy meal slows absorption and may reduce the drug's effectiveness in inducing sleep.

12. b. *Rationale:* Zaleplon should not be taken concurrently with alcohol or other CNS depressant drugs because of the increased risk of excessive sedation and respiratory depression.

13. b. *Rationale:* Cimetidine inhibits both the aldehyde oxidase and the cytochrome P450 CYP3A4 enzymes that metabolize zaleplon. If cimetidine is taken, zaleplon dosage should be reduced to 5 mg. It is very important that clients taking zaleplon be taught about this interaction, because cimetidine is available without prescription, and the client may not inform the healthcare provider who prescribes zaleplon about taking cimetidine.

14. d. *Rationale:* A newer controlled release form of zolpidem (Ambien CR) contains a rapid-releasing layer of medication, which aids a person in falling asleep and a second layer, which is released more slowly to promote sleep all night.

15. c. *Rationale:* Adverse effects of zolpidem include daytime drowsiness, dizziness, nausea, diarrhea, and anterograde amnesia. Rebound insomnia may occur for a night or two after stopping the drug, and withdrawal symptoms may occur if it is stopped abruptly after approximately 1 week of regular use.

16. a. *Rationale:* Alprazolam is the most commonly prescribed benzodiazepine; its dose should be reduced by 50% if it is given concurrently with the antidepressant fluvoxamine.

17. b. *Rationale:* In older adults, most benzodiazepines are metabolized more slowly, and half-lives are longer than in younger adults. Exceptions are lorazepam and oxazepam, whose half-lives and dosages are the same for older adults as for younger ones. The recommended initial dose of zaleplon or zolpidem is 5 mg, one half of the initial dose recommended for younger adults. Dosages of eszopiclone should also be reduced for older adults, beginning with 1 mg initially, not to exceed 2 mg at bedtime.

18. b. *Rationale:* When benzodiazepines are used with opioid analgesics, the analgesic dose should be reduced initially and increased gradually to avoid excessive CNS depression.

19. c. *Rationale:* The antianxiety benzodiazepines are often given in three or four daily doses. This is necessary for the short-acting agents, but there is no pharmacologic basis for multiple daily doses of the long-acting drugs. Because of their prolonged actions, all or most of the daily dose can be given at bedtime. This schedule promotes sleep, and there is usually enough residual sedation to maintain antianxiety effects throughout the next day.

20. Flumazenil (Romazicon)

Chapter 9: Antipsychotic Drugs

SECTION II: ASSESSING YOUR UNDERSTANDING

ACTIVITY A
FILL IN THE BLANKS
1. psychosis
2. Hallucinations
3. Delusions
4. paranoia
5. neuroleptics

ACTIVITY B
MATCHING
1. B   2. E   3. A   4. C   5. D

ACTIVITY C
SHORT ANSWERS
1. Psychosis is a severe mental disorder characterized by disordered thought processes (disorganized and often bizarre thinking); blunted or inappropriate emotional responses; bizarre behavior ranging from hypoactivity to hyperactivity with agitation, aggressiveness, hostility, and combativeness; social withdrawal, in which a person pays less than normal attention to the environment and other people; deterioration from previous levels of occupational and social functioning (poor self-care and interpersonal skills); hallucinations; and paranoid delusions.
2. Acute psychotic episodes, also called confusion or delirium, have a sudden onset over hours to days and may be precipitated by physical disorders (e.g., brain damage related to cerebrovascular disease or head injury, metabolic disorders, infections); drug intoxication (e.g., adrenergics, antidepressants, some anticonvulsants, amphetamines, cocaine); or drug withdrawal after chronic use (e.g., alcohol; benzodiazepine antianxiety or sedative-hypnotic agents).

3. The neurodevelopmental model proposes that schizophrenia results when abnormal brain synapses are formed in response to an intrauterine insult during the second trimester of pregnancy, when neuronal migration is normally taking place. Intrauterine events such as upper respiratory tract infection, obstetric complications, and neonatal hypoxia have been associated with schizophrenia. The emergence of psychosis in response to the formation of these abnormal circuits in adolescence or early adulthood corresponds to the time period of neuronal maturation.

4. Genetics is strongly suspected to play a role in the development of schizophrenia. Family studies identify increased risk if a first-degree relative has the illness (10%), if a second-degree relative has the illness (3%), if both parents have the illness (40%), and if a monozygotic twin has the illness (48%). Adoption studies of twins suggest that heredity, rather than environment, is a key factor in the development of schizophrenia. Many genetic studies are underway to identify the gene or genes responsible for schizophrenia. Possible genes linked to schizophrenia include *WKL1* on chromosome 22, which is thought to play a role in catatonic schizophrenia; *DISC1*, mutations of which cause delays in migration of brain neurons in mouse models; and the gene responsible for the glutamate receptor, which regulates the amount of glutamine in synapses.

5. Negative symptoms of schizophrenia include lack of pleasure (anhedonia), lack of motivation, blunted affect, poor grooming and hygiene, poor social skills, poverty of speech, and social withdrawal.

SECTION III: APPLYING YOUR KNOWLEDGE

ACTIVITY D
CASE STUDIES
CASE STUDY 1

1. Advantages of clozapine include improvement of negative symptoms without the extrapyramidal side effects associated with older antipsychotic drugs. However, despite these advantages, it is a second-line drug, recommended only for clients who have not responded to treatment with at least two other antipsychotic drugs or who exhibit recurrent suicidal behavior.

2. Clozapine is associated with agranulocytosis, a life-threatening decrease in white blood cells (WBCs) that usually occurs during the first 3 months of therapy. A black box warning alerts health practitioners to this dangerous side effect. Weekly WBC counts are required during the first 6 months of therapy; if acceptable WBC counts are maintained, then WBC counts can be monitored every 2 weeks thereafter.

3. Black box warnings for clozapine (especially in the first months of treatment) include increased risk for fatal myocarditis, orthostatic hypotension with or without syncope, and, rarely, cardiopulmonary arrest. Clozapine is also more likely to cause constipation, drowsiness, and weight gain than other atypical drugs. Clozapine is metabolized primarily by CYP1A2 enzymes and, to a lesser degree, by CYP2D6 and CYP3A4 enzymes.

CASE STUDY 2

1. For clients who are unable or unwilling to take the oral drug as prescribed, a slowly absorbed, long-acting formulation (haloperidol decanoate) may be given IM, once monthly.

2. The signs and symptoms of extrapyramidal side effects include twisting and rhythmic movements (acute dystonia), tremors (parkinsonism), and inability to sit or remain still (akathisia).

SECTION IV: PRACTICING FOR NCLEX

1. a and b. *Rationale:* Neuroleptic malignant syndrome (a potentially fatal adverse effect characterized by rigidity, severe hyperthermia, agitation, confusion, delirium, dyspnea, tachycardia, respiratory failure, and acute renal failure); is treated with hydration, cooling measures and antipyretics to reduce fever, benzodiazepines to reduce agitation, dantrolene to directly relax muscles, and bromocriptine or amantadine (dopamine agonists) to reduce CNS depression.

2. d. *Rationale:* Tardive dyskinesia, a late extrapyramidal effect, may occur with all phenothiazine and typical nonphenothiazine drugs and is generally considered to be irreversible. It may be treated by reducing the dosage or switching to a second-generation antipsychotic. Prevention through early detection is key.

3. c. *Rationale:* Early extrapyramidal effects are treated by reducing dosage, changing to a second-generation antipsychotic, or using anticholinergic medications. Akathisia may also be treated with benzodiazepines and beta-blockers to reduce the urge to move.

4. a. *Rationale:* Antipsychotics may take several weeks to achieve maximum therapeutic effect.

5. b. *Rationale:* The home care nurse must assist and support caregivers' efforts to maintain medications and manage adverse drug effects, other aspects of daily care, and follow-up psychiatric care. In addition, the home care nurse may need to coordinate the efforts of several health and social service agencies or providers

6. d. *Rationale:* If haloperidol is used, it is usually given IV, by bolus injection. The initial dose is 0.5 to 10 mg, depending on the severity of the agitation. It should be injected at a rate no faster than 5 mg/min; the dose may be repeated every 30 to 60 minutes, up to a total amount of 30 mg, if necessary.

7. c. *Rationale:* Some clients become acutely agitated or delirious and need sedation to prevent their injuring themselves by thrashing about, removing tubes and intravenous (IV) catheters, and so forth. Some physicians prefer a benzodiazepine-type sedative, whereas others may use haloperidol. Before giving either drug, causes of delirium (e.g., drug intoxication or withdrawal) should be identified and eliminated if possible.

8. c. *Rationale:* Antipsychotic drugs undergo extensive hepatic metabolism and then elimination in urine. In the presence of liver disease (e.g., cirrhosis, hepatitis), metabolism may be slowed and drug elimination half-lives prolonged, with resultant accumulation and increased risk of adverse effects. Therefore, these drugs should be used cautiously in clients with hepatic impairment.

9. a. *Rationale:* Because most antipsychotic drugs are extensively metabolized in the liver and the metabolites are excreted through the kidneys, the drugs should be used cautiously in clients with impaired renal function. Renal function should be monitored periodically during long-term therapy. If renal function test results (e.g., blood urea nitrogen) become abnormal, the drug may need to be lowered in dosage or discontinued.

10. b. *Rationale:* Jaundice has been associated with phenothiazines, usually after 2 to 4 weeks of therapy. It is considered a hypersensitivity reaction, and clients should not be re-exposed to a phenothiazine.

11. c. *Rationale:* African Americans tend to respond more rapidly; experience a higher incidence of adverse effects, including tardive dyskinesia; and metabolize antipsychotic drugs more slowly than whites. When compared with haloperidol, olanzapine has been associated with fewer extrapyramidal reactions in African Americans.

12. d. *Rationale:* Clients with dementia may become agitated because of environmental or medical problems. Alleviating such causes, when possible, is safer and more effective than administering antipsychotic drugs. Inappropriate use of antipsychotic drugs exposes clients to adverse drug effects and does not resolve underlying problems.

13. d. *Rationale:* If antipsychotic drugs are used to control acute agitation in older adults, they should be used in the lowest effective dose for the shortest effective duration. If the drugs are used to treat dementia, they may relieve some symptoms (e.g., agitation, hallucinations, hostility, suspiciousness, uncooperativeness), but they do not improve memory loss and may further impair cognitive functioning.

14. d. *Rationale:* Children usually have a faster metabolic rate than adults and may therefore require relatively high doses of antipsychotics for their size and weight.

15. a. *Rationale:* A major concern about giving traditional antipsychotic drugs perioperatively is their potential for adverse interactions with other drugs. For example, antipsychotic drugs potentiate the effects of general anesthetics and other CNS depressants that are often used before, during, and after surgery. As a result, risks of hypotension and excessive sedation are increased unless doses of other drugs are reduced.

16. a, b, and c. *Rationale:* Acute dystonia (manifested by severe spasms of muscles of the face, neck, tongue, or back) typically occurs early in treatment and constitutes an emergency. Severe manifestations of acute dystonia include oculogyric crisis (severe involuntary upward rotation of the eyes) and opisthotonus (severe spasm of back muscles causing head and heels to bend backward with the body bowed forward).

17. b. *Rationale:* Acute dystonia is treated with intramuscular or intravenous administration of anticholinergic medications such as benztropine or diphenhydramine.

18. Aripiprazole (Abilify)

19. partial agonist

20. b. *Rationale:* Clinically significant drug interactions may occur with drugs that induce or inhibit the liver enzymes, and dosage of quetiapine (Seroquel) may need to be increased in clients who are taking enzyme inducers (e.g., carbamazepine, phenytoin, rifampin) or decreased in clients who are taking enzyme inhibitors (e.g., cimetidine, erythromycin).

Chapter 10: Antidepressants and Mood Stabilizers

SECTION II: ASSESSING YOUR UNDERSTANDING

ACTIVITY A
FILL IN THE BLANKS
1. Postpartun depression
2. Major depression
3. Bipolar disorder type I
4. Bipolar disorder type II
5. 5 months

ACTIVITY B
MATCHING
1. E   2. B   3. A   4. C   5. D

ACTIVITY C
SHORT ANSWERS
1. Toxicity is most likely to occur in depressed clients who intentionally ingest large amounts of drug in suicide attempts and in young children who accidentally gain access to medication containers. Measures to prevent acute poisoning from drug overdose include dispensing only a few days' supply (i.e., 5 to 7 days) to clients with suicidal tendencies and storing the drugs in places that are inaccessible to young children. General measures to treat acute poisoning include early detection of signs and symptoms, stopping the drug, and instituting treatment if indicated.

2. For clients with certain concurrent medical conditions, antidepressants may have adverse effects. For clients with cardiovascular disorders, most antidepressants can cause hypotension, but the SSRIs, bupropion, and venlafaxine are rarely associated with cardiac dysrhythmias. Duloxetine, venlafaxine, and MAOIs can increase blood pressure. For clients with seizure disorders, bupropion, clomipramine, and duloxetine should be avoided. SSRIs, MAOIs, and desipramine are less likely to cause seizures. For clients with diabetes mellitus, SSRIs may have a hypoglycemic effect. Duloxetine may slightly increase fasting glucose levels, and bupropion and venlafaxine have little effect on blood sugar levels. Duloxetine can cause mydriasis, increasing intraocular pressure in patients with narrow-angle glaucoma.

3. Lithium is the drug of choice for clients with bipolar disorder. When used therapeutically, lithium is effective in controlling mania in 65% to 80% of clients. When used prophylactically, the drug decreases the frequency and intensity of manic cycles.

4. With SSRIs and venlafaxine, therapy is begun with once-daily oral administration of the manufacturer's recommended dosage. Dosage may be increased after 3 or 4 weeks if depression is not relieved. As with most other drugs, smaller doses may be indicated in older adults and in clients taking multiple medications. Duloxetine is initiated with twice-a-day oral administration without regard to food.

5. Serotonin syndrome, a serious and sometimes fatal reaction characterized by hypertensive crisis, hyperpyrexia, extreme agitation progressing to delirium and coma, muscle rigidity, and seizures, may occur due to combined therapy with an SSRI and an MAOI or other drugs that potentiate serotonin neurotransmission. An SSRI or SNRI and an MAOI should not be given concurrently or within 2 weeks of each other. In most cases, if a client taking an SSRI is to be transferred to an MAOI, the SSRI should be discontinued at least 14 days before starting the MAOI. However, because of its prolonged half-life, fluoxetine should be discontinued at least 5 weeks before starting an MAOI.

SECTION III: APPLYING YOUR KNOWLEDGE

ACTIVITY D
CASE STUDIES
CASE STUDY 1
1. If an antidepressant medication was recently started, the nurse may need to remind the client that it usually takes 2 to 4 weeks to take effect. The nurse should encourage the client to continue taking the medication.

2. The family should be taught to report any change in the client's behavior, especially anxiety, agitation, panic attacks, insomnia, irritability, hostility, impulsivity, akathisia, hypomania, or mania. A client who has one or more of these symptoms may be at greater risk for worsening depression or suicidality.

CASE STUDY 2

1. Adverse effects include a high incidence of gastrointestinal (GI) symptoms (e.g., nausea, diarrhea, weight loss) and sexual dysfunction (e.g., delayed ejaculation in men, impaired orgasmic ability in women). Most SSRIs also cause some degree of CNS stimulation (e.g., anxiety, nervousness, insomnia), which is most prominent with fluoxetine.
2. Fluoxetine also forms an active metabolite with a half-life of 7 to 9 days. Therefore, steady-state blood levels are achieved slowly, over several weeks, and drug effects decrease slowly (over 2 to 3 months) when fluoxetine is discontinued.

SECTION IV: PRACTICING FOR NCLEX

1. a. *Rationale:* Third-trimester intrauterine exposure to fluoxetine or other SSRIs may result in a *neonatal withdrawal syndrome*, which shares some similarity to a mild serotonin syndrome. Common symptoms include irritability, prolonged crying, respiratory distress, rigidity, and possibly seizures. Care for an infant with neonatal withdrawal syndrome is supportive; symptoms usually abate within a few days.
2. serotonin syndrome. *Rationale:* Serotonin syndrome, a serious and sometimes fatal reaching characterized by hypertensive crisis, hyperpyrexia, extreme agitation progressing to delirium and coma, muscle rigidity, and seizures may occur due to combined therapy with an SSRI or SNRI and an MAOI or other drug that potentiates serotonin neurotransmission.
3. b. *Rationale:* A black box warning alerts health care providers to the increased risk of suicidal ideation in children, adolescents, and young adults 18 to 24 years of age when taking antidepressant medications.
4. c. *Rationale:* Bipolar disorder type II is characterized by episodes of major depression plus hypomanic episodes and occurs more frequently in women.
5. d. *Rationale:* Critically ill clients may be receiving an antidepressant when the critical illness develops, or they may need a drug to combat the depression that often develops with major illness. The decision to continue or start an antidepressant should be based on a thorough assessment of the client's condition, other drugs being given, potential adverse drug effects, and other factors. If an antidepressant is given, its use must be cautious and slow, and the client's responses must be carefully monitored, because critically ill clients are often frail and unstable, with multiple organ dysfunctions.
6. b. *Rationale:* Hepatic impairment leads to reduced first-pass metabolism of most antidepressant drugs, resulting in higher plasma levels. The drugs should be used cautiously in clients with severe liver impairment. Cautious use means lower doses, longer intervals between doses, and slower dose increases than usual.
7. a. *Rationale:* SSRIs are the drugs of choice in older adults, as in younger ones, because they produce fewer sedative, anticholinergic, cardiotoxic, and psychomotor adverse effects than the TCAs and related antidepressants.

8. b. *Rationale:* A TCA probably is not a drug of first choice for adolescents, because TCAs are more toxic in overdose than other antidepressants, and suicide is a leading cause of death in adolescents.
9. d. *Rationale:* Amitriptyline, desipramine, imipramine, and nortriptyline are the TCAs most commonly prescribed to treat depression in children older than 12 years of age. Because of potentially serious adverse effects, blood pressure, ECG, and plasma drug levels should be monitored.
10. b. *Rationale:* For most children and adolescents, it is probably best to reserve drug therapy for those who do not respond to nonpharmacologic treatments such as cognitive behavioral therapy.
11. a. *Rationale:* African Americans tend to have higher plasma drug levels for a given dose, respond more rapidly, experience a higher incidence of adverse effects, and metabolize TCAs more slowly than whites. To decrease adverse effects, initial doses may need to be lower than those given to whites, and later doses should be titrated according to clinical response and serum drug levels.
12. c. *Rationale:* Lithium should be stopped 1 to 2 days before surgery and resumed when full oral intake of food and fluids is allowed. Lithium may prolong the effects of anesthetics and neuromuscular blocking drugs.
13. a, b, d, and e. *Rationale:* The most clearly defined withdrawal syndromes are associated with SSRIs and TCAs. With SSRIs, withdrawal symptoms include dizziness, gastrointestinal upset, lethargy or anxiety/hyperarousal, dysphoria, sleep problems, and headache. Symptoms can last from several days to several weeks.
14. a and b. *Rationale:* Toxic manifestations of lithium overdosage occur at serum lithium levels greater than 2.5 mEq/L. Treatment involves supportive care to maintain vital functions, including correction of fluid and electrolyte imbalances. With severe overdoses, hemodialysis is preferred, because it removes lithium from the body.
15. d. *Rationale:* When lithium therapy is being initiated, the serum drug concentration should be measured two or three times weekly in the morning, 12 hours after the last dose of lithium.
16. clinical response
17. b. *Rationale:* Bupropion does not cause orthostatic hypotension or sexual dysfunction.
18. a, b, d, and e. *Rationale:* Because the available drugs have similar efficacy in treating depression, the choice of an antidepressant depends on the client's age; medical conditions; previous history of drug response, if any; and the specific drug's adverse effects. Cost also needs to be considered.
19. a. *Rationale:* St John's wort may reduce the effectiveness of cyclosporine, HIV protease inhibitors, oral contraceptives, digoxin, warfarin, and theophylline through interactions mediated by CYP3A4, CYP2C9, CYP1A2, and CYP2C19 enzyme systems as well as other mechanisms.
20. Lithium carbonate (Eskalith)

Chapter 11: Antiseizure Drugs

SECTION II: ASSESSING YOUR UNDERSTANDING

ACTIVITY A

FILL IN THE BLANKS

1. seizure
2. convulsion
3. antiseizure drug
4. epilepsy
5. Partial seizures

ACTIVITY B
MATCHING
1. B   2. D   3. A   4. C   5. E

ACTIVITY C
SHORT ANSWERS
1. Seizures may occur as single events in response to hypoglycemia, fever, electrolyte imbalances, overdoses of numerous drugs (e.g., amphetamine, cocaine, isoniazid, lidocaine, lithium, methylphenidate, antipsychotics, theophylline), and withdrawal of alcohol or sedative-hypnotic drugs.
2. Epilepsy is characterized by sudden, abnormal, hypersynchronous firing of neurons; it is diagnosed by clinical signs and symptoms of seizure activity and by the presence of abnormal brain wave patterns on the electroencephalogram.
3. Epilepsy can be classified as idiopathic or attributable to a secondary cause. Secondary causes in infancy include developmental defects, metabolic disease, and birth injury. Fever is a common cause during late infancy and early childhood, and inherited forms usually begin in childhood or adolescence. When epilepsy begins in adulthood, it is often caused by an acquired neurologic disorder (e.g., head injury, stroke, brain tumor) or by the effects of alcohol or other drugs. The incidence of epilepsy is higher in young children and older adults than in other age groups.
4. The tonic phase involves sustained contraction of skeletal muscles; abnormal postures such as opisthotonos; and absence of respiration, during which the person becomes cyanotic. The clonic phase is characterized by rapid rhythmic and symmetric jerking movements of the body.
5. An absence seizure is characterized by abrupt alterations in consciousness that last only a few seconds.

SECTION III: APPLYING YOUR KNOWLEDGE

ACTIVITY D
CASE STUDIES
CASE STUDY 1
1. Status epilepticus is a life-threatening emergency characterized by generalized tonic-clonic convulsions lasting for several minutes or occurring at close intervals during which the client does not regain consciousness. Hypotension, hypoxia, and cardiac dysrhythmias may also occur.
2. In a person taking medications for a diagnosed seizure disorder, the most common cause of status epilepticus is abruptly stopping AEDs.

CASE STUDY 2
1. With oral phenytoin, the rate and extent of absorption vary with the drug formulation. Peak plasma drug levels occur in 2 to 3 hours with prompt-acting forms and in about 12 hours with long-acting forms. Intramuscular (IM) phenytoin is poorly absorbed and not recommended. The drug is metabolized in the liver to inactive metabolites that are excreted in the urine.
2. The most common adverse effects of phenytoin affect the CNS (e.g., ataxia, drowsiness, lethargy) and the gastrointestinal (GI) tract (e.g., nausea, vomiting). *Gingival hyperplasia*, an overgrowth of gum tissue, is also common, especially in children. Long-term use may lead to an increased risk of osteoporosis because of its effect on vitamin D metabolism. Serious reactions are uncommon but may include allergic reactions, hepatitis, nephritis, bone marrow depression, and mental confusion.

3. Clients should not switch between generic and trade name formulations of phenytoin because of differences in absorption and bioavailability. If a client is stabilized on a generic formulation and switches to Dilantin, there is a risk of higher serum phenytoin levels and toxicity.

SECTION IV: PRACTICING FOR NCLEX
1. a, b, and d. *Rationale:* Seizures are classified as idiopathic or secondary (caused by tumors, metabolic disorders, overdoses of numerous drugs, or withdrawal of alcohol or sedative-hypnotic drugs).
2. a. *Rationale:* The home care nurse must work with clients and family members to implement and monitor AED therapy. When an AED is started, a few weeks may be required to titrate the dosage and determine whether the chosen drug is effective in controlling seizures. The nurse can play an important role in clinical assessment of the client by interviewing the family about the occurrence of seizures (using a log of date, time, duration, and characteristics of seizures).
3. c. *Rationale:* The community health nurse may assist the physician to titrate drug doses by ensuring that the client keeps appointments for serum drug level testing and follow-up care
4. b. *Rationale:* The use of continuous nasogastric enteral feedings may decrease the absorption of phenytoin administered through the same route, predisposing the client to the risk of seizure activity.
5. d. *Rationale:* The occurrence of nystagmus (abnormal movements of the eyeball) indicates phenytoin toxicity; the drug should be reduced in dosage or discontinued until serum levels decrease.
6. a and d. *Rationale:* Most AEDs are metabolized in the liver and may accumulate in the presence of liver disease or impaired liver function. Doses may need to be reduced or given at less frequent intervals.
7. a. *Rationale:* Oral drugs are absorbed slowly and inefficiently in newborns. If an antiseizure drug is necessary during the first 7 to 10 days of life, IM phenobarbital is effective.
8. c. *Rationale:* AEDs must be used cautiously to avoid excessive sedation and interference with learning and social development.
9. a, b, and c. *Rationale:* Older adults often have multiple medical conditions, take multiple drugs, and have decreases in protein binding and liver and kidney function. As a result, older adults are at high risk for adverse drug effects and adverse drug–drug interactions with AEDs.
10. a. *Rationale:* In older adults, decreased elimination by the liver and kidneys may lead to drug accumulation, with subsequent risks of dizziness, impaired coordination, and injuries due to falls.
11. hyponatremia
12. d. *Rationale:* An IV benzodiazepine (e.g., lorazepam 0.1 mg/kg at 2 mg/minute) is the drug of choice for rapid control of tonic–clonic seizures.
13. d. *Rationale:* Oxcarbazepine decreases effectiveness of felodipine and oral contraceptives, and a barrier type of contraception is recommended during oxcarbazepine therapy.
14. a. *Rationale:* The effectiveness of drug therapy is evaluated primarily by client response in terms of therapeutic or adverse effects. Periodic measurements of serum drug levels are recommended, especially when multiple AEDs are being given.

15. b. *Rationale:* Sexually active adolescent girls and women of childbearing potential who require an AED must be evaluated and monitored very closely, because all of the AEDs are considered teratogenic. In general, infants exposed to one AED have a significantly higher risk of birth defects than those who are not exposed, and infants exposed to two or more AEDs have a significantly higher risk than those exposed to one AED.

16. Zonisamide (Zonegran)

17. b. *Rationale:* Valproic acid preparations (Depakene, Depakote, and Depacon) are chemically unrelated to other AEDs. They are thought to enhance the effects of GABA in the brain and are also used to treat manic reactions in bipolar disorder and to prevent migraine headache.

18. a. *Rationale:* Topiramate (Topamax), which has a broad spectrum of antiseizure activity, may act by increasing the effects of GABA and other mechanisms. It is rapidly absorbed and produces peak plasma levels about 2 hours after oral administration. The average elimination half-life is about 21 hours, and steady-state concentrations are reached in about 4 days with normal renal function.

19. b. *Rationale:* Levetiracetam is well and rapidly absorbed with oral administration; peak plasma levels occur in about 1 hour. Food reduces peak plasma levels by 20%, and these levels do not occur until 1.5 hours; however, this does not affect the extent of drug absorption. The drug is minimally bound (10%) to plasma proteins and reaches steady-state plasma concentrations after 2 days of twice-daily administration. This rapid attainment of therapeutic effects is especially useful for clients with frequent or severe seizures.

20. Gabapentin (Neurontin)

Chapter 12: Antiparkinson Drugs

SECTION II: ASSESSING YOUR UNDERSTANDING

ACTIVITY A
FILL IN THE BLANKS
1. Parkinson's disease (also called parkinsonism)
2. substantia nigra of the basal ganglia
3. resting tremor
4. increasing
5. increase

ACTIVITY B
MATCHING
1. C   2. A   3. E   4. B   5. D

ACTIVITY C
SHORT ANSWERS
1. The basal ganglia in the brain normally contain substantial amounts of the neurotransmitters dopamine and acetylcholine. The correct balance of dopamine and acetylcholine is important in regulating posture, muscle tone, and voluntary movement. People with Parkinson's disease have an imbalance in these neurotransmitters, resulting in a decrease in inhibitory brain dopamine and a relative increase in excitatory acetylcholine.

2. The first symptom of Parkinson's disease is often a resting tremor that begins in the fingers and thumb of one hand (pill-rolling movements); eventually it spreads over one side of the body and progresses to the contralateral limbs. Other common symptoms include slow movement (*bradykinesia*), inability to move (*akinesia*), rigid limbs, shuffling gait, stooped posture, mask-like facial expression, and a soft speaking voice. Less common symptoms may include depression, personality changes, loss of appetite, sleep disturbances, speech impairment, or sexual difficulty.

3. Drugs used in Parkinson's disease help correct the neurotransmitter imbalance by increasing levels of dopamine (*dopaminergic drugs*) or inhibiting the actions of acetylcholine in the brain (*anticholinergic drugs*).

4. The FDA has issued a black box warning regarding an increased risk of suicidality in children and adolescents when treated with antidepressants including selegiline-transdermal.

5. Because levodopa can dilate pupils and raise intraocular pressure, it is contraindicated in narrow-angle glaucoma.

SECTION III: APPLYING YOUR KNOWLEDGE
ACTIVITY D
CASE STUDIES
CASE STUDY 1
1. Rasagiline is the newest irreversible MAO inhibitor. It is indicated for initial treatment of idiopathic parkinsonism and, as an adjunct therapy with levodopa, to reduce "off time" when movements are poorly controlled.
2. Because rasagiline has not been determined to be selective for MAO-B in humans, care must be taken to avoid tyramine-containing foods.
3. Rasagiline has the potential to increase serotonin neurotransmission. When it is given with other drugs that enhance stimulation of serotonergic receptors (e.g. antidepressants, St. John's wort, dextromethorphan, and meperidine), serotonin syndrome, a potential fatal CNS toxicity reaction characterized by hyperpyrexia and death, can occur. Rasagiline should be discontinued at least 14 days before beginning treatment with most antidepressants or other MAO inhibitors. Fluoxetine should be discontinued at least 5 weeks before initiating rasagiline, because of its long half-life. Rasagiline is well absorbed orally, metabolized in the liver, and excreted primarily by the kidneys.

CASE STUDY 2
1. Individuals with RLS, also known as Ekbom's syndrome, experience paresthesias of the muscles, particularly in the calf and thighs, creating the urge to move. The paresthesia is relieved by movement and returns when the individual is at rest or trying to sleep. The disorder may result in insomnia, mental distress, and in some cases suicide.
2. Dopaminergic drugs (e.g., levodopa, cabergoline, pramipexole, ropinirole, rotigotine-transdermal) may be prescribed to reduce the symptoms of restless leg syndrome (RLS).

SECTION IV: PRACTICING FOR NCLEX
1. a, c, d, and e. *Rationale:* Classic symptoms of Parkinson's disease include resting tremor, bradykinesia, rigidity, and postural instability.
2. Amantadine
3. dopamine receptors
4. dopamine; acetylcholine
5. a. *Rationale:* The home care nurse can help clients and caregivers understand that the purpose of drug therapy for Parkinson's disease is to control symptoms and that noticeable improvement may not occur for several weeks.
6. a, c, and d. *Rationale:* the nurse can encourage clients to consult physical therapists, speech therapists, and dietitians to help maintain their ability to perform activities of daily living. In addition, teaching about preventing or managing adverse drug effects may be necessary. Caregivers may need to be informed that most activities (e.g., eating, dressing) take longer and require considerable effort by clients with parkinsonism.

7. b. *Rationale:* Tolcapone therapy should not be initiated for any individual with liver disease or elevated liver enzymes. Liver transaminase enzymes should be monitored frequently on the schedule described in the text.
8. d. *Rationale:* With amantadine, excretion is primarily via the kidneys, and the drug should be used with caution in clients with renal failure.
9. b. *Rationale:* Dosage of levodopa/carbidopa may need to be reduced because of an age-related decrease in peripheral AADC, the enzyme that carbidopa inhibits.
10. a. *Rationale:* When centrally active anticholinergics are given for Parkinson's disease, agitation, mental confusion, hallucinations, and psychosis may occur.
11. c. *Rationale:* The optimal dose is the lowest one that allows the client to function adequately. Optimal dosage may not be established for 6 to 8 weeks with levodopa.
12. b. *Rationale:* The levodopa/carbidopa combination is probably the most effective drug when bradykinesia and rigidity become prominent. However, because levodopa becomes less effective after approximately 5 to 7 years, many clinicians use other drugs first and reserve levodopa for use when symptoms become more severe.
13. a and c. *Rationale:* For advanced idiopathic parkinsonism, a combination of medications is used. Two advantages of combination therapy are better control of symptoms and reduced dosage of individual drugs.
14. d. *Rationale:* Pramipexole (Mirapex), ropinirole (Requip), and rotigotine-transdermal (Neupro) stimulate dopamine receptors in the brain. They are approved for both beginning and advanced stages of Parkinson's disease. In early stages, one of these drugs can be used alone to improve motor performance, improve ability to participate in usual activities of daily living, and delay levodopa therapy.
15. b. *Rationale:* Because of adverse effects and recurrence of parkinsonian symptoms after a few years of levodopa therapy, levodopa is usually reserved for clients with significant symptoms and functional disabilities.
16. dopamine
17. a. *Rationale:* Levodopa is the most effective drug available for the treatment of Parkinson's disease. It relieves all major symptoms, especially bradykinesia and rigidity. Levodopa does not alter the underlying disease process, but it may improve a client's quality of life.
18. glaucoma
19. memory function
20. a, c, and d. *Rationale:* Anticholinergic drugs decrease the effects of acetylcholine, which decreases the relative excess of acetylcholine in relation to the amount of dopamine that occurs in Parkinson's disease. The effect is to decrease salivation, spasticity, and tremors.

Chapter 13: Skeletal Muscle Relaxants

SECTION II: ASSESSING YOUR UNDERSTANDING

ACTIVITY A

FILL IN THE BLANKS

1. Skeletal muscle relaxants
2. Muscle spasm
3. clonic
4. tonic
5. Spasticity

ACTIVITY B

MATCHING

1. B 2. A 3. D 4. E 5. C

ACTIVITY C

SHORT ANSWERS

1. MS involves destruction of portions of the myelin sheath that covers nerves in the brain, spinal cord, and optic nerve. Myelin normally insulates the neuron from electrical activity and conducts electrical impulses rapidly along nerve fibers. When myelin is destroyed (a process called demyelination, which probably results from inflammation), fibrotic lesions are formed and nerve conduction is slowed or blocked around the lesions. Lesions in various states of development (e.g., acute, subacute, chronic) often occur at multiple sites in the central nervous system
2. People with minimal symptoms do not require treatment but should be encouraged to maintain a healthy lifestyle. Those with more extensive symptoms should try to avoid emotional stress, extremes of environmental temperature, infections, and excessive fatigue.
3. Drug therapy for MS may involve various medications for different stages of the disease. Corticosteroids, which are potent anti-inflammatory drugs, are used to treat acute exacerbations (see Chap. 23); interferon-beta, glatiramer, and mitoxantrone suppress the immune system and are given to prevent relapses (see Chap. 41). Other drugs (e.g., antibiotics, antidepressants, anticonvulsants for neuropathic pain) are used to treat symptoms. A skeletal muscle relaxant (e.g., baclofen, tizanidine, dantrolene) is used to treat the symptom of spasticity.
4. All skeletal muscle relaxants except dantrolene are centrally active drugs. Pharmacologic action is usually attributed to general depression of the CNS but may involve blockage of nerve impulses that cause increased muscle tone and contraction.
5. Skeletal muscle relaxants are used primarily as adjuncts to other treatment measures such as physical therapy. Occasionally, parenteral agents are given to facilitate orthopedic procedures and examinations. In spastic disorders, skeletal muscle relaxants are indicated when spasticity causes severe pain or for inability to tolerate physical therapy, sit in a wheelchair, or participate in self-care activities of daily living (e.g., eating, dressing). The drugs should not be given if they cause excessive muscle weakness and impair rather than facilitate mobility and function.

SECTION III: APPLYING YOUR KNOWLEDGE

ACTIVITY D

CASE STUDIES

CASE STUDY 1

1. Physical therapy may help maintain muscle tone, and occupational therapy may help maintain ability to perform activities of daily living.
2. Oral baclofen begins to act in 1 hour, peaks in 2 hours, and lasts 4 to 8 hours. It is metabolized in the liver and excreted in urine; its half-life is 3 to 4 hours. Dosage must be reduced in clients with impaired renal function.
3. When oral baclofen is discontinued, dosage should be tapered and the drug withdrawn over 1 to 2 weeks.

CASE STUDY 2

1. Malignant hyperthermia is a rare but life-threatening complication of anesthesia characterized by hypercarbia, metabolic acidosis, skeletal muscle rigidity, fever, and cyanosis.
2. For preoperative prophylaxis in people with previous episodes of malignant hyperthermia, the drug is given orally for 1 to 2 days before surgery.
3. For intraoperative malignant hyperthermia, the drug is given intravenously (IV). After an occurrence during surgery, the drug is given orally for 1 to 3 days to prevent recurrence of symptoms. Common adverse effects include drowsiness, dizziness, diarrhea, and fatigue.

SECTION IV: PRACTICING FOR NCLEX

1. baclofen; tizanidine
2. a and c. *Rationale:* Physical therapy and other nonpharmacologic treatments are useful in treating muscle spasm and spasticity.
3. a and c. *Rationale:* Both muscle spasms and spasticity can cause pain and disability.
4. Spasticity
5. c. *Rationale:* Muscle spasms usually result from trauma to the affected skeletal muscle.
6. b. *Rationale:* Baclofen is metabolized in the liver and excreted in urine. The patient must be monitored for adverse effects on liver function.
7. a, b, and c. *Rationale:* Clients may need continued assessment of drug effects, monitoring of functional abilities, assistance in arranging, and other care. Caregivers may need instruction about nonpharmacologic interventions to help prevent or relieve spasticity.
8. d. *Rationale:* The skeletal muscle relaxants should be used cautiously in clients with renal impairment. Dosage of baclofen must be reduced.
9. b. *Rationale:* Any CNS depressant or sedating drug should be used cautiously in older adults. Risks of falls, mental confusion, and other adverse effects are higher because of impaired drug metabolism and excretion.
10. a. *Rationale:* For most of the skeletal muscle relaxants, safety and effectiveness for use in children 12 years of age and younger have not been established. The drugs should be used only when clearly indicated; for short periods; when close supervision is available for monitoring drug effects (especially sedation); and when mobility and alertness are not required.
11. b. *Rationale:* For spasticity in people with MS, baclofen (Lioresal) and tizanidine (Zanaflex) are approved. The two drugs are similarly effective, but tizanidine may cause fewer adverse effects.
12. c. *Rationale:* Tizanidine (Zanaflex) is given orally, and it begins to act within 30 to 60 minutes, peaks in 1 to 2 hours, and lasts 3 to 4 hours.
13. d. *Rationale:* Common adverse effects with methocarbamol drug include drowsiness, dizziness, nausea, urticaria, fainting, incoordination, and hypotension.
14. d. *Rationale:* Metaxalone (Skelaxin) is used to relieve discomfort from acute, painful musculoskeletal disorders. It is contraindicated in clients with anemias or severe renal or hepatic impairment.
15. cardiovascular
16. c. *Rationale:* With cyclobenzaprine (Flexeril), duration of use should not exceed 3 weeks.
17. a. *Rationale:* Carisoprodol (Soma) is used to relieve discomfort from acute, painful musculoskeletal disorders. It is not recommended for long-term use. If used long term or in high doses, it can cause physical dependence, and it may cause symptoms of withdrawal if stopped abruptly.
18. a. *Rationale:* Most skeletal muscle relaxants cause CNS depression and have the same contraindications as other CNS depressants. They should be used cautiously in clients with impaired renal or hepatic function or respiratory depression and in clients who must be alert.
19. Dantrolene
20. Baclofen; diazepam

Chapter 14: Substance Abuse Disorders

SECTION II: ASSESSING YOUR UNDERSTANDING

ACTIVITY A
FILL IN THE BLANKS
1. Substance abuse
2. CNS
3. tolerance
4. pleasure (or reward)
5. dependence

ACTIVITY B
MATCHING
1. B   2. D   3. A   4. C   5. E

ACTIVITY C
SHORT ANSWERS
1. Substance abuse is defined as self-administration of a drug for prolonged periods or in excessive amounts to the point of producing physical or psychological dependence; impairing functions of body organs; reducing the ability to function in usual activities of daily living; and decreasing the ability and motivation to function as a productive member of society.
2. Commonly abused drugs include CNS depressants (e.g., alcohol, antianxiety and sedative-hypnotic agents, opioid analgesics), CNS stimulants (e.g., cocaine, methamphetamine, methylphenidate, nicotine), and other mind-altering drugs (e.g., marijuana, "ecstasy").
3. Although these drugs produce different effects, they are associated with feelings of pleasure, positive reinforcement, and compulsive self-administration.
4. Drugs of abuse seem to be readily available. Internet websites have become an important source of the drugs. In some instances, instructions for manufacturing particular drugs are available. Although patterns of drug abuse vary in particular populations and geographic areas, continuing trends seem to include increased use of methamphetamine, "club drugs," prescription drugs, and using multiple drugs at the same time.
5. Characteristics of drug dependence include craving a drug, often with unsuccessful attempts to decrease its use; compulsive drug-seeking behavior; physical dependence (withdrawal symptoms if drug use is decreased or stopped); and continuing to take a drug despite adverse consequences (e.g., drug-related illnesses, mental or legal problems, job loss or decreased ability to function in an occupation, impaired family relationships).

SECTION III: APPLYING YOUR KNOWLEDGE

ACTIVITY D

CASE STUDIES

CASE STUDY 1

1. Physical dependence involves physiologic adaptation to chronic use of a drug so that unpleasant symptoms occur when the drug is stopped, when its action is antagonized by another drug, or when its dosage is decreased. The withdrawal or abstinence syndrome produces specific manifestations according to the type of drug and does not occur as long as adequate dosage is maintained. Attempts to avoid withdrawal symptoms reinforce psychological dependence and promote continuing drug use and relapses to drug-taking behavior.

2. Psychological dependence involves feelings of satisfaction and pleasure from taking the drug. These feelings, perceived as extremely desirable by the drug-dependent person, contribute to acute intoxication, development and maintenance of drug-abuse patterns, and return to drug-taking behavior after periods of abstinence.

3. Tolerance means that the body adjusts to the drugs so that higher doses are needed to achieve feelings of pleasure ("reward") or stave off withdrawal symptoms ("punishment"). Both reward and punishment serve to reinforce continued substance abuse.

CASE STUDY 2

1. One theory is that drugs stimulate or inhibit neurotransmitters in the brain to produce pleasure and euphoria or to decrease unpleasant feelings such as anxiety. For example, dopaminergic neurons in the limbic system are associated with the brain's reward system and are thought to be sites of action of alcohol, amphetamines, cocaine, nicotine, and opiates. These major drugs of abuse increase dopaminergic transmission and the availability of dopamine.

2. For example, amphetamines promote dopamine release and inhibit its reuptake, and cocaine inhibits dopamine reuptake. These actions are believed to stimulate the brain's reward system and lead to compulsive drug administration and abuse.

3. Substance abusers who inject drugs intravenously (IV) are prey to serious problems because they use impure drugs of unknown potency, contaminated needles, poor hygiene, and other dangerous practices. Specific problems include overdoses, death, and numerous infections (e.g., hepatitis, human immunodeficiency virus infection, endocarditis, phlebitis, cellulitis at injection sites).

SECTION IV: PRACTICING FOR NCLEX

1. a and c. *Rationale:* With disulfiram (Antabuse), alcohol produces significant distress (flushing, tachycardia, bronchospasm, sweating, nausea and vomiting). This reaction may be used to treat alcohol dependence.

2. d. *Rationale:* With oral anticoagulants (e.g., warfarin), alcohol interactions vary. Acute ingestion increases anticoagulant effects and the risk of bleeding.

3. d. *Rationale:* Chronic ingestion decreases anticoagulant effects by inducing drug-metabolizing enzymes in the liver and increasing the rate of warfarin metabolism. However, if chronic ingestion has caused liver damage, metabolism of warfarin may be slowed. This increases the risk of excessive anticoagulant effect and bleeding.

4. c. *Rationale:* With oral antidiabetic drugs that decrease blood sugar, alcohol potentiates hypoglycemic effects. These drugs include acarbose (Precose), exenatide (Byetta), glipizide (Glucotrol), glyburide (DiaBeta), glimepiride (Amaryl), miglitol (Glyset), nateglinide (Starlix), pioglitazone (Actos), pramlintide (Symlin), repaglinide (Prandin), and rosiglitazone (Avandia).

5. b. *Rationale:* With antihypertensive agents, alcohol potentiates vasodilation and hypotensive effects.

6. b. *Rationale:* With other CNS depressants (e.g., sedative-hypnotics, opioid analgesics, antianxiety agents, antipsychotic agents, general anesthetics, tricyclic antidepressants), alcohol potentiates CNS depression and increases risks of excessive sedation, respiratory depression, and impaired mental and physical functioning. Combining alcohol with these drugs may be lethal and should be avoided.

7. a and b. *Rationale:* Smoking or inhaling drug vapors is a preferred route of administration for cocaine, marijuana, and nicotine because the drugs are rapidly absorbed from the large surface area of the lungs. Then, they rapidly circulate to the heart and brain without dilution by the systemic circulation or metabolism by enzymes.

8. d. *Rationale:* Abusers of alcohol and other drugs are not reliable sources of information about the types or amounts of drugs used. Most abusers understate the amount and frequency of substance use.

9. a. *Rationale:* Heroin addicts may overstate the amount used in attempts to obtain higher doses of methadone.

10. Alcohol, marijuana, opioids, and sedatives

11. a. *Rationale:* Health care professionals (e.g., physicians, pharmacists, nurses) are considered to be at high risk for development of substance abuse disorders, at least partly because of easy access.

12. b. *Rationale:* Psychological rehabilitation efforts should be part of any treatment program for a drug-dependent person.

13. d. *Rationale:* Inhalants can harm the brain, liver, heart, kidneys, and lungs, and abuse of any drug during adolescence may interfere with brain development. Substances containing gasoline, benzene, or carbon tetrachloride are especially likely to cause serious damage to the liver, kidneys, and bone marrow. Inhalants can also produce psychological dependence, and some produce tolerance.

14. d. *Rationale:* Usage of GHB has increased in recent years, mainly in the party or dance-club setting, and GHB is increasingly involved in poisonings, overdoses, date rapes, visits to hospital emergency departments, and fatalities.

15. d. *Rationale:* Phencyclidine (PCP) produces excitement, delirium, hallucinations, and other profound psychological and physiologic effects, including a state of intoxication similar to that produced by alcohol; altered sensory perceptions; impaired thought processes; impaired motor skills; psychotic reactions; sedation and analgesia; nystagmus and diplopia; and pressor effects that can cause hypertensive crisis, cerebral hemorrhage, convulsions, coma, and death. Death from overdose also has occurred as a result of respiratory depression. Bizarre murders, suicides, and self-mutilations have been attributed to the schizophrenic reaction induced by PCP, especially in high doses. The drug also produces flashbacks.

16. b. *Rationale:* Nicotine is available in transdermal patches, chewing gum, an oral inhaler, and a nasal spray. The gum, inhaler, and spray are used intermittently during the day; the transdermal patch is applied once daily. Transdermal patches produce a steady blood level of nicotine and clients seem to use them more consistently than they use the other products. The patches and gum are available over the counter; the inhaler and nasal spray require a prescription. The products are contraindicated in people with significant cardiovascular disease (angina pectoris, dysrhythmias, or recent myocardial infarction).

17. a, c, and d. *Rationale:* Drug therapy for cocaine dependence is largely symptomatic. Agitation and hyperactivity may be treated with a benzodiazepine antianxiety agent; psychosis may be treated with haloperidol (Haldol) or another antipsychotic agent; cardiac dysrhythmias may be treated with usual antidysrhythmic drugs; myocardial infarction may be treated by standard methods; and so forth. Initial detoxification and long-term treatment are best accomplished in centers or units that specialize in substance-abuse disorders. Long-term treatment of cocaine abuse usually involves psychotherapy, behavioral therapy, and 12-step programs.

18. c. *Rationale:* Heroin may be taken by IV injection, smoking, or nasal application (snorting). IV injection produces intense euphoria, which occurs within seconds, lasts a few minutes, and is followed by a period of sedation. Effects diminish over approximately 4 hours, depending on the dose. Addicts may inject several times daily, cycling between desired effects and symptoms of withdrawal. Tolerance to euphoric effects develops rapidly, leading to dosage escalation and continued use to avoid withdrawal. Like other opioids, heroin causes severe respiratory depression with overdose and produces a characteristic abstinence syndrome.

19. c. *Rationale:* Convulsions are more likely to occur during the first 48 hours of withdrawal and delirium after 48 to 72 hours for clients with benzodiazepine dependence.

20. Alcohol

Chapter 15: Central Nervous System Stimulants

SECTION II: ASSESSING YOUR UNDERSTANDING

ACTIVITY A
FILL IN THE BLANKS
1. ADHD
2. Narcolepsy
3. ADHD, narcolepsy
4. ADHD
5. learning disabilities

ACTIVITY B
MATCHING
1. B   2. A   3. D   4. E   5. C

ACTIVITY C
SHORT ANSWERS
1. ADHD is the most common psychiatric or neurobehavioral disorder in children. It is usually diagnosed between 3 and 7 years of age and may affect as many as 6% or 7% of school-age children. It is characterized by persistent hyperactivity, short attention span, difficulty completing assigned tasks or schoolwork, restlessness, and impulsiveness. Such behaviors make it difficult for the child to get along with others (e.g., family members, peer groups, teachers) and to function in situations requiring controlled behavior (e.g., classrooms).

2. Narcolepsy is a sleep disorder characterized by daytime "sleep attacks" in which the person goes to sleep at any place or at any time. Signs and symptoms also include excessive daytime drowsiness, fatigue, muscle weakness and hallucinations at onset of sleep, and disturbances of nighttime sleep patterns.

3. In addition to drug therapy, prevention of sleep deprivation, regular sleeping and waking times, avoiding shift work, and short naps may be helpful in reducing daytime sleepiness.

4. CNS stimulants act by facilitating initiation and transmission of nerve impulses that excite other cells. The drugs are somewhat selective in their actions at lower doses but tend to involve the entire CNS at higher doses. In ADHD, the drugs improve academic performance, behavior, and interpersonal relationships.

5. Amphetamines increase the amounts of norepinephrine, dopamine, and possibly serotonin in the brain, thereby producing mood elevation or euphoria, increasing mental alertness and capacity for work, decreasing fatigue and drowsiness, and prolonging wakefulness.

SECTION III: APPLYING YOUR KNOWLEDGE
ACTIVITY D
CASE STUDIES
CASE STUDY 1
1. Acceptable nursing diagnoses are
   - Sleep Pattern Disturbance related to hyperactivity, nervousness, insomnia
   - Risk for Injury: Adverse drug effects (excessive cardiac and CNS stimulation, drug dependence)
   - Deficient Knowledge: Drug effects on children and adults
2. Try to identify potentially significant sources of caffeine intake.
3. The client will take CNS stimulants safely and accurately.

CASE STUDY 2
1. This statement by Jane's mother indicates that she requires further education regarding the administration of stimulants to her child. You should include in your education of the patient's parents the following points:
   - Stimulant drugs should be taken only as prescribed.
   - These drugs have a high potential for abuse.
   - The risks of serious health problems and drug dependence are lessened if they are taken correctly.
   - The likelihood of medical problems is greatly increased when ADHD medication is used improperly or in combination with other drugs.
2. Jane's weight should be recorded at least weekly, and excessive losses should be reported. The drugs may cause weight loss; caloric intake (of nutritional foods) may need to be increased, especially in children. Alterations in attention span and task performance should be noted.
3. Monitor for symptoms of drug dependence and stunted growth. You should assist parents in scheduling drug administration to increase beneficial effects and help prevent drug dependence and stunted growth. In addition, ask parents to control drug distribution and monitor the number of pills or capsules available and the number prescribed. The goals are to prevent overuse by the child for whom the drug is prescribed and to prevent the child from sharing the medication with other children who wish to take the drug for nonmedical purposes.

SECTION IV: PRACTICING FOR NCLEX

1. a. *Rationale:* All of the CNS stimulants, including caffeine, can cause life-threatening health problems with excessive intake.

2. b and d. *Rationale:* Narcolepsy is characterized by daytime drowsiness and unpredictable "sleep attacks."

3. c. *Rationale:* CNS stimulants improve behavior and attention in patients with ADHD.

4. d. *Rationale:* ADHD usually starts in childhood and may persist through adulthood.

5. a, c, and d. *Rationale:* ADHD is characterized by hyperactivity, impulsivity, and a short attention span.

6. b. *Rationale:* Older adults are likely to experience anxiety, confusion, insomnia, and nervousness from excessive CNS stimulation. In addition, older adults often have cardiovascular disorders (e.g., angina, dysrhythmias, hypertension) that may be aggravated by the cardiac-stimulating effects of the drugs, including dietary caffeine. In general, reduced doses are safer in older adults.

7. b. *Rationale:* A drug holiday (i.e., stopping drug therapy) is recommended at least annually to evaluate the child's treatment regimen. Dosage adjustments are usually needed as the child grows and hepatic metabolism slows. Also, drug holidays decrease weight loss and growth suppression.

8. d. *Rationale:* Methylphenidate is commonly prescribed and is usually given daily for the first 3 to 4 weeks of treatment to allow caregivers to assess beneficial and adverse effects.

9. b, d, and e. *Rationale:* Drug therapy is indicated when symptoms are moderate to severe; are present for several months; and interfere in social, academic, or behavioral functioning.

10. b and d. *Rationale:* Treatment is largely symptomatic and supportive. In general, place the client in a cool room, monitor cardiac function and body temperature, and minimize external stimulation. Activated charcoal (1 g/kg of body weight) may be given.

11. a. *Rationale:* Caffeine is well absorbed from the GI tract and reaches a peak blood level within 30-45 minutes after oral ingestion. It easily crosses the blood–brain barrier and has a half-life of 3.5 to 5 hours. It is extensively metabolized, mainly in the liver, and excreted mainly in urine.

12. d. *Rationale:* Caffeine is an ingredient in some nonprescription analgesic preparations and may increase analgesia. It is combined with an ergot alkaloid to treat migraine headaches (e.g., Cafergot).

13. b. *Rationale:* Theophylline preparations are xanthines used in the treatment of respiratory disorders, such as asthma and bronchitis. In these conditions, the desired effect is bronchodilation and improvement of breathing; CNS stimulation is then an adverse effect.

14. b. *Rationale:* Modafinil is not recommended for clients with a history of left ventricular hypertrophy or ischemic changes on electrocardiograms.

15. a. *Rationale:* In general, the caffeine content of a guarana product is unknown, and guarana may not be listed as an ingredient. As a result, consumers may not know how much caffeine they are ingesting in products containing guarana.

16. c. *Rationale:* The main goal of therapy with CNS stimulants is to relieve symptoms of the disorders for which they are given. A secondary goal is to have clients use the drugs appropriately.

17. a, b, and c. *Rationale:* CNS stimulants are dangerous for drivers and those involved in similar activities and have no legitimate use in athletics.

18. b. *Rationale:* When a CNS stimulant is prescribed, it is started with a low dose that is then increased as necessary, usually at weekly intervals, until an effective dose (i.e., decreased symptoms) or the maximum daily dose is reached. In addition, the number of doses that can be obtained with one prescription should be limited. This action reduces the likelihood of drug dependence or diversion (use by people for whom the drug is not prescribed).

19. d. *Rationale:* CNS stimulants are not recommended for ADHD in children younger than 3 years of age.

20. 250 mg

Chapter 16: Physiology of the Autonomic Nervous System

SECTION II: ASSESSING YOUR UNDERSTANDING

ACTIVITY A
FILL IN THE BLANKS
1. nervous system
2. CNS
3. PNS
4. Afferent
5. efferent

ACTIVITY B
MATCHING
1. C   2. D   3. B   4. E   5. A

ACTIVITY C
SHORT ANSWERS
1. Norepinephrine is synthesized in adrenergic nerve endings and released into the synapse when adrenergic nerve endings are stimulated. It exerts intense but brief effects on presynaptic and postsynaptic adrenergic receptors. The effects of norepinephrine are terminated by reuptake of most of the neurotransmitter back into the nerve endings, where it is packaged into vesicles for reuse as a neurotransmitter. This reuptake and termination process can be inhibited by cocaine and tricyclic antidepressant medications and is responsible for the activation of the sympathetic nervous system seen with these drugs. The remainder of the norepinephrine, which was not taken back into the nerve endings, diffuses into surrounding tissue fluids and blood, or it is metabolized by monoamine oxidase (MAO) or catechol-O-methyltransferase.

2. Norepinephrine functions as a circulating neurohormone, along with epinephrine. In response to adrenergic nerve stimulation, norepinephrine and epinephrine are secreted into the bloodstream by the adrenal medullae and transported to all body tissues. They are continually present in arterial blood in amounts that vary according to the degree of stress present and the ability of the adrenal medullae to respond to stimuli.

3. Functions stimulated by the parasympathetic nervous system are often described as resting, reparative, or vegetative functions. They include digestion, excretion, cardiac deceleration, anabolism, and near vision.

4. When acetylcholine acts on body cells that respond to parasympathetic nerve stimulation, it interacts with two types of cholinergic receptors: nicotinic and muscarinic. Nicotinic receptors are located in motor nerves and skeletal muscle. When they are activated by acetylcholine, the cell membrane depolarizes and produces muscle contraction. Muscarinic receptors are located in most internal organs, including the cardiovascular, respiratory, gastrointestinal, and genitourinary systems. When muscarinic receptors are

activated by acetylcholine, the affected cells may be excited or inhibited in their functions.
5. Dopamine is an adrenergic neurotransmitter and catecholamine. In the brain, dopamine is essential for normal function.

SECTION III: APPLYING YOUR KNOWLEDGE

ACTIVITY D

CASE STUDIES

CASE STUDY 1

1. Sympathomimetic, adrenergic, and alpha- and beta-adrenergic agonists are drugs that have the same effects on the human body as stimulation of the sympathetic nervous system.
2. Parasympathomimetic, cholinomimetic, and cholinergic are drugs that have the same effects on the body as stimulation of the parasympathetic nervous system.
3. Sympatholytic, antiadrenergic, and alpha- and beta-adrenergic blocking drugs inhibit sympathetic stimulation.
4. Parasympatholytic, anticholinergic, and cholinergic blocking drugs inhibit parasympathetic stimulation.

CASE STUDY 2

1. Increased capacity for vigorous muscle activity in response to a perceived threat, whether real or imaginary, is often called the fight-or-flight reaction.
2. Increased arterial blood pressure and cardiac output are some of the primary responses to a perceived threat. Other responses include increased rate of cellular metabolism, such as increased oxygen consumption and carbon dioxide production; increased breakdown of muscle glycogen for energy; and increased rate of blood coagulation.

SECTION IV: PRACTICING FOR NCLEX

1. c. *Rationale:* The number of receptors in the ANS is dynamic and can be upregulated or downregulated as needed.
2. muscarinic, nicotinic
3. c. *Rationale:* Adrenergic receptors include alpha and beta receptors as well as dopamine receptors; there are several subtypes.
4. agonists
5. d. *Rationale:* Drugs that activate ANS receptors function like endogenous neurotransmitters to stimulate the ANS.
6. a. *Rationale:* Stimulation of receptors in the parasympathetic nervous system produces cholinergic effects.
7. b. *Rationale:* Stimulation of receptors in the sympathetic nervous system produces adrenergic effects.
8. effector
9. c. *Rationale:* Drugs that act on the ANS usually affect the entire body rather than certain organs and tissues.
10. c. *Rationale:* Muscarinic$_1$ receptors are expressed primarily in the CNS, autonomic ganglia, and the gastric and salivary glands.
11. Inositol phosphate
12. a, b, and c. *Rationale:* Specific body responses to parasympathetic stimulation include dilation of blood vessels in the skin; decreased heart rate, possibly bradycardia; increased secretion of digestive enzymes and motility of the gastrointestinal tract; constriction of smooth muscle of bronchi; increased secretions from glands in the lungs, stomach, intestines, and skin (sweat glands).
13. vagus

14. d. *Rationale:* Activation of alpha$_1$ receptors in smooth muscle cells is thought to open ion channels, allow calcium ions to move into the cell and produce muscle contraction (e.g., vasoconstriction, gastrointestinal and bladder-sphincter contraction).
15. a. *Rationale:* In the brain, some of the norepinephrine released into the synaptic cleft between neurons returns to the nerve endings from which it was released and stimulates presynaptic alpha$_2$ receptors. This negative feedback prevents calcium-mediated release of norepinephrine from storage vesicles into the synapse, resulting in decreased sympathetic outflow and an antiadrenergic effect.
16. alpha, beta
17. c. *Rationale:* Dopamine receptors are located in the brain, in blood vessels of the kidneys and other viscera, and probably in presynaptic sympathetic nerve terminals. Activation (agonism) of these receptors may result in stimulation or inhibition of cellular function.
18. antagonistic
19. tyrosine
20. a, b, and c. *Rationale:* The functions of the ANS can be broadly described as activities designed to maintain a constant internal environment (homeostasis), to respond to stress or emergencies, and to repair body tissues.

Chapter 17: Adrenergic Drugs

SECTION II: ASSESSING YOUR UNDERSTANDING

ACTIVITY A

FILL IN THE BLANKS

1. Adrenergic
2. isoproterenol
3. receptor
4. exogenous
5. heart

ACTIVITY B

MATCHING

1. E   2. A   3. B   4. C   5. D

ACTIVITY C

SHORT ANSWERS

1. Clinical indications for the use of adrenergic drugs stem mainly from their effects on the heart, blood vessels, and bronchi. They are often used as emergency drugs in the treatment of acute cardiovascular, respiratory, and allergic disorders.
2. In cardiac arrest, Stokes-Adams syndrome (sudden attacks of unconsciousness caused by heart block), and profound bradycardia, adrenergic drugs may be used as cardiac stimulants. In hypotension and shock, they may be used to increase blood pressure. In hemorrhagic or hypovolemic shock, the drugs are second-line agents that may be used if adequate fluid volume replacement does not restore sufficient blood pressure and circulation to maintain organ perfusion.
3. In bronchial asthma and other obstructive pulmonary diseases, the drugs are used as bronchodilators to relieve bronchoconstriction and bronchospasm. In upper respiratory infections, including the common cold and sinusitis, they may be given orally or applied topically to the nasal mucosa to reduce nasal congestion (decongestant effect).

4. Adrenergic drugs are useful in treating a variety of symptoms of allergic disorders. Severe allergic reactions are characterized by hypotension, bronchoconstriction, and laryngoedema. As vasoconstrictors, the drugs are useful in correcting the hypotension that often accompanies severe allergic reactions. The drug-induced vasoconstriction of blood vessels in mucous membranes produces a decongestant effect to relieve edema in the respiratory tract, skin, and other tissues. As bronchodilators, the drugs also help relieve the bronchospasm of severe allergic reactions. Adrenergic drugs may be used to treat allergic rhinitis; acute hypersensitivity (anaphylactoid reactions to drugs, animal serums, insect stings, and other allergens); serum sickness; urticaria; and angioneurotic edema.

5. Other clinical uses of adrenergic drugs include relaxation of uterine musculature and inhibition of uterine contractions in preterm labor. They also may be added to local anesthetics for their vasoconstrictive effect, thus preventing unwanted systemic absorption of the anesthetic, prolonging anesthesia, and reducing bleeding. Topical uses include application to skin and mucous membranes for vasoconstriction and hemostatic effects and to the eyes for vasoconstriction and mydriasis.

SECTION III: APPLYING YOUR KNOWLEDGE

ACTIVITY D
CASE STUDIES

1. The physician's treatment of choice to reduce broncho-spasm would be epinephrine. In bronchial asthma and other obstructive pulmonary diseases, epinephrine is used as a bronchodilator to relieve bronchoconstriction and bronchospasm.

2. Over-the-counter epinephrine preparations have a short duration of action, which promotes frequent and excessive use. Prolonged use may cause adverse effects and result in the development of tolerance to the therapeutic effects of the drug. There is also concern by some health professionals that reliance on OTC medications may delay the asthmatic patient from seeking medical care. Supporters point out that OTC bronchodilators are much less costly than prescription medications and are an affordable "rescue treatment" option for patients who do not have insurance coverage for prescription medications.

3. Treatment guidelines for asthma recommend use of anti-inflammatory medications (e.g., corticosteroids) and prescription bronchodilators (e.g., beta$_2$-adrenergic agonists) for the optimal treatment of asthma.

4. Another area of concern is the ozone-depleting propellants used in OTC inhalation products such as Primatene Mist. At this time, however, these medications have "essential use designation" by the FDA, because they constitute the only over-the-counter inhalation products available to individuals with asthma.

5. Ephedrine is a common ingredient in OTC anti-asthma tablets (e.g., Bronkaid, Primatene). The tablets contain 12.5 to 25 mg of ephedrine and 100 to 130 mg of theophylline, a xanthine bronchodilator.

6. People who have heart disease or are elderly should not use over-the-counter asthma treatments on a regular basis.

SECTION IV: PRACTICING FOR NCLEX

1. ephedra (ephedrine alkaloids)
2. d. *Rationale:* Phenylephrine stimulates alpha$_1$ receptors.
3. a, b, and c. *Rationale:* Contraindications to adrenergic drugs include cardiac dysrhythmias, angina, hypertension, hyperthyroidism, cerebrovascular disease, narrow-angle glaucoma, and hypersensitivity to sulfites.

4. d. *Rationale:* Local anesthetics containing adrenergics should not be used in any area of the body with a single blood supply (fingers, toes, nose, and ears).

5. b. *Rationale:* A benefit of epinephrine in arrest situations due to asystole or pulseless electrical activity is the added ability to stimulate electrical and mechanical activity and produce myocardial contraction.

6. vasopressin

7. c. *Rationale:* Use of beta-adrenergic blocking drugs (e.g., propranolol) may decrease the effectiveness of epinephrine in cases of anaphylaxis.

8. a. *Rationale:* Higher doses of epinephrine and use of intravenous fluids may be required to maintain a patent airway and restore blood pressure.

9. auto-injector (such as EpiPen or EpiPen Jr.)

10. Epinephrine

11. a. *Rationale:* Adrenergic drugs are used as cardiac stimulants, vasopressors, bronchodilators, nasal decongestants, uterine relaxants, adjuncts to local anesthetics, and topically for hemostatic and mydriatic effects.

12. d. *Rationale:* A major function of the home care nurse is to teach clients to use the drugs correctly (especially metered-dose inhalers); to report excessive CNS or cardiac stimulation to a health care provider; and not to take OTC drugs or herbal preparations with the same or similar ingredients as prescription drugs.

13. b. *Rationale:* The liver is rich in the enzymes MAO and COMT, which are responsible for metabolism of circulating epinephrine and other adrenergic drugs (e.g., norepinephrine, dopamine, isoproterenol). However, other tissues in the body also possess these enzymes and are capable of metabolizing natural and synthetic catecholamines. Any unchanged drug can be excreted in the urine. Many noncatecholamine adrenergic drugs are excreted largely unchanged in the urine. Therefore, liver disease is not usually considered a contraindication to administration of adrenergic drugs.

14. c. *Rationale:* Adrenergic drugs exert effects on the renal system that may cause problems for clients with renal impairment. For example, adrenergic drugs with alpha$_1$ activity cause constriction of renal arteries, thereby diminishing renal blood flow and urine production. These drugs also constrict urinary sphincters, causing urinary retention and painful urination, especially in men with prostatic hyperplasia.

15. d. *Rationale:* Ophthalmic preparations of adrenergic drugs should be used cautiously. For example, phenylephrine is used as a vasoconstrictor and mydriatic. Applying larger-than-recommended doses to the normal eye or usual doses to the traumatized, inflamed, or diseased eye may result in systemic absorption of the drug sufficient to cause increased blood pressure and other adverse effects.

16. Phenylephrine

17. c. *Rationale:* Epinephrine is mainly used in children for treatment of bronchospasm due to asthma or allergic reactions. Parenteral epinephrine may cause syncope when given to asthmatic children.

18. a and b. *Rationale:* Ephedrine and ephedra-containing herbal preparations (e.g., ma huang, herbal ecstasy) are often abused as an alternative to amphetamines.

19. a. *Rationale:* Adrenergic drugs are given topically and systemically to constrict blood vessels in nasal mucosa and decrease the nasal congestion associated with the common cold, allergic rhinitis, and sinusitis. Topical

agents are effective, undergo little systemic absorption, are available OTC, and are widely used. However, overuse leads to decreased effectiveness (tolerance); irritation and ischemic changes in the nasal mucosa; and rebound congestion. These effects can be minimized by using small doses only when necessary and for no longer than 3 to 5 days.

20. d. *Rationale:* The usual goal of vasopressor drug therapy is to maintain tissue perfusion and a mean arterial blood pressure of at least 80 to 100 mm Hg.

Chapter 18: Antiadrenergic Drugs

SECTION II: ASSESSING YOUR UNDERSTANDING

ACTIVITY A
FILL IN THE BLANKS
1. Antiadrenergic
2. blood pressure
3. pathologic
4. antagonists
5. antagonist

ACTIVITY B
MATCHING
1. A   2. E   3. D   4. B   5. C

ACTIVITY C
SHORT ANSWERS
1. Alpha$_2$-adrenergic agonists such as clonidine (Catapres) inhibit the release of norepinephrine in the brain, thereby decreasing the effects of sympathetic nervous system stimulation throughout the body. A major clinical effect is decreased blood pressure. Although clinical effects are attributed mainly to drug action at presynaptic alpha$_2$ receptors in the brain, postsynaptic alpha$_2$ receptors in the brain and peripheral tissues (e.g., vascular smooth muscle) may also be involved. Activation of alpha$_2$ receptors in the pancreatic islets suppresses insulin secretion.
2. Alpha$_1$-adrenergic blocking drugs such as tamsulosin can prevent alpha-mediated contraction of smooth muscle in nonvascular tissues. This action makes these drugs useful in the treatment of benign prostatic hyperplasia (BPH), a condition characterized by obstructed urine flow as the enlarged prostate gland presses on the urethra. Alpha$_1$-blocking agents can decrease urinary retention and improve urine flow by relaxing muscles in the prostate and urinary bladder.
3. Beta-adrenergic blocking agents occupy beta-adrenergic receptor sites and prevent the receptors from responding to sympathetic nerve impulses, circulating catecholamines, and beta-adrenergic drugs.
4. Nonselective alpha-adrenergic blocking drugs such as phentolamine occupy peripheral alpha$_1$ receptors, causing vasodilation, and presynaptic alpha$_2$ receptors, causing cardiac stimulation. Consequently, decreased blood pressure is accompanied by tachycardia and perhaps other dysrhythmias.
5. Beta$_1$ receptor blockade has an inhibitory effect on the cardiovascular system resulting in decreased heart rate (negative *chronotropy*); decreased force of myocardial contraction (negative *inotropy*); slowed conduction through the atrioventricular (AV) node (negative *dromotropy*); decreased automaticity of ectopic pacemakers; decreased cardiac output at rest and with exercise; and decreased blood pressure in supine and standing positions, especially in people with hypertension.

SECTION III: APPLYING YOUR KNOWLEDGE
ACTIVITY D
CASE STUDIES
1. Alfuzosin (Uroxatral) is an alpha$_1$-blocking drug specifically indicated for BPH.
2. This is a moderately protein bound, extended-release medication similar to prazosin, but it has the advantage of once-a-day dosing. It has a half-life of 10 hours and a duration of action of 24 hours. Alfuzosin should be taken after meals to promote absorption.
3. Mr. Jenks likely has alfuzosin toxicity. The drug is metabolized extensively in the liver by cytochrome P450 3A4 enzymes and should not be given with potent inhibitors of this enzyme such as ketoconazole, itraconazole, or ritonavir. Because the drug is metabolized in the liver, the presence of moderate to severe liver insufficiency will cause drug toxicity to develop.
4. Common adverse effects include dizziness, headache, fatigue, and increased incidence of upper respiratory infections.

SECTION IV: PRACTICING FOR NCLEX
1. b. *Rationale:* Clinical indications for beta-blocking agents are mainly cardiovascular disorders such as angina pectoris, cardiac tachydysrhythmias, hypertension, myocardial infarction, heart failure, and glaucoma.
2. a. *Rationale:* Selective Alpha$_1$-adrenergic blocking drugs are used in the treatment of hypertension, BPH, and vasospastic disorders.
3. d. *Rationale:* Alpha$_2$ agonists are used in the treatment of hypertension
4. b. *Rationale:* Alpha$_2$-adrenergic agonists such as clonidine (Catapres) inhibit the release of norepinephrine in the brain, thereby decreasing the effects of sympathetic nervous system stimulation throughout the body.
5. a, b, and c. *Rationale:* Antiadrenergic drugs decrease or block the effects of sympathetic nerve stimulation, endogenous catecholamines (e.g., epinephrine), and adrenergic drugs.
6. c. *Rationale:* Antiadrenergic drugs are one of several families of medications that may be used to treat urgent or malignant hypertension. An alpha$_2$ agonist such as clonidine might be prescribed under such conditions. A loading dose of clonidine 0.2 mg, followed by 0.1 mg/hour until the diastolic blood pressure falls below 110 mm Hg, may be administered.
7. 0.7 mg
8. a. *Rationale:* Beta-blockers may be used in the treatment of acute MI. Early administration of a beta-blocker after an acute MI results in a lower incidence of reinfarction, ventricular dysrhythmias, and mortality.
9. b. *Rationale:* Patients must be carefully monitored for hypotension and HF when receiving beta-blockers after an MI.
10. d. *Rationale:* With alpha$_1$-adrenergic blocking drugs, the home care nurse may need to teach patients ways to avoid orthostatic hypotension
11. b. *Rationale:* With beta-adrenergic blocking drugs, the home care nurse may need to assist patients and caregivers in assessing for therapeutic and adverse drug effects. It is helpful to have the patient or someone else in the household count and record the radial pulse daily, preferably at about the same time interval before or after taking a beta-blocker.

12. c. *Rationale:* In the presence of hepatic disease (e.g., cirrhosis) or impaired blood flow to the liver (e.g., reduced cardiac output from any cause), dosages of some beta-blockers such as propranolol, metoprolol, and timolol should be substantially reduced, because these drugs are extensively metabolized in the liver.
13. kidneys
14. b. *Rationale:* Many beta-blockers are eliminated primarily in the urine and pose potentially serious problems for patients with renal failure. In renal failure, dosage of acebutolol, atenolol, and nadolol must be reduced, because they are eliminated mainly through the kidneys.
15. 50
16. c. *Rationale:* Alpha$_2$-adrenergic agonists may be used to treat hypertension in older adults, and alpha$_1$-adrenergic antagonists may be used to treat hypertension and BPH. Dosage of these drugs should be reduced, because older adults are more likely to experience adverse drug effects, especially with impaired renal or hepatic function. As with other populations, these drugs should not be stopped suddenly. Instead, they should be tapered in dosage and discontinued gradually, over 1 to 2 weeks.
17. floppy iris
18. d. *Rationale:* When beta-blockers are given to children, general guidelines indicate that the dosage should be adjusted according to body weight.
19. d. *Rationale:* Beta-adrenergic blocking drugs are used in children for disorders similar to those in adults. However, safety and effectiveness have not been established, and manufacturers of most of the drugs do not recommend pediatric use or suggest dosages. The drugs are probably contraindicated in young children with a resting heart rate of less than 60 beats per minute.
20. d. *Rationale:* It is important to note that bronchodilation does not occur in a patient taking beta-blockers when given epinephrine to treat an allergic reaction to an allergen or during allergy testing. This absence of the normal response to epinephrine is due to drug-induced beta$_2$ blockade.

Chapter 19: Cholinergic Drugs

SECTION II: ASSESSING YOUR UNDERSTANDING

ACTIVITY A
FILL IN THE BLANKS
1. Cholinergic
2. acetylcholine
3. Myasthenia gravis
4. glutamatergic
5. cholinergic

ACTIVITY B
MATCHING
1. B   2. E   3. C   4. D   5. A

ACTIVITY C
SHORT ANSWERS
1. Cholinergic drugs stimulate the parasympathetic nervous system in the same manner as acetylcholine. Some drugs act directly to stimulate cholinergic receptors; others act indirectly by inhibiting the enzyme acetylcholinesterase, thereby slowing acetylcholine metabolism at autonomic nerve synapses.
2. In normal brain function, acetylcholine is an essential neurotransmitter and plays an important role in cognitive functions, including memory storage and retrieval.

3. Acetylcholine stimulates cholinergic receptors in the gut to promote normal secretory and motor activity. Cholinergic stimulation results in increased peristalsis and relaxation of the smooth muscle in sphincters to facilitate movement of flatus and feces. The secretory functions of the salivary and gastric glands are also stimulated.
4. Acetylcholine stimulates cholinergic receptors in the urinary system to promote normal urination. Cholinergic stimulation results in contraction of the detrusor muscle and relaxation of the urinary sphincter to facilitate emptying the urinary bladder.
5. Direct-acting cholinergic drugs are synthetic derivatives of choline. Most direct-acting cholinergic drugs are quaternary amines, carry a positive charge, and are lipid insoluble. Because they do not readily enter the central nervous system, their effects occur primarily in the periphery. Direct-acting cholinergic drugs are highly resistant to metabolism by acetylcholinesterase, the enzyme that normally metabolizes acetylcholine.

SECTION III: APPLYING YOUR KNOWLEDGE
ACTIVITY D
CASE STUDIES
1. Myasthenia gravis is an autoimmune disorder in which autoantibodies are thought to destroy nicotinic receptors for acetylcholine on skeletal muscle. As a result, acetylcholine is less able to stimulate muscle contraction, and muscle weakness occurs.
2. The anticholinesterase agents are used in the diagnosis and treatment of myasthenia gravis. Neostigmine (Prostigmin) is an anticholinesterase agent. Neostigmine, like bethanechol, is a quaternary amine and carries a positive charge. This reduces its lipid solubility and results in poor absorption from the GI tract.
3. Oral doses of neostigmine are much larger than parenteral doses. When neostigmine is used for long-term treatment of myasthenia gravis, resistance to its action may occur and larger doses may be required.

SECTION IV: PRACTICING FOR NCLEX
1. d. *Rationale:* Pralidoxime, a cholinesterase reactivator, is the specific treatment for neuromuscular blockade due to overdose with irreversible indirect cholinergic drugs.
2. b. *Rationale:* Atropine will reverse muscarinic effects due to overdose of cholinergic drugs but will not reverse the nicotinic effects of skeletal-muscle weakness or paralysis due to overdose of indirect cholinergic drugs.
3. Edrophonium
4. c. *Rationale:* Indirect-acting cholinergic or anticholinesterase drugs are indicated to treat myasthenia gravis and Alzheimer's disease.
5. b. *Rationale:* The direct-acting cholinergic drug, bethanechol, is used to treat urinary retention due to urinary bladder atony and postoperative abdominal distention due to paralytic ileus.
6. c. *Rationale:* Indirect-acting cholinergic drugs also stimulate nicotinic receptors in skeletal muscles, resulting in improved skeletal muscle tone and strength.
7. parasympathetic
8. a. *Rationale:* The patient with myasthenia gravis may have diplopia or diminished muscle strength that makes it difficult to self-administer medications. Pre-pouring medications in an easy-to-open device facilitates medication administration.

9. b. *Rationale:* The hepatic metabolism of neostigmine and pyridostigmine may be impaired by liver disease, resulting in increased adverse effects.

10. d. *Rationale:* Cholinergic drugs are contraindicated in urinary or GI tract obstruction because they increase the contractility of smooth muscle in the urinary and GI systems and may result in injury to structures proximal to the obstruction.

11. gastric acid

12. d. *Rationale:* Individuals with coronary artery disease should not take cholinergics because they can result in bradycardia, vasodilation, and hypotension.

13. d. *Rationale:* Patients with hyperthyroidism should avoid cholinergic drugs. In the individual with hyperthyroidism, the initial response to cholinergic medications (bradycardia and hypotension) triggers the baroreceptor reflex. As this reflex attempts to resolve the hypotension, norepinephrine is secreted from sympathetic nerves regulating the heart. Norepinephrine may trigger reflex tachycardia and other cardiac dysrhythmias.

14. d. *Rationale:* Cholinergic drugs are contraindicated in individuals with asthma because they may cause bronchoconstriction and increased respiratory secretions.

15. bethanechol

16. a and b. *Rationale:* Direct-acting cholinergic drugs cause increased tone and contractility of smooth muscle (detrusor) in the urinary bladder and relaxation of the sphincter.

17. increased

18. acetylcholine

19. a. *Rationale:* Indirect-acting cholinergic medications for Alzheimer's disease are widely distributed, including to the central nervous system. Thus, indirect-acting cholinergic drugs are able to improve cholinergic neurotransmission in the brain.

20. acetylcholinesterase

Chapter 20: Anticholinergic Drugs

SECTION II: ASSESSING YOUR UNDERSTANDING

ACTIVITY A
FILL IN THE BLANKS
1. Anticholinergic
2. Tertiary
3. quaternary
4. nicotinic
5. muscarinic

ACTIVITY B
MATCHING
1. C   2. A   3. E   4. B   5. D

ACTIVITY C
SHORT ANSWERS
1. Most anticholinergic medications are either *tertiary amines* or *quaternary amines* Tertiary amines are uncharged, lipid-soluble molecules. Atropine and scopolamine are tertiary amines and therefore are able to cross cell membranes readily. They are well absorbed from the gastrointestinal (GI) tract and conjunctiva, and they cross the blood–brain barrier. Tertiary amines are excreted in the urine.

2. Some belladonna derivatives and synthetic anticholinergics are quaternary amines. These drugs carry a positive charge and are lipid insoluble. Consequently, they do not readily cross cell membranes. They are poorly absorbed from the GI tract and do not cross the blood–brain barrier. Quaternary amines are excreted largely in the feces.

3. In general, anticholinergic drugs act by occupying receptor sites on target organs innervated by the parasympathetic nervous system, thereby leaving fewer receptor sites free to respond to acetylcholine. Parasympathetic response is absent or decreased, depending on the number of receptors blocked by anticholinergic drugs and the underlying degree of parasympathetic activity. Because cholinergic *muscarinic receptors* are widely distributed in the body, anticholinergic drugs produce effects in a variety of locations, including the central nervous system (CNS), heart, smooth muscle, glands, and the eye.

4. Anticholinergic drugs cause decreased cardiovascular response to the parasympathetic (vagal) stimulation that slows heart rate. Atropine is the anticholinergic drug most often used for its cardiovascular effects. According to Advanced Cardiac Life Support (ACLS) protocol, atropine is the drug of choice to treat symptomatic sinus bradycardia. Low doses (<0.5 mg) may produce a slight and temporary decrease in heart rate; however, moderate to large doses (0.5-1 mg) increase heart rate by blocking parasympathetic vagal stimulation. Although the increase in heart rate may be therapeutic in bradycardia, it can be an adverse effect in patients with other types of heart disease, because atropine increases the myocardial oxygen demand. Atropine usually has little or no effect on blood pressure. Large doses cause facial flushing because of dilation of blood vessels in the neck.

5. Anticholinergic drugs cause bronchodilation and decreased respiratory tract secretions. Anticholinergics block the action of acetylcholine in bronchial smooth muscle when given by inhalation. This action reduces intracellular GMP, a bronchoconstrictive substance. When anticholinergic drugs are given systemically, respiratory secretions decrease and may become viscous, resulting in mucous plugging of small respiratory passages. Administering the medications by inhalation decreases this effect while preserving the beneficial bronchodilation effect

SECTION III: APPLYING YOUR KNOWLEDGE

ACTIVITY D
CASE STUDIES
1. An appropriate response is, "Your medication will dilate your bronchi, which will help you to breathe better." Tiotropium bromide (Spiriva HandiHaler) is a long-acting, antimuscarinic and anticholinergic, quaternary ammonium compound that inhibits M3 receptors in smooth muscle, resulting in bronchodilation.

2. This statement indicates the need for more patient teaching. Tiotropium bromide (Spiriva HandiHaler) is a dry powder in capsule form intended for oral inhalation with the HandiHaler inhalation device. The capsule is to be used with the inhalation device only. Tiotropium bromide is not used in place of a rescue inhaler. It is indicated for daily maintenance treatment of bronchospasm associated with COPD. It is not indicated for acute episodes of bronchospasm (i.e., rescue therapy).

3. The proper response should be, "Your medication dose should not be modified; it is ordered once a day." Tiotropium bromide (Spiriva HandiHaler) is indicated for daily maintenance treatment of bronchospasm associated with COPD. The patient should be taught to follow the prescription.

4. You would expect the physician to monitor the client routinely for drug toxicity. Tiotropium is eliminated via the renal system, and patients with moderate to severe renal dysfunction should be carefully monitored for drug toxicity. No dosage adjustments are required for older patients or patients with hepatic impairment or mild renal impairment.

SECTION IV: PRACTICING FOR NCLEX

1. Atropine
2. a, c, and d. *Rationale:* Anticholinergic overdose is characterized by hyperthermia, hot dry flushed skin, dry mouth, mydriasis, delirium, tachycardia, paralytic ileus, urinary retention, myoclonic movements, seizures, coma, and respiratory arrest.
3. Physostigmine
4. d. *Rationale:* Anticholinergic drugs are contraindicated for patients with BPH, myasthenia gravis, hyperthyroidism, narrow-angle glaucoma, tachydysrhythmias, myocardial infarction, heart failure, or conditions associated with esophageal reflux.
5. b. *Rationale:* Anticholinergic drugs are given preoperatively to prevent anesthesia-associated complications such as bradycardia, excessive respiratory secretions, and hypotension.
6. b. *Rationale:* Anticholinergic medications are indicated in the relief of central nervous system symptoms of Parkinson's disease or extrapyramidal symptoms associated with some antipsychotic drugs.
7. Atropine
8. a. *Rationale:* Ipratropium and tiotropium are anticholinergic medications given by inhalation for bronchodilation effects in the treatment of asthma and chronic bronchitis
9. mydriatic, cycloplegic
10. c. *Rationale:* Anticholinergic drugs (e.g., dicyclomine, glycopyrrolate) are indicated for antispasmodic effects in GI disorders. Historically, they have also been used to treat peptic ulcer disease; however, they are weak inhibitors of gastric acid secretion and have been largely replaced other, more effective medications (e.g., proton pump inhibitors)
11. b, c, and d. *Rationale:* Cholinergic (muscarinic) receptors are widespread throughout the body, producing effects in a variety of locations. including the central nervous system, heart, smooth muscle, glands, and eyes.
12. antimuscarinic
13. b. *Rationale:* Anticholinergic drugs block the action of acetylcholine on the parasympathetic nervous system.
14. d. *Rationale:* Anticholinergic drugs are commonly used in home care with children and adults. The home care nurse may need to teach older patients or caregivers that the drugs prevent sweating and heat loss and increase risks of heat stroke if precautions to avoid overheating are not taken.
15. a. *Rationale:* Atropine is an important drug in the emergency drug box. According to ACLS guidelines, atropine is the first drug to be administered in the emergency treatment of bradydysrhythmias. Atropine 0.5 mg should be administered IV every 3-5 minutes and may be repeated up to 3 mg (0.03-0.04 mg/kg) total dose.
16. a. *Rationale:* Older adults are especially likely to have significant adverse reactions because of slowed drug metabolism and the frequent presence of several disease processes. A patient who complains of blurred vision may need help with ambulation, especially with stairs or in other potentially hazardous environments. Obstacles and hazards should be removed if possible.

17. d. *Rationale:* Normally, anticholinergics do not change intraocular pressure, but with narrow-angle glaucoma, they may increase intraocular pressure and precipitate an episode of acute glaucoma.
18. c. *Rationale:* Anticholinergics may be helpful in reducing the frequency of bowel movements and abdominal discomfort associated with irritable colon or colitis.
19. a. *Rationale:* In infections such as cystitis, urethritis, and prostatitis, anticholinergic drugs decrease the frequency and pain of urination. The drugs are also given to increase bladder capacity in enuresis, paraplegia, or neurogenic bladder.
20. b. *Rationale:* Anticholinergic drugs are given for their central effects in decreasing salivation, spasticity, and tremors. They are used mainly in patients who have minimal symptoms, who do not respond to levodopa, or who cannot tolerate levodopa because of adverse reactions or contraindications. An additional use of anticholinergic drugs is to relieve parkinson-like symptoms that occur with older antipsychotic drugs.

Chapter 21: Physiology of the Endocrine System

SECTION II: ASSESSING YOUR UNDERSTANDING

ACTIVITY A
FILL IN THE BLANKS
1. hypothalamus
2. negative feedback system
3. Hormones
4. Protein
5. Hormones

ACTIVITY B
MATCHING
1. C   2. D   3. A   4. B   5. E

ACTIVITY C
SHORT ANSWERS
1. The endocrine system is comprises the hypothalamus of the brain, pituitary gland, thyroid gland, parathyroid glands, pancreas, adrenal glands, ovaries, and testes.
2. The endocrine system participates in the regulation of essentially all body activities, including metabolism of nutrients and water, reproduction, growth and development, and adapting to changes in internal and external environments.
3. Hormones are substances that are synthesized and secreted into body fluids by one group of cells and have physiologic effects on other body cells. Hormones act as chemical messengers to transmit information between body cells and organs. Most hormones from the traditional endocrine glands are secreted into the bloodstream and act on distant organs.
4. The kidneys produce erythropoietin, a hormone that stimulates the bone marrow to produce red blood cells.
5. White blood cells produce cytokines that function as messengers among leukocytes in inflammatory and immune processes.

SECTION III: APPLYING YOUR KNOWLEDGE

ACTIVITY D
CASE STUDIES
1. Hypofunction may be associated with a variety of circumstances. A congenital defect may result in the absence of an endocrine gland, the presence of an abnormally developed gland, or the absence of an enzyme

required for glandular synthesis of its specific hormone. An endocrine gland may be damaged or destroyed by impaired blood flow, infection or inflammation, autoimmune disorders, or neoplasms. An endocrine gland may atrophy and become less able to produce its hormone because of aging, drug therapy, disease, or unknown reasons.

2. An endocrine gland may produce adequate hormone, but the hormone may not be able to function normally because of receptor defects.

3. An endocrine gland may atrophy and become less able to produce its hormone because of aging, drug therapy, disease, or unknown reasons.

4. Excessive stimulation and enlargement of an endocrine gland may result from a hormone-producing tumor of the gland or from a hormone-producing tumor of nonendocrine tissues. Hyperfunction is usually characterized by excessive hormone production.

SECTION IV: PRACTICING FOR NCLEX

1. d. *Rationale:* Receptors are capable of increasing (upregulation) or decreasing (downregulation) with chronic exposure to abnormal levels of hormones.
2. activates
3. c. *Rationale:* The endocrine and nervous systems are closely connected, anatomically and physiologically, and work in harmony to integrate and regulate body functions.
4. c. *Rationale:* Water-soluble, protein-derived hormones have a short duration of action and are inactivated by enzymes mainly in the liver and kidneys.
5. b, c, and d. *Rationale:* Hormones given for therapeutic purposes may be natural hormones from human or animal sources or synthetic hormones.
6. Addison's
7. b. *Rationale:* Adrenal corticosteroids are widely used for anti-inflammatory effects in endocrine and nonendocrine disorders.
8. a. *Rationale:* Hormones are given for physiologic or pharmacologic effects and are more often given for disorders resulting from endocrine gland hypofunction than for those related to hyperfunction.
9. small
10. a and b. *Rationale:* Many of the most important hormones have been synthesized, and synthetic preparations may have more potent and prolonged effects than naturally occurring hormones.
11. alter
12. a, b, and d. *Rationale:* Malfunction of an endocrine organ is usually associated with hyposecretion, hypersecretion, or inappropriate secretion of its hormones.
13. c. *Rationale:* Steroid hormones are lipid soluble and therefore cross cell membranes easily. Inside the cell cytoplasm, the hormone molecules bind with specific receptor proteins. The hormone–receptor complex then enters the nucleus of the cell, where it activates nucleic acids (DNA and RNA) and the genetic code to synthesize new proteins.
14. leukotrienes
15. d. *Rationale:* Phospholipids are major components of the cell membrane portion of all body cells.
16. a, b, and c. *Rationale:* The gastrointestinal mucosa produces hormones that are important in the digestive process (e.g., gastrin, enterogastrone, secretin, and cholecystokinin).
17. b. *Rationale:* The kidneys produce erythropoietin, a hormone that stimulates the bone marrow to produce red blood cells.

18. c. *Rationale:* Lung tumors may produce corticotropin (adrenocorticotropic hormone, or ACTH), antidiuretic hormone, or parathyroid hormone; kidney tumors may produce parathyroid hormone.
19. leukocytes
20. hypothalamus

Chapter 22: Hypothalamic and Pituitary Hormones

SECTION II: ASSESSING YOUR UNDERSTANDING
ACTIVITY A
FILL IN THE BLANKS
1. homeostasis
2. hypophyseal
3. hypothalamus
4. target tissues
5. nerve

ACTIVITY B
MATCHING
1. E   2. C   3. A   4. B   5. D

ACTIVITY C
SHORT ANSWERS
1. FSH, one of the gonadotropins, stimulates functions of sex glands. FSH is produced by the anterior pituitary gland of both sexes, beginning at puberty. It acts on the ovaries in a cyclical fashion during the reproductive years, stimulating growth of ovarian follicles. These follicles then produce estrogen, which prepares the endometrium for implantation of a fertilized ovum. FSH acts on the testes to stimulate the production and growth of sperm (spermatogenesis), but it does not stimulate secretion of male sex hormones.
2. LH (also called interstitial cell–stimulating hormone) is another gonadotropin that stimulates hormone production by the gonads of both sexes. In women, LH is important in the maturation and rupture of the ovarian follicle (ovulation). After ovulation, LH acts on the cells of the collapsed follicular sac to produce the corpus luteum, which then produces progesterone during the last half of the menstrual cycle. When blood progesterone levels rise, a negative feedback effect is exerted on hypothalamic and anterior pituitary secretion of gonadotropins. Decreased pituitary secretion of LH causes the corpus luteum to die and stop producing progesterone. Lack of progesterone causes slough and discharge of the endometrial lining as menstrual flow. (Of course, if the ovum has been fertilized and attached to the endometrium, menstruation does not occur.) In men, LH stimulates the Leydig's cells in the spaces between the seminiferous tubules to secrete androgens, mainly testosterone.
3. Prolactin plays a part in milk production by nursing mothers. It is not usually secreted in nonpregnant women because of the hypothalamic hormone PIF. During late pregnancy and lactation, various stimuli, including suckling, inhibit the production of PIF, allowing prolactin to be synthesized and released.
4. Melanocyte-stimulating hormone (MSH) plays a role in skin pigmentation and has recently been found to play important roles in feeding and energy metabolism as well as in inflammation. Recently, MSH, particularly gamma-MSH, has been linked to cardiovascular regulation and sodium metabolism.
5. Oxytocin functions in childbirth and lactation. It initiates uterine contractions at the end of gestation to induce childbirth, and it causes milk to move from breast glands to nipples so the infant can obtain the milk by suckling.

SECTION III: APPLYING YOUR KNOWLEDGE

ACTIVITY D

CASE STUDIES

1. The drugs goserelin (Zoladex), histrelin (Vantas), leuprolide (Lupron), nafarelin (Synarel), and triptorelin (Trelstar) are equivalent to GnRH. After initial stimulation of LH and FSH secretion, chronic administration of therapeutic doses inhibits gonadotropin secretion.

2. After initial stimulation of LH and FSH secretion, chronic administration of therapeutic doses inhibits gonadotropin secretion. This action results in decreased production of testosterone and estrogen, which is reversible when administration is stopped.

3. These GnRH equivalents cannot be given orally, because they would be destroyed by enzymes in the GI tract. Goserelin (Zoladex), histrelin (Vantas), leuprolide (Lupron), nafarelin (Synarel), and triptorelin (Trelstar) are given by injection and are available in depot preparations that can be given once monthly or less often.

4. Adverse effects of Lupron are basically those of testosterone or estrogen deficiency. When given for prostate cancer, the drug may cause increased bone pain and increased difficulty in urinating during the first few weeks of treatment.

SECTION IV: PRACTICING FOR NCLEX

1. vasopressin

2. c and d. *Rationale:* The posterior pituitary gland stores and releases two hormones that are synthesized by nerve cells in the hypothalamus: ADH and oxytocin.

3. c and d. *Rationale:* Conditions resulting from excessive amounts of pituitary hormones (hyperpituitarism) are most often treated with surgery or radiation.

4. a. *Rationale:* Dosage of all pituitary hormones must be individualized, because the responsiveness of affected tissues varies.

5. d. *Rationale:* Middle-aged and older adults may use GH to combat the effects of aging, such as decreased energy, weaker muscles and joints, and wrinkled skin. Possible adverse effects associated with GH, especially with high doses or chronic use, include acromegaly, diabetes, hypertension, and increased risk of serious cardiovascular disease (e.g., heart failure).

6. a. *Rationale:* There is concern about a possible link between GH, which stimulates tumor growth, and cancer. GH stimulates the release of IGF-1 (also called somatomedin), a substance that circulates in the blood and stimulates cell division. Most tumor cells have receptors that recognize IGF-1, bind it, and allow it to enter the cell, where it could trigger uncontrolled cell division. This concern may be greater for middle-aged and older adults, because malignancies are more common in these groups than in adolescents and young adults.

7. oxytocin (Pitocin)

8. d. *Rationale:* Oxytocin (Pitocin) is a synthetic drug that exerts the same physiologic effects as the posterior pituitary hormone. It promotes uterine contractility and is used clinically to induce labor and in the postpartum period to control bleeding. Oxytocin must be used only when clearly indicated and when the recipient can be supervised by well-trained personnel, as in a hospital.

9. Vasopressin

10. c. *Rationale:* Desmopressin (DDAVP, Stimate), and vasopressin Pitressin) are synthetic equivalents of ADH. A major clinical use is the treatment of neurogenic diabetes insipidus, a disorder characterized by a deficiency of ADH and the excretion of large amounts of dilute urine.

11. a. *Rationale:* Pegvisomant (Somavert) is a GH receptor antagonist used in the treatment of acromegaly in adults who are unable to tolerate or are resistant to other management strategies. The drug selectively binds to GH receptors, blocking the binding of endogenous GH. In general, dosage should be individualized according to response. Dosage reduction of hypoglycemic agents may be required, because the drug may increase glucose tolerance.

12. endogenous

13. b and d. *Rationale:* Octreotide (Sandostatin) has pharmacologic actions similar to those of somatostatin. Indications for use include acromegaly, in which the drug reduces blood levels of GH and insulin-like growth factor-1 (IGF-1); carcinoid tumors, in which it inhibits diarrhea and flushing; and vasoactive intestinal peptide tumors, in which it relieves diarrhea (by decreasing GI secretions and motility). It is also used to treat diarrhea in acquired immunodeficiency syndrome (AIDS) and other conditions.

14. Cosyntropin (Cortrosyn)

15. d. *Rationale:* Antidiuretic hormone (ADH), also called *vasopressin*, functions to regulate water balance. When ADH is secreted, it makes renal tubules more permeable to water.

16. Thyrotropin

17. a, b, and c. *Rationale:* GH, also called *somatotropin*, stimulates growth of body tissues. It regulates cell division and protein synthesis required for normal growth and promotes an increase in cell size and number, including growth of muscle cells and lengthening of bone.

18. a. *Rationale:* GH is often considered an insulin antagonist because it suppresses the abilities of insulin to stimulate uptake of glucose in peripheral tissues and enhance glucose synthesis in the liver. Paradoxically, administration of GH produces hyperinsulinemia by stimulating insulin secretion.

19. 20s

20. anabolism

Chapter 23: Corticosteroids

SECTION II: ASSESSING YOUR UNDERSTANDING

ACTIVITY A

FILL IN THE BLANKS

1. Corticosteroids
2. Exogenous
3. slows, stops
4. negative feedback mechanism
5. Corticosteroids

ACTIVITY B

MATCHING

1. C   2. D   3. A   4. B   5. E

ACTIVITY C

SHORT ANSWERS

1. Corticosteroid secretion is controlled by the hypothalamus, the anterior pituitary, and adrenal cortex (the hypothalamic–pituitary–adrenal, or HPA, axis). Various stimuli (e.g., low plasma levels of corticosteroids, pain, anxiety, trauma, illness, anesthesia) activate the system. These stimuli cause the hypothalamus of the brain to secrete corticotropin-releasing hormone or factor (CRH or CRF), which stimulates the anterior pituitary gland to secrete corticotropin, and corticotropin then stimulates the adrenal cortex to secrete corticosteroids.

2. The stress response activates the sympathetic nervous system (SNS) to produce more epinephrine and norepinephrine and the adrenal cortex to produce as much as 10 times the normal amount of cortisol. The synergistic interaction of these hormones increases the person's ability to respond to stress. However, the increased SNS activity continues to stimulate cortisol production (the main glucocorticoids secreted as part of the body's response to stress) and overrules the negative feedback mechanism. Excessive and prolonged corticosteroid secretion damages body tissues.

3. Glucocorticoids are important in metabolic, inflammatory, and immune processes. Glucocorticoids include cortisol, corticosterone, and cortisone. Cortisol accounts for at least 95% of glucocorticoid activity; corticosterone and cortisone account for a small amount of activity. Glucocorticoids are secreted cyclically, with the largest amount being produced in the early morning and the smallest amount during the evening hours (in people with a normal day–night schedule). At the cellular level, glucocorticoids account for most of the characteristics and physiologic effects of the corticosteroids

4. Mineralocorticoids are a class of steroids that play a vital role in the maintenance of fluid and electrolyte balance through their influence on salt and water metabolism. Aldosterone is the main mineralocorticoid and is responsible for approximately 90% of mineralocorticoid activity.

5. The adrenal cortex secretes male (androgens) and female (estrogens and progesterone) sex hormones. Compared with the effect of hormones produced by the testes and ovaries, the adrenal sex hormones have an insignificant effect on normal body function. Adrenal androgens, secreted continuously in small quantities by both sexes, are responsible for most of the physiologic effects exerted by the adrenal sex hormones. They increase protein synthesis (anabolism), which increases the mass and strength of muscle and bone tissue; they affect development of male secondary sex characteristics; and they increase hair growth and libido in women.

SECTION III: APPLYING YOUR KNOWLEDGE

ACTIVITY D

CASE STUDIES

1. Systemic lupus erythematosus is a collagen disorder, as are scleroderma and periarteritis nodosa. Collagen is the basic structural protein of connective tissue, tendons, cartilage, and bone, and it is therefore present in almost all body tissues and organ systems. The collagen disorders are characterized by inflammation of various body tissues, particularly tendons, cartilage, and connective tissues. Signs and symptoms depend on which body tissues or organs are affected and the severity of the inflammatory process.

2. Dermatologic disorders that may be treated with systemic corticosteroids include acute contact dermatitis, erythema multiforme, herpes zoster (prophylaxis of postherpetic neuralgia), lichen planus, pemphigus, skin rashes caused by drugs, and toxic epidermal necrolysis.

3. The effectiveness of corticosteroids in neoplastic diseases, such as acute and chronic leukemias, Hodgkin's disease, other lymphomas, and multiple myelomas, probably stems from their ability to suppress lymphocytes and other lymphoid tissue.

4. Corticosteroids suppress cellular and humoral immune responses and help prevent rejection of transplanted tissue. Drug therapy is usually continued as long as the transplanted tissue is in place.

5. In patients with asthma, corticosteroids increase the number of beta-adrenergic receptors and increase or restore the responsiveness of beta receptors to beta-adrenergic bronchodilating drugs. In cases of asthma, COPD, and rhinitis, the drugs decrease mucus secretion and inflammation. In anaphylactic shock resulting from an allergic reaction, corticosteroids may increase or restore cardiovascular responsiveness to adrenergic drugs.

SECTION IV: PRACTICING FOR NCLEX

1. d. *Rationale:* A black box warning has been issued by the FDA for individuals who are transferred from systemically active corticosteroids to flunisolide inhaler; deaths from adrenal insufficiency have been reported.

2. b and c. *Rationale:* Adverse effects of systemic corticosteroids may include infections, hypertension, glucose intolerance, obesity, cosmetic changes, bone loss, growth retardation in children, cataracts, pancreatitis, peptic ulcerations, and psychiatric disturbances

3. b. *Rationale:* Strategies to minimize HPA suppression and risks of acute adrenal insufficiency include administering a systemic corticosteroid during high-stress situations in clients who are on long-term systemic therapy (i.e., are steroid dependent).

4. a. *Rationale:* Strategies to minimize HPA suppression and risks of acute adrenal insufficiency include giving short courses of systemic therapy for acute disorders.

5. c. *Rationale:* Strategies to minimize HPA suppression and risks of acute adrenal insufficiency include gradually tapering the dose of any systemic corticosteroid.

6. d. *Rationale:* Strategies to minimize HPA suppression and risks of acute adrenal insufficiency include using local rather than systemic therapy when possible, alone or in combination with low doses of systemic drugs.

7. corticotropin

8. d. *Rationale:* Daily administration of corticosteroids and mineralocorticoids is required in cases of chronic adrenocortical insufficiency (Addison's disease).

9. androgenic

10. a, b, and d. *Rationale:* The most frequently desired pharmacologic effects of exogenous corticosteroids are anti-inflammatory, immunosuppressive, antiallergic, and antistress effects.

11. a. *Rationale:* Because of potentially serious adverse effects, especially with oral drugs, it is extremely important that corticosteroids be used as prescribed. A major responsibility of home care nurses is to teach, demonstrate, supervise, monitor, or do whatever is needed to facilitate correct use.

12. b. *Rationale:* Corticosteroids improve survival and decrease the risk of respiratory failure with pneumocystosis, a common cause of death in patients with AIDS.

13. b. *Rationale:* Sepsis may be complicated by impaired corticosteroid production. There is sufficient evidence to support the idea that giving a long course of low-dose corticosteroids in patients with septic shock can improve survival without causing harm. However, overall, corticosteroids do not affect mortality.

14. d. *Rationale:* Although corticosteroids have been widely used, several well-controlled studies demonstrated that the drugs are not beneficial in early treatment or in prevention of adult respiratory distress syndrome (ARDS).

15. a. *Rationale:* Some studies support the use of IV methylprednisolone. So, if other medications do not produce adequate bronchodilation, it seems reasonable to try an IV corticosteroid during the first 72 hours of the

illness. However, corticosteroid therapy increases the risks of pulmonary infection.

16. b. *Rationale:* In adrenal insufficiency, hypotension is a common symptom in critically ill patients, and hypotension caused by adrenal insufficiency may mimic either hypovolemic or septic shock. If adrenal insufficiency is the cause of the hypotension, administration of corticosteroids can eliminate the need for vasopressor drugs to maintain adequate tissue perfusion.

17. slowed

18. hypercorticism

19. a, c, and d. *Rationale:* Corticosteroids are used for the same conditions in older adults as in younger ones. Older adults are especially likely to have conditions that are aggravated by the drugs (e.g., congestive heart failure, hypertension, diabetes mellitus, arthritis, osteoporosis, increased susceptibility to infection, concomitant drug therapy that increases risks of gastrointestinal ulceration and bleeding). Consequently, risk–benefit ratios of systemic corticosteroid therapy should be carefully considered, especially for long-term therapy.

20. moderate

Chapter 24: Thyroid and Antithyroid Drugs

SECTION II: ASSESSING YOUR UNDERSTANDING

ACTIVITY A
FILL IN THE BLANKS
1. thyroxine
2. iodine and tyrosine
3. cellular metabolism
4. Primary hypothyroidism
5. Congenital hypothyroidism

ACTIVITY B
MATCHING
1. A   2. D   3. E   4. B   5. C

ACTIVITY C
SHORT ANSWERS
1. Hyperthyroidism is characterized by excessive secretion of thyroid hormone and usually involves an enlarged thyroid gland that has an increased number of cells and an increased rate of secretion. It may be associated with Graves' disease, nodular goiter, thyroiditis, overtreatment with thyroid drugs, functioning thyroid carcinoma, or a pituitary adenoma that secretes excessive amounts of TSH. The hyperplasic thyroid gland may secrete 5 to 15 times the normal amount of thyroid hormone. As a result, body metabolism is greatly increased.

2. Thyroid storm or thyrotoxic crisis is a rare but severe complication characterized by extreme symptoms of hyperthyroidism, such as severe tachycardia, fever, dehydration, heart failure, and coma. It is most likely to occur in patients with hyperthyroidism that has been inadequately treated, especially when stressful situations occur (e.g., trauma, infection, surgery, emotional upset).

3. Thyroid drugs such as the synthetic drug levothyroxine provide an exogenous source of thyroid hormone. Antithyroid drugs act by decreasing production or release of thyroid hormones. The thioamide drugs inhibit synthesis of thyroid hormone. Iodine preparations inhibit the release of thyroid hormones and cause them to be stored within the thyroid gland. Radioactive iodine emits rays that destroy the thyroid gland tissue.

4. Thyroid drugs are indicated for primary or secondary hypothyroidism, cretinism, and myxedema. Antithyroid drugs may be necessary for hyperthyroidism associated with Graves' disease, nodular goiter, thyroiditis, overtreatment with thyroid drugs, functioning thyroid carcinoma, or a pituitary adenoma that secretes excessive amounts of TSH. Antithyroid drugs may also be indicated for thyroid storm.

5. Iodine preparations and thioamide antithyroid drugs are contraindicated in pregnancy, because they can lead to goiter and hypothyroidism in the fetus or newborn. Radioactive iodine is contraindicated during lactation as well. Because radioactive iodine may cause cancer and chromosome damage in children, it should be used only for hyperthyroidism that cannot be controlled by other drugs or surgery.

SECTION III: APPLYING YOUR KNOWLEDGE

ACTIVITY D
CASE STUDIES
CASE STUDY 1
1. Subclinical hypothyroidism involves a mildly elevated serum TSH and normal serum thyroxine levels.
2. Thyroid replacement therapy in the patient with hypothyroidism is lifelong; no clearcut guidelines exist regarding duration of antithyroid drug therapy because of exacerbations and remissions. Replacement therapy usually continues until the patient has been euthyroid for 6 to 12 months.

CASE STUDY 2
1. Subclinical hyperthyroidism is defined as a reduced TSH level (<0.1 microunit/L) and normal T_3 and T_4 levels.
2. The most common cause of hyperthyroidism is excess thyroid hormone therapy. Subclinical hyperthyroidism is a risk factor for osteoporosis in postmenopausal women who do not take estrogen replacement therapy, because it leads to reduced bone mineral density. Subclinical hyperthyroidism also greatly increases the risk for atrial fibrillation in patients older than 60 years of age.

SECTION IV: PRACTICING FOR NCLEX
1. a. *Rationale:* The FDA has issued a black box warning regarding the use of thyroid hormones for the treatment of obesity or for weight loss, either alone or with other therapeutic agents. Significant and serious complications may develop in euthroid individuals talking thyroid hormones.

2. c. *Rationale:* Individuals with hypothyroidism are especially likely to experience respiratory depression and myxedema coma with opioid analgesics and other sedating drugs.

3. b. *Rationale:* For congenital hypothyroidism (cretinism), drug therapy should be started within 6 weeks of after birth.

4. d. *Rationale:* For congenital hypothyroidism (cretinism), drug therapy should be started within 6 weeks of birth and continued for life, or mental retardation may result.

5. a. *Rationale:* Thyroid replacement therapy in the patient with hypothyroidism is lifelong; no clearcut guidelines exist regarding duration of antithyroid drug therapy because of exacerbations and remissions. Replacement therapy usually continues until the patient has been euthyroid for 6 to 12 months.

6. Levothyroxine (Synthroid, Levothroid)
7. a. *Rationale:* Patients who are taking antithyroid drugs should be monitored closely for hypothyroidism, which usually develops within 1 year after starting treatment for hyperthyroidism.
8. Propylthiouracil (PTU)
9. a, b, and d. *Rationale:* The home care nurse may be involved in a wide range of activities, including assessing the patient's response to therapy, teaching about the disease process, managing of symptoms, and preventing and managing adverse drug effects. The nurse would not modify medications without a physician's order.
10. b. *Rationale:* Individuals in thyroid storm or thyrotoxic crisis are commonly managed in the critical care unit. Increased rates of cellular metabolism and oxygen consumption occur, with a resultant increase in heat production. The hypermetabolic state increases the metabolism of medications, so increased or more frequent dosing may be necessary.
11. c. *Rationale:* Drug metabolism in the liver is delayed in patients with hypothyroidism and liver disease, so most drugs given to these patients have a prolonged effect.
12. euthyroidism
13. a. *Rationale:* For hypothyroidism, levothyroxine is given. Thyroid hormone replacement increases the workload of the heart and may cause serious adverse effects in older adults, especially those with cardiovascular disease.
14. a and b. *Rationale:* For hyperthyroidism, PTU or methimazole is used. Potential risks for adverse effects are similar to those in adults. Radioactive iodine may cause cancer and chromosome damage in children; therefore, this agent should be used only for hyperthyroidism that cannot be controlled by other antithyroid drugs or surgery.
15. d. *Rationale:* Treatment of hyperthyroidism changes the rate of body metabolism, including the rate of metabolism of many drugs. In the hyperthyroid state, drug metabolism may be very rapid, and higher doses of most drugs may be necessary to achieve therapeutic results. When the patient becomes euthyroid, the rate of drug metabolism is decreased. Consequently, doses of all medications should be evaluated and probably reduced to avoid severe adverse effects.
16. b. *Rationale:* Diagnostic tests to evaluate thyroid function or a trial withdrawal may be implemented to determine whether the patient is likely to remain euthyroid without further drug therapy. If a drug is to be discontinued, this is usually done gradually over weeks or months.
17. c. *Rationale:* When hypothyroidism and adrenal insufficiency coexist, the adrenal insufficiency should be treated with a corticosteroid drug before starting thyroid replacement. Thyroid hormones increase tissue metabolism and tissue demands for adrenocortical hormones. If adrenal insufficiency is not treated first, administration of thyroid hormone may cause acute adrenocortical insufficiency, a life-threatening condition.
18. levothyroxine
19. exogenous
20. euthyroid

Chapter 25: Hormones That Regulate Calcium and Bone Metabolism

SECTION II: ASSESSING YOUR UNDERSTANDING

ACTIVITY A
FILL IN THE BLANKS
1. parathyroid hormone (PTH)
2. PTH
3. hypoparathyroidism
4. hyperparathyroidism
5. hypocalcemia

ACTIVITY B
MATCHING
1. E   2. B   3. A   4. C   5. D

ACTIVITY C
SHORT ANSWERS
1. PTH secretion is stimulated by low serum calcium levels and inhibited by normal or high levels (a negative feedback system). Because phosphate is closely related to calcium in body functions, PTH also regulates phosphate metabolism. In general, when serum calcium levels increase, serum phosphate levels decrease, and vice versa. Thus, an inverse relationship exists between calcium and phosphate.
2. When the serum calcium level falls below the normal range, PTH raises the level by acting on bone, intestines, and kidneys. In bone, breakdown is increased, so that calcium moves from bone into the serum. In the intestines, there is increased absorption of calcium ingested in food (PTH activates vitamin D, which increases intestinal absorption). In the kidneys, there is increased reabsorption of calcium in the renal tubules and less urinary excretion. The opposite effects occur with phosphate (e.g., PTH decreases serum phosphate and increases urinary phosphate excretion).
3. Hyperparathyroidism is most often caused by a tumor or hyperplasia of a parathyroid gland. It also may result from ectopic secretion of PTH by malignant tumors (e.g., carcinomas of the lung, pancreas, kidney, ovary, prostate gland, or bladder). Clinical manifestations and treatment of hypoparathyroidism are the same as those of hypocalcemia. Clinical manifestations and treatment of hyperparathyroidism are the same as those of hypercalcemia.
4. Calcitonin is a hormone from the thyroid gland whose secretion is controlled by the concentration of ionized calcium in the blood flowing through the thyroid gland. When the serum level of ionized calcium is increased, secretion of calcitonin is increased. The function of calcitonin is to lower serum calcium in the presence of hypercalcemia, which it does by decreasing movement of calcium from bone to serum and increasing urinary excretion of calcium. The action of calcitonin is rapid but of short duration. Therefore, this hormone has little effect on long-term calcium metabolism.
5. Vitamin D (*calciferol*) is a fat-soluble vitamin that includes both ergocalciferol (obtained from foods) and cholecalciferol (formed by exposure of skin to sunlight). It functions as a hormone and plays an important role in calcium and bone metabolism. The main action of vitamin D is to raise serum calcium levels by increasing intestinal absorption of calcium and mobilizing calcium from bone. It also promotes bone formation by providing adequate

serum concentrations of minerals. Vitamin D is not physiologically active in the body. It must be converted to an intermediate metabolite in the liver, then to an active metabolite (1,25-dihydroxyvitamin D or calcitriol) in the kidneys. PTH and adequate hepatic and renal function are required to produce the active metabolite.

SECTION III: APPLYING YOUR KNOWLEDGE

ACTIVITY D

CASE STUDIES

1. Osteoporosis results when bone strength (bone density and bone quality) is impaired, leading to increased porousness and vulnerability to fracture.
2. Hormonal deficiencies, some diseases, and some medications (e.g., glucocorticoids) can also increase resorption, resulting in loss of bone mass and osteoporosis.
3. Bone tissue is constantly being formed and broken down in a process called *remodeling*. During childhood, adolescence, and early adulthood, formation usually exceeds breakdown (resorption) as the person attains adult height and peak bone mass. After approximately 35 years of age, resorption is greater than formation.
4. Alendronate (Fosamax), ibandronate (Boniva), pamidronate (Aredia), risedronate (Actonel), and zoledronate (Zometa) are drugs that bind to bone and inhibit calcium resorption from bone. Bisphosphonates are poorly absorbed from the intestinal tract. Bisphosphonates must be taken on an empty stomach, with water, at least 30 minutes before any other fluid, food, or medication. The drugs are not metabolized. The drug bound to bone is slowly released into the bloodstream. Most of the drug that is not bound to bone is excreted in the urine.

SECTION IV: PRACTICING FOR NCLEX

1. a. *Rationale:* For men, corticosteroids decrease testosterone levels by approximately one half, and replacement therapy may be needed.
2. b. *Rationale:* Both men and women who take corticosteroids are at risk for osteoporosis.
3. d. *Rationale:* Postmenopausal women are at high risk for osteoporosis.
4. a, c, and d. *Rationale:* Calcium deficiency commonly occurs in the elderly because of long-term dietary deficiencies of calcium and vitamin D, impaired absorption of calcium from the intestine, lack of exposure to sunlight, and impaired liver or kidney metabolism of vitamin D to its active form.
5. 2500
6. 400
7. d. *Rationale:* Deficiency of vitamin D causes inadequate absorption of calcium and phosphorus.
8. a and c. *Rationale:* Hyperparathyroidism is most often caused by a tumor or hyperplasia of a parathyroid gland.
9. a. *Rationale:* Patients with renal impairment or failure often have disturbances in calcium and bone metabolism. If hypercalcemia develops in patients with severely impaired renal function, hemodialysis or peritoneal dialysis with calcium-free solution is effective and safe. Calcium acetate may be used to prevent or treat hyperphosphatemia. The calcium reduces blood levels of phosphate by reducing its absorption from foods.
10. a, b, and c. *Rationale:* Calcium deficiency commonly occurs because of long-term dietary deficiencies of calcium and vitamin D, impaired absorption of calcium from the intestine, lack of exposure to sunlight, and impaired liver or kidney metabolism of vitamin D to its active form.

11. d. *Rationale:* Patients diagnosed with osteoporosis require adequate calcium and vitamin D (at least the recommended dietary allowance), whether obtained from the diet or from supplements. Calcium 600 mg and vitamin D 200 international units once or twice daily are often recommended for postmenopausal women with osteoporosis, and pharmacologic doses of vitamin D are sometimes used to treat patients with serious osteoporosis. If such doses are used, caution should be exercised, because excessive amounts of vitamin D can cause hypercalcemia and hypercalciuria.
12. c. *Rationale:* Preventive measures are necessary for patients taking phenytoin (Dilantin) and phenobarbital, because these drugs may contribute to osteoporosis through their effects on calcium metabolism. These anticonvulsant medications increase hepatic metabolism of vitamin D, which leads to a decrease in calcium absorption in the intestine. Supplemental calcium and vitamin D as well as specific drugs for osteoporosis should be considered if bone density is low.
13. a, c, and d. *Rationale:* Preventive measures are necessary for patients on chronic corticosteroid therapy (e.g., prednisone 7.5 mg daily; equivalent amounts of other systemic drugs; high doses of inhaled drugs). For both men and women, most of the guidelines for prevention of osteoporosis apply (e.g., calcium supplements, regular exercise, a bisphosphonate drug). In addition, low doses and nonsystemic routes help prevent osteoporosis and other adverse effects. For men, corticosteroids decrease testosterone levels by approximately one half, and replacement therapy may be needed.
14. calcitriol
15. 12 mg/dL
16. a and c. *Rationale:* Calcium preparations and digoxin have similar effects on the myocardium. Therefore, if calcium is given to a patient taking digoxin, the risks of digitalis toxicity and cardiac dysrhythmias are increased. This combination must be used very cautiously. Oral calcium preparations decrease effects of oral tetracycline drugs by combining with the antibiotic and preventing its absorption. They should not be given at the same time or within 2 to 3 hours of each other.
17. osteoporosis
18. a. *Rationale:* Sodium chloride (0.9%) injection (normal saline) is an IV solution that contains water, sodium, and chloride. It is included here because it is the treatment of choice for hypercalcemia and is usually effective. The sodium contained in the solution inhibits the reabsorption of calcium in renal tubules and thereby increases urinary excretion of calcium.
19. d. *Rationale:* Phosphates should be given only when hypercalcemia is accompanied by hypophosphatemia (serum phosphorus <3 mg/dL) and renal function is normal, to minimize the risk of soft-tissue calcification.
20. renal tubules

Chapter 26: Antidiabetic Drugs

SECTION II: ASSESSING YOUR UNDERSTANDING

ACTIVITY A

FILL IN THE BLANKS

1. Insulin
2. Amylin
3. liver
4. fat
5. glomeruli

ACTIVITY B
MATCHING
1. D   2. B   3. A   4. E   5. C

ACTIVITY C
SHORT ANSWERS

1. Metformin increases the use of glucose by muscle and fat cells, decreases hepatic glucose production, and decreases intestinal absorption of glucose. It is preferably called an antihyperglycemic rather than a hypoglycemic agent, because it does not cause hypoglycemia, even in large doses, when used alone. Metformin is absorbed from the small intestine, circulates without binding to plasma proteins, and has a serum half-life of 1.3 to 4.5 hours. It is not metabolized in the liver and is excreted unchanged in the urine.

2. Thiazolidinediones include pioglitazone and rosiglitazone. They are sometimes called "glitazones" and are also referred to as insulin sensitizers. Thiazolidinediones decrease insulin resistance, a major factor in the pathophysiology of type 2 diabetes. The drugs stimulate receptors on muscle, fat, and liver cells. This stimulation increases or restores the effectiveness of circulating insulin and results in increased uptake of glucose by peripheral tissues and decreased production of glucose by the liver. Thiazolidinediones may be used as monotherapy with diet and exercise or in combination with insulin, metformin, a sulfonylurea, an amylin analog (pramlintide), or an incretin mimetic (extenatide).

3. Pramlintide (Symlin) is a synthetic analog of amylin, a peptide hormone secreted with insulin by the beta cells of the pancreas that is important in the regulation of glucose control during the postprandial period. Pramlintide is used as an adjunctive treatment with mealtime insulin for adult patient with type 1 or type 2 diabetes who have not achieved optimal glucose control with insulin therapy alone. Pramlintide slows gastric emptying, helping to regulate the postprandial rise in blood glucose. The drug also suppresses postprandial glucagon secretion, thus helping maintain better blood glucose control. Pramlintide increases the sense of satiety, possibly reducing food intake and promoting weight loss. Pramlintide and insulin therapy may be combined with metformin or sulfonylureas for patients with type 2 diabetes.

4. Extenatide acts as a natural helper hormone by stimulating the pancreas to secrete the right amount of insulin based on the food that was just eaten. This helps to reduce the problem of high blood glucose after meals. Extenatide also halts gluconeogenesis by the liver, keeping it from making too much glucose after a meal. Extenatide slows gastric emptying, which serves to reduce the sudden rise of blood glucose after a meal and also quickly stimulates a feeling of satiety when eating. This fosters a sense of fullness, which causes the patient to eat less and potentially lose weight. Extenatide may reduce the absorption of concurrently administered oral medications.

5. Certain supplements may increase blood glucose levels. Bee pollen may cause hyperglycemia and decrease the effects of antidiabetic medications; it should not be used by people with diabetes. Ginkgo biloba extract is thought to increase blood sugar in patients with diabetes by increasing hepatic metabolism of insulin and oral hypoglycemic drugs, thereby making the drugs less effective. It is not recommended for use. Glucosamine, as indicated by animal studies, may cause impaired beta-cell function and insulin secretion similar to that observed in humans with type 2 diabetes. Long-term effects in humans are unknown, but the product

is considered potentially harmful to people with diabetes or prediabetes. Adverse effects on blood sugar and drug interactions with antidiabetic medications have not been reported. However, blood sugar should be monitored carefully. With chondroitin, which is often taken with glucosamine for osteoarthritis, there is no information about effects on blood sugar, use by diabetic patients, or interactions with antidiabetic drugs.

SECTION III: APPLYING YOUR KNOWLEDGE
ACTIVITY D
CASE STUDIES

1. Type 2 is a heterogenous disease, and its etiology probably involves multiple factors such as a genetic predisposition and environmental factors. Obesity is a major cause. With obesity and chronic ingestion of excess calories, along with a sedentary lifestyle, more insulin is required. The increased need leads to prolonged stimulation and eventual "fatigue" of pancreatic beta cells. As a result, the cells become less responsive to elevated blood glucose levels and less able to produce enough insulin to meet metabolic needs. Therefore, insulin is secreted but is inadequate or ineffective, especially when insulin demand is increased by obesity, pregnancy, aging, or other factors.

2. Most signs and symptoms stem from a lack of effective insulin and the subsequent metabolic abnormalities. Their incidence and severity depend on the amount of effective insulin, and they may be precipitated by infection, rapid growth, pregnancy, or other factors that increase demand for insulin. Most early symptoms result from disordered carbohydrate metabolism, which causes excess glucose to accumulate in the blood (hyperglycemia). Hyperglycemia produces glucosuria, which, in turn, produces polydipsia, polyuria, dehydration, and polyphagia.

3. When large amounts of glucose are present, as in the hyperglycemic state of diabetes, water is pulled into the renal tubule. This results in a greatly increased urine output (polyuria). The excessive loss of fluid in urine leads to increased thirst (polydipsia) and, if fluid intake is inadequate, to dehydration. Dehydration also occurs because high blood glucose levels increase osmotic pressure in the bloodstream, and fluid is pulled out of the cells in the body's attempt to regain homeostasis.

4. Extenatide is administered subcutaneously twice a day and has been approved to be administered with oral medications such as sulfonylureas, metformin, and/or thiazolidinediones. Major advantages of exenatide over insulin are increased satiety and weight loss. Extenatide is available via a pre-filled injection pen in two doses (5 or 10 mcg) and does not need to be adjusted base on blood glucose levels or the amount of food a patient was able to consume. The drug should be taken twice a day within 60 minutes of the morning and evening meal (at least 6 hours apart). Extenatide can be injected into the subcutaneous tissue of the upper arm or leg or the abdominal area. It should be stored at all times in the original packaging in a refrigerator at 36 to 46 degrees F, protected from light, kept dry, and discarded once opened after 30 days.

SECTION IV: PRACTICING FOR NCLEX

1. b and d. *Rationale:* Individuals with impaired glucose tolerance can significantly reduce the risk of developing type 2 diabetes through intervention with diet and exercise.

2. d. *Rationale:* A FPG result (126 mg/dL on two separate occasions is diagnostic of diabetes; values of 100 to

125 mg/dL are termed impaired fasting glucose, and values <100 mg/dL are considered normal.

3. a. *Rationale:* fasting plasma glucose test (FPG) is the simplest and least expensive screening test.

4. The American Diabetes Association (ADA) suggests a target A1C of <7 percent. A1C should be measured every 3 to 6 months.

5. b, c, and d. *Rationale:* Aspects of the home care nursing role include mobilizing and coordinating health care providers and community resources; teaching and supporting patients and caregivers; monitoring the patient's health status and progress in disease management; assisting the patient to obtain diabetic supplies for monitoring and medication administration; and preventing or solving problems.

6. A and B. *Rationale:* Hyperglycemia may complicate the progress of the critically ill patient, resulting in increased complications such as postoperative infections, poor recovery, and increased mortality. Tight glycemic control is a key factor in preventing complications and improving mortality in diabetic patients in the intensive care unit.

7. a. *Rationale:* Sulfonylureas and their metabolites are excreted mainly by the kidneys; renal impairment may lead to accumulation and hypoglycemia. They should be used cautiously, with close monitoring of renal function, in patients with mild to moderate renal impairment and are contraindicated in severe renal impairment.

8. d. *Rationale:* Renal insufficiency may increase risks of adverse effects with antidiabetic drugs; and treatment with thiazide diuretics, corticosteroids, estrogens, and other drugs may cause hyperglycemia, thereby increasing dosage requirements for antidiabetic drugs.

9. c. *Rationale:* Type 2 diabetes is being increasingly identified in children. This trend is attributed mainly to obesity and inadequate exercise, because most children with type 2 are seriously overweight and have poor eating habits.

10. a and c. *Rationale:* In young children, hypoglycemia may be manifested by changes in behavior, including severe hunger, irritability, and lethargy. In addition, mental functioning may be impaired in all age groups, even with mild hypoglycemia. Anytime hypoglycemia is suspected, blood glucose should be tested.

11. b. *Rationale:* Recognition of hypoglycemia may be delayed because signs and symptoms are vague and the children may be unable to communicate them to parents or caregivers. Because of these difficulties, most pediatric diabetologists recommend maintaining blood glucose levels between 100 and 200 mg/dL to prevent hypoglycemia. In addition, the bedtime snack and blood glucose measurement should never be skipped.

12. c. *Rationale:* Avoiding hypoglycemia is a major goal in infants and young children because of potentially damaging effects on growth and development. For example, the brain and spinal cord do not develop normally without an adequate supply of glucose.

13. d. *Rationale:* Administration of insulin for infants and toddlers who weigh less than 10 kg or require less than 5 units of insulin per day can be difficult because small doses are hard to measure in a U-100 syringe. Use of diluted insulin allows more accurate administration. The most common dilution strength is U-10 (10 units/mL), and a diluent is available from insulin manufacturers for this purpose. Vials of diluted insulin should be clearly labeled and should be discarded after 1 month.

14. a. *Rationale:* During illness, children are highly susceptible to dehydration, and an adequate fluid intake is very important. Many clinicians recommend sugar-containing liquids (e.g., regular sodas, clear juices, regular gelatin desserts) if blood glucose values are lower than 250 mg/dL. If blood glucose values are above 250 mg/dL, diet soda, unsweetened tea, and other fluids without sugar should be given.

15. a and c. *Rationale:* Insulin is the only drug indicated for use in type 1 diabetes; it is required as replacement therapy because affected children cannot produce insulin. Effective management requires a consistent schedule of meals, snacks, blood glucose monitoring, insulin injections and dose adjustments, and exercise.

16. Insulin

17. d. *Rationale:* IV fluids, the first step in treating DKA, usually consist of 0.9% sodium chloride, an isotonic solution. Hypotonic solutions are usually avoided because they allow intracellular fluid shifts and may cause cerebral, pulmonary, and peripheral edema.

18. c. *Rationale:* Studies indicate that insulin is absorbed fastest from the abdomen, followed by the deltoid, thigh, and hip.

19. b. *Rationale:* With regular insulin before meals, it is very important that the medication be injected 30 to 45 minutes before meals so that the insulin will be available when blood sugar increases after the meal.

20. blood glucose

Chapter 27: Estrogens, Progestins, and Hormonal Contraceptives

SECTION II: ASSESSING YOUR UNDERSTANDING

ACTIVITY A
FILL IN THE BLANKS
1. Estrogens and progestins
2. estrogens
3. amenorrhea
4. anorexia nervosa
5. cholesterol

ACTIVITY B
MATCHING
1. B   2. C   3. A   4. E   5. D

ACTIVITY C
SHORT ANSWERS
1. Like other steroid hormones, estrogens and progestins are synthesized from cholesterol. The ovaries and adrenal glands can manufacture cholesterol or extract it from the blood. Through a series of chemical reactions, cholesterol is converted to progesterone and then to androgens, testosterone, and androstenedione. The ovaries use these male sex hormones to produce estrogens. After formation, the hormones are secreted into the bloodstream in response to stimulation by the anterior pituitary gonadotropic hormones, follicle-stimulating hormone (FSH), and luteinizing hormone (LH). In the bloodstream, the hormones combine with serum proteins and are transported to target tissues, where they enter body cells. They cross cell membranes easily because of their steroid structure and lipid solubility. Inside the cells, the hormones bind to estrogen or progestin receptors and regulate intracellular protein synthesis.
2. The main function of the estrogens is to promote growth in tissues related to reproduction and sexual characteristics in women

3. In nonpregnant women, between puberty and menopause, estrogens are secreted in a monthly cycle called the menstrual cycle. During the first half of the cycle, before ovulation, estrogens are secreted in progressively larger amounts. During the second half of the cycle, estrogens and progesterone are secreted in increasing amounts until 2 to 3 days before the onset of menstruation. At that time, secretion of both hormones decreases abruptly. When the endometrial lining of the uterus loses its hormonal stimulation, it is discharged vaginally as menstrual flow.

4. Estrogens are deactivated in the liver and readily excreted through the kidneys. Metabolites are also formed in the gastrointestinal tract, brain, skin, and other steroid target tissues. Most of the conjugates are excreted in urine, and some are excreted in bile and recirculated to the liver or excreted in feces.

5. In the nonpregnant woman, progesterone is secreted by the corpus luteum during the last half of the menstrual cycle, which occurs after ovulation. This hormone continues the changes in the endometrial lining of the uterus begun by estrogens during the first half of the menstrual cycle. These changes provide for implantation and nourishment of a fertilized ovum. When fertilization does not take place, the estrogen and progesterone levels decrease and menstruation occurs.

SECTION III: APPLYING YOUR KNOWLEDGE

ACTIVITY D
CASE STUDIES

1. Black cohosh is an herb used to self-treat symptoms of menopause. It is reportedly effective in relieving vasomotor instability.

2. Black cohosh apparently exerts a nonhormonal effect and does not affect the endometrium or estrogen-dependent cancers; however, its effects on bone and osteoporosis are unknown.

3. Black cohosh may increase the hypotensive effects of antihypertensive drugs, so blood pressure should be monitored closely in hypertensive patients. Adverse effects of black cohosh may include nausea, vomiting, dizziness, hypotension, and visual disturbances.

4. If Remifemin is taken, the recommended dosage is 1 tablet (standardized to contain 20 mg of herbal drug) twice daily. Other dosage forms are available, and dosage depends on the method of preparation. Black cohosh is not recommended for use longer than 6 months for menopausal symptoms.

SECTION IV: PRACTICING FOR NCLEX

1. a. *Rationale:* The FDA recommended that HRT be used only for women with symptoms severe enough to warrant its use, at the lowest dose and for the shortest duration possible, to ease the menopausal transition.

2. b. *Rationale:* Studies have demonstrated no evidence for HRT in secondary prevention of heart disease and have shown increased rates of CHD, thromboembolic stroke, venous thromboembolism, dementia, and breast cancer, which outweigh the benefits of decreased risks of fracture and colon cancer.

3. d. *Rationale:* Thromboembolic disorders are most likely to occur during the first year of use; risks of developing breast cancer increase with the duration of drug use.

4. uterus

5. a and b. *Rationale:* Most interactions with antimicrobials have been reported with oral contraceptives. To prevent pregnancy from occurring during antimicrobial therapy, a larger dose of oral contraceptive or an additional or alternative form of birth control is probably advisable.

6. c. *Rationale:* When estrogens are used alone in postmenopausal women, they cause endometrial hyperplasia and may cause endometrial cancer. Women with an intact uterus should also be given a progestin, which opposes the effects of estrogen on the endometrium.

7. epiphyseal closure

8. b. *Rationale:* Cigarette smoking in individuals who use oral contraceptives increases the risk for blood clots in the legs, lungs, heart, or brain.

9. d. *Rationale:* Oral contraceptives are very effective at preventing pregnancy, but they do not prevent transmission of sexually transmitted diseases.

10. endogenous

11. a and c. *Rationale:* In families that include postmenopausal women, home care nurses may need to teach about nonhormonal strategies for preventing or treating osteoporosis and cardiovascular disease.

12. b. *Rationale:* When visiting families that include adolescent girls or young women, home care nurses may need to teach about birth control measures or about preventing osteoporosis by improving diet and exercise patterns.

13. d. *Rationale:* Estrogens are contraindicated in impaired liver function, liver disease, or liver cancer. Impaired liver function may lead to impaired estrogen metabolism, with resultant accumulation and adverse effects.

14. smallest

15. a and c. *Rationale:* Estrogen and progestin may be used less often for osteoporosis in future for two main reasons. First, recent evidence indicates that the risks of estrogen–progestin and estrogen-only hormonal therapy outweigh the benefits. Second, there are other effective measures for prevention and treatment of osteoporosis, including calcium and vitamin D supplements, bisphosphonate drugs (e.g., alendronate, risedronate), and weight-bearing exercise. ERT is still considered for fracture prevention among women who are at high risk of fracture and who are unable to take other preventive medications.

16. a. *Rationale:* The main function of the progestin is to decrease the risk of endometrial cancer; therefore, women who have had a hysterectomy do not need it.

17. Plan B (levonorgestrel)

18. a, b, and c. *Rationale:* Oral contraceptives decrease effects of some benzodiazepines (e.g., lorazepam, oxazepam, temazepam), insulin, sulfonylurea antidiabetic drugs, and warfarin.

19. intramuscularly

20. b. *Rationale:* There is no evidence to suggest that use of progestins in the first trimester of pregnancy to prevent habitual abortion is safe. There is evidence that fetal harm is possible if the drug is given during the first 4 months of pregnancy.

Chapter 28: Androgens and Anabolic Steroids

SECTION II: ASSESSING YOUR UNDERSTANDING

ACTIVITY A
FILL IN THE BLANKS

1. Androgens
2. cholesterol
3. estrogens
4. androstenedione
5. Testosterone

ACTIVITY B
MATCHING
1. A 2. D 3. C 4. E 5. B

ACTIVITY C
SHORT ANSWERS
1. The main functions of testosterone are related to the development of male sexual characteristics, reproduction, and metabolism.
2. Anabolic steroids are synthetic drugs with increased anabolic activity and decreased androgenic activity compared with testosterone. They were developed during attempts to modify testosterone so that its tissue-building and growth-stimulating effects could be retained while its masculinizing effects could be eliminated or reduced.
3. Athletes are considered a high-risk group because some start taking the drugs as early as middle school and continue for years. The use of performance-enhancing drugs in non-athletes is also on the rise to improve performance outside of sports.
4. Anabolic steroids can stop bone growth and damage the heart, kidneys, and liver of adolescents.
5. Liver disorders include benign and malignant neoplasms, cholestatic hepatitis and jaundice, and peliosis hepatis, a disorder in which blood-filled cysts develop in the liver and may lead to hemorrhage or liver failure.

SECTION III: APPLYING YOUR KNOWLEDGE

ACTIVITY D
CASE STUDIES
1. Androstenedione and DHEA, androgens produced by the adrenal cortex, are also available as over-the-counter (OTC) dietary supplements. They are marketed as safe, natural, alternative androgens for building muscles.
2. These products, which have weak androgenic activity, act mainly as precursors for the production of sex hormones. DHEA may stimulate growth of prostate gland and breast and uterine tissues, so it is contraindicated in men with prostate cancer or benign prostatic hypertrophy (BPH) and in women with estrogen-responsive breast or uterine cancer. Clients older than 40 years of age should be aggressively screened for hormonally sensitive cancers before taking DHEA.
3. Adverse effects of DHEA include aggressiveness, hirsutism, insomnia, and irritability.
4. Androstenedione may be converted to testosterone by way of an enzyme found in most body tissues. However, it may also be converted to estrogens, and the testosterone that is produced may be further converted to estrogen (estradiol). Researchers have found little effect on serum testosterone levels or muscle development with resistance training in people taking androstenedione. They did find increased serum levels of estrone and estradiol, which indicate that a significant proportion of the androstenedione was converted to estrogens. Thus, taking a supplement for masculinizing effects may produce feminizing effects instead.
5. Whether large doses of the OTC products can produce some of the serious adverse effects associated with standard anabolic steroids is unknown.

SECTION IV: PRACTICING FOR NCLEX
1. b. *Rationale:* Because androgens cause premature epiphyseal closure, boys with established deficiency states receiving androgens should undergo x-ray examination every 6 months to detect bone maturation and prevent loss of adult height.
2. adrenal cortex
3. d. *Rationale:* Because of their abuse potential, androgens and anabolic steroids are classified as Schedule III controlled substances.
4. b. *Rationale:* Androgens and anabolic steroids are used to enhance athletic performance and are termed *ergogenic* (causing an increase in muscular work capacity); they are widely abused in attempts to enhance muscle development, muscle strength, and athletic performance.
5. c. *Rationale:* The main functions of testosterone are related to the development of male sexual characteristics, reproduction, and metabolism.
6. a. *Rationale:* The androgens produced by the ovaries have little androgenic activity and are used mainly as precursor substances for the production of naturally occurring estrogens.
7. b. *Rationale:* Androgens and anabolic steroids are contraindicated in clients with preexisting liver disease. Prolonged use of high doses may cause potentially life-threatening conditions such as peliosis hepatis, hepatic neoplasms, and hepatocellular carcinoma. In addition, androgen therapy should be discontinued if cholestatic hepatitis with jaundice occurs or if liver function tests become abnormal.
8. a. *Rationale:* Drug-induced jaundice is reversible when androgens are stopped.
9. d. *Rationale:* In older men, androgens may increase prostate size and interfere with urination, increase the risk of prostatic cancer, and cause excessive sexual stimulation and priapism.
10. b. *Rationale:* Older adults often have hypertension and other cardiovascular disorders that may be aggravated by the sodium and water retention associated with androgens and anabolic steroids.
11. deficiency
12. a. *Rationale:* The main indication for use of androgens is for boys with established deficiency states. Because the drugs cause epiphyseal closure, hands and wrists should undergo x-ray examination every 6 months to detect bone maturation and prevent loss of adult height.
13. b. *Rationale:* Androgens may increase effects of cyclosporine and warfarin, apparently by slowing their metabolism and increasing their concentrations in the blood. These combinations should be avoided if possible. However, if required, serum creatinine and cyclosporine levels should be monitored with cyclosporine, and prothrombin time or international normalized ratio (INR) with warfarin.
14. c. *Rationale:* Androgens also increase effects of sulfonylurea antidiabetic drugs. Concurrent use should be avoided if possible. If required, smaller doses of sulfonylureas may be needed, blood glucose levels should be monitored closely, and clients should be assessed for signs of hypoglycemia.
15. increases
16. c. *Rationale:* Androgens and anabolic steroids are contraindicated during pregnancy (because of possible masculinizing effects on a female fetus), in clients with preexisting liver disease, and in men with prostate-gland disorders.
17. endometriosis
18. a, c, and d. *Rationale:* With male sex hormones, the most clearcut indication for use is to treat androgen deficiency states (e.g., hypogonadism, cryptorchidism, impotence, oligospermia) in boys and men.

19. c. *Rationale:* All synthetic anabolic steroids are weak androgens. Consequently, giving these drugs for anabolic effects also produces masculinizing effects. This characteristic limits the clinical usefulness of these drugs in women and children. Profound changes in growth and sexual development may occur if these drugs are given to young children.

20. 24

Chapter 29: General Characteristics of Antimicrobial Drugs

SECTION II: ASSESSING YOUR UNDERSTANDING

ACTIVITY A
FILL IN THE BLANKS
1. Antimicrobial
2. microorganisms
3. Viruses
4. adenoviruses
5. Fungi

ACTIVITY B
MATCHING
1. B   2. E   3. A   4. C   5. D

ACTIVITY C
SHORT ANSWERS
1. The human body and the environment contain many microorganisms, most of which do not cause disease and live in a state of balance with the human host. When the balance is upset and infection occurs, the characteristics of the infecting microorganisms and the adequacy of host defense mechanisms are major factors in the severity of the infection and the person's ability to recover. Conditions that impair defense mechanisms increase the incidence and severity of infections and impede recovery. In addition, use of antimicrobial drugs may lead to serious infections caused by drug-resistant microorganisms.
2. Normal flora protects the human host by occupying space and consuming nutrients. This interferes with the ability of potential pathogens to establish residence and proliferate. If the normal flora is suppressed by antimicrobial drug therapy, potential pathogens may thrive. For example, the yeast *Candida albicans* is a normal resident of the vagina and the intestinal tract. An antibacterial drug may destroy the normal bacterial flora without affecting the fungal organism. As a result, *C. albicans* can proliferate and cause infection. Much of the normal flora can cause disease under certain conditions, especially in elderly, debilitated, or immune-suppressed people. Normal bowel flora also synthesize vitamin K and vitamin B complex.
3. Colonization involves the presence of normal microbial flora or transient environmental organisms that do not harm the host. Infectious disease involves the presence of a pathogen plus clinical signs and symptoms indicative of an infection. These microorganisms are usually spread by direct contact with an infected person or contaminated hands, food, water, or objects.
4. Opportunistic infections are likely to occur in people with severe burns, cancer, human immunodeficiency virus (HIV) infection, indwelling intravenous (IV) or urinary catheters, and antibiotic or corticosteroid drug therapy.
5. Broad-spectrum antibiotics affect the bacteria for which they are prescribed, transient organisms, other pathogens, and normal flora.

SECTION III: APPLYING YOUR KNOWLEDGE

ACTIVITY D
CASE STUDIES
1. The human body normally has areas that are sterile and areas that are colonized with microorganisms. Sterile areas are body fluids and cavities, the lower respiratory tract (trachea, bronchi, lungs), much of the gastrointestinal (GI) and genitourinary tracts, and the musculoskeletal system. Colonized areas include the skin, upper respiratory tract, and colon.
2. Microorganisms that are part of the normal flora and nonpathogenic in one area of the body may be pathogenic in other parts of the body; for example, *Escherichia coli* often causes urinary tract infections. Normal flora protects the human host by occupying space and consuming nutrients. This interferes with the ability of potential pathogens to establish residence and proliferate. Normal bowel flora synthesize vitamin K and vitamin B complex.
3. If the normal flora is suppressed by antimicrobial drug therapy, pathogens may thrive. Normal flora may cause disease when antibiotics are used. For example, *Candida albicans* is a normal resident of the vagina and the intestinal tract. An antibacterial drug may destroy the normal bacterial flora without affecting the fungal organism. As a result, *C. albicans* can proliferate and cause infection. Much of the normal flora can cause disease under certain conditions, especially in elderly, debilitated, or immunosuppressed people.

SECTION IV: PRACTICING FOR NCLEX
1. a. *Rationale:* Patient education related to antibiotic therapy should stress the importance of completing a full course of antibiotics as prescribed.
2. a and b. *Rationale:* Inappropriate use of antibiotics increases adverse drug effects, infections with drug-resistant microorganisms, and health care costs as well as reducing the number of available effective drugs for serious or antibiotic-resistant infections.
3. c. *Rationale:* Check specific recommendations with regard to the administration of the antibiotic with food and other medications to decrease binding to food and drugs and prevent inactivation.
4. evenly spaced
5. a. *Rationale:* Antimicrobial drug therapy requires close monitoring in patients with renal impairment, because many drugs are excreted primarily by the kidneys and some are nephrotoxic and may further damage the kidneys.
6. d. *Rationale:* For most surgeries involving an incision through the skin, a first-generation cephalosporin such as cefazolin (Kefzol) with activity against *Staphylococcus aureus* or *Streptococcus* species is commonly used.
7. a. *Rationale:* The amount and frequency of anti-infective and antimicrobial agents should be individualized according to characteristics of the causative organism, the chosen drug, and the patient's size and condition (e.g., type and severity of infection, ability to use and excrete the chosen drug).
8. presence
9. b. *Rationale:* Some infections that require relatively long-term IV antibiotic therapy include endocarditis, osteomyelitis, and some surgical-wound infections.
10. b, c, and d. *Rationale:* The role of the home care nurse includes teaching the patient and caregiver how to store and administer the medication, monitor the IV site, monitor the infection, manage problems, and report patient responses.

11. c. *Rationale:* General infection-control practices include frequent and thorough hand hygiene, use of gloves when indicated, and appropriate handling and disposal of body substances (e.g., blood, urine, feces, sputum, vomitus, wound drainage).

12. c. *Rationale:* Measurement of plasma drug levels and dosage adjustment are often necessary to accommodate the changing physiology of a critically ill patient. Drug levels are usually measured after four or five doses are given so that steady-state concentrations have been reached.

13. d. *Rationale:* Patients in critical care units are at high risk for acquiring nosocomial pneumonia because of the severity of their illness, duration of hospitalization, and antimicrobial drug therapy. The strongest predisposing factor is mechanical ventilation, which bypasses airway defenses against movement of microorganisms from the upper to the lower respiratory tract. Organisms often associated with nosocomial pneumonia are *Staphylococcus aureus* and gram-negative bacilli.

14. a. *Rationale:* Bacterial pneumonia is usually treated with a broad-spectrum antibiotic until culture and susceptibility reports become available.

15. a. *Rationale:* Selection of antibacterial drugs may be difficult because of frequent changes in antibiotic resistance patterns. Antibiotic rotation (i.e., switching preferred antibiotic or antibiotic classes used to treat infections, on a scheduled basis) has been successful in reducing rates of ventilator-associated pneumonia and mortality.

16. a, c, and d. *Rationale:* Antimicrobial therapy in patients with liver impairment is not well defined. Some drugs are metabolized by the liver (e.g., cefoperazone, chloramphenicol, clindamycin, erythromycin), and dosage must be reduced in patients with severe liver impairment. Some are associated with elevations of liver enzymes and/or hepatotoxicity (e.g., certain fluoroquinolones, tetracyclines, isoniazid, and rifampin). Laboratory monitoring may be helpful in high-risk populations.

17. c. *Rationale:* A laboratory value that indicates severe renal impairment is CrCl <15-30 mL/minute.

18. tetracyclines (except doxycycline) and flucytosine

19. b. *Rationale:* Dosing of antibiotics is important in patients with acute or chronic renal failure who are receiving hemodialysis or peritoneal dialysis. Some drugs are removed by dialysis, and an extra dose may be needed during or after dialysis.

20. Penicillins

Chapter 30: Beta-Lactam Antibacterials: Penicillins, Cephalosporins, and Other Drugs

SECTION II: ASSESSING YOUR UNDERSTANDING

ACTIVITY A
FILL IN THE BLANKS
1. penicillin
2. penicillins
3. cross-allergenicity
4. dicloxacillin, nafcillin, and oxacillin
5. carbenicillin (Geocillin), ticarcillin, and piperacillin

ACTIVITY B
MATCHING
1. D   2. A   3. B   4. C   5. E

ACTIVITY C
SHORT ANSWERS
1. Patients on hemodialysis usually require an additional dose of penicillin after treatment, because hemodialysis removes substantial amounts and produces subtherapeutic serum drug levels.

2. Amoxicillin-clavulanate (Augmentin) should be used with caution in patients with hepatic impairment. It is contraindicated in patients who have had cholestatic jaundice and hepatic dysfunction with previous use of the drug. Cholestatic liver impairment usually subsides when the drug is stopped. Hepatotoxicity is attributed to the clavulanate component and has also occurred with ticarcillin-clavulanate (Timentin).

3. Many beta-lactam antibiotics are given in the home setting. With oral agents, the role of the home care nurse is mainly to teach accurate administration and observation for therapeutic and adverse effects. With liquid suspensions for children, shaking to resuspend the medication and measuring with a measuring spoon or calibrated device are required for safe dosing. Household spoons should not be used, because they vary widely in capacity.

4. Metabolic and electrolyte imbalances may occur in patients receiving penicillins who have renal impairment or congestive heart failure. Hypernatremia and hypokalemic metabolic acidosis are most likely to occur with ticarcillin, and hyperkalemia with large IV doses of penicillin G potassium.

5. Beta-lactam antimicrobials are commonly used in critical care units to treat pneumonia, bloodstream infections, wound infections, and other infections.

SECTION III: APPLYING YOUR KNOWLEDGE

ACTIVITY D
CASE STUDIES
CASE STUDY 1
1. Central nervous system toxicity, including seizures, has been reported. Seizures are more likely in patients with a seizure disorder or when recommended doses are exceeded; however, they have occurred in other patients as well.

2. Lidocaine is mixed in preparation of the solution for IM injection to decrease pain with administration, and the same cautions should be used as with imipenem. Unlike imipenem and meropenem, ertapenem does not have in vitro activity against *Pseudomonas aeruginosa* or *Acinetobacter baumannii*. The drug would be discontinued.

CASE STUDY 2
1. "The physician orders aztreonam because it is effective against *P. aeruginosa,* which caused your infection." Aztreonam (Azactam) is active against gram-negative bacteria, including Enterobacteriaceae and *P. aeruginosa,* and many strains that are resistant to multiple antibiotics.

2. Activity of aztreonam against gram-negative bacteria is similar to that of the aminoglycosides, but the drug does not cause kidney damage or hearing loss.

SECTION IV: PRACTICING FOR NCLEX
1. a. *Rationale:* Probenecid (Benemid) blocks renal excretion of the penicillins and can be given concurrently with penicillins to increase serum drug levels.

2. c. *Rationale:* In the rare instance in which penicillin is considered essential, a skin test may be helpful in assessing hypersensitivity.

3. b. *Rationale:* As a class, penicillins usually are more effective in infections caused by gram-positive bacteria than those caused by gram-negative bacteria.

4. a and b. *Rationale:* Choice of a beta-lactam antibacterial depends on the organism causing the infection, the severity of the infection, and other factors.

5. a, b, and c. *Rationale:* Beta-lactam antibiotics include penicillins, cephalosporins, carbapenems, and monobactams.

6. c. *Rationale:* Beta-lactam antimicrobials are commonly used in critical care units to treat pneumonia, bloodstream infections, wound infections, and other infections. Renal, hepatic, and other organ functions should be monitored in critically ill patients, and drug dosages should be reduced when indicated.

7. d. *Rationale:* The beta-lactam drugs are frequently given concomitantly with other antimicrobial drugs because critically ill patients often have multiorganism or nosocomial infections.

8. d. *Rationale:* Aztreonam, imipenem, meropenem, and ertapenem may cause abnormalities in liver function test results (i.e., elevated alanine and aspartate aminotransferases [ALT and AST] and alkaline phosphatase), but hepatitis and jaundice rarely occur.

9. a. *Rationale:* For serious or life-threatening infections in patients on hemodialysis, give 12.5% of the initial dose after each hemodialysis session, in addition to maintenance doses.

10. b. *Rationale:* After an initial loading dose, the dosage of aztreonam should be reduced by 50% or more in patients with CrCl of 30 mL/minute or less. Give at the usual intervals of 6, 8, or 12 hours.

11. d. *Rationale:* Dosage of imipenem should be reduced in most patients with renal impairment, and the drug is contraindicated in patients with severe renal impairment (CrCl of 5 mL/minute or less) unless hemodialysis is started within 48 hours. For patients already on hemodialysis, the drug may cause seizures and should be used very cautiously, if at all.

12. c. *Rationale:* Penicillins and cephalosporins are widely used to treat infections in children and are generally safe. They should be used cautiously in neonates, because immature kidney function slows their elimination. Dosages should be based on age, weight, severity of the infection being treated, and renal function.

13. c. *Rationale:* Some cephalosporins are used in surgical prophylaxis. The particular drug depends largely on the type of organism likely to be encountered in the operative area. First-generation drugs, mainly cefazolin, are used for procedures associated with gram-positive postoperative infections, such as prosthetic implant surgery.

14. b. *Rationale:* Aminoglycosides are often given concomitantly with penicillins for serious infections, such as those caused by *Pseudomonas aeruginosa*. The drugs should not be admixed in a syringe or in an IV solution, because the penicillin inactivates the aminoglycoside.

15. penicillins

16. a, c, and d. *Rationale:* Because anaphylactic shock may occur with administration of the penicillins, especially by parenteral routes, emergency drugs and equipment must be readily available. Treatment may require parenteral epinephrine, oxygen, and insertion of an endotracheal or tracheostomy tube if laryngeal edema occurs.

17. Penicillin

18. penicillins

19. dehydropeptidase

20. a. *Rationale:* Imipenem is formulated with cilastatin, which inhibits the destruction of imipenem by the enzyme. The addition of cilastatin increases the urinary

concentration of imipenem and reduces the potential renal toxicity of the antibacterial agent. Recommended doses indicate the amount of imipenem; the solution contains an equivalent amount of cilastatin.

Chapter 31: Aminoglycosides and Fluoroquinolones

SECTION II: ASSESSING YOUR UNDERSTANDING

ACTIVITY A
FILL IN THE BLANKS
1. aminoglycosides
2. quinolones
3. fluoroquinolones
4. bactericidal
5. parenteral

ACTIVITY B
MATCHING
1. B   2. A   3. C   4. E   5. D

ACTIVITY C
SHORT ANSWERS
1. The fluoroquinolones are synthesized by adding a fluorine molecule to the quinolone structure. This addition increases drug activity against gram-negative microorganisms, broadens the antimicrobial spectrum to include several other microorganisms, and allows use of the drugs in treating systemic infections.

2. Aminoglycosides are bactericidal agents with similar pharmacologic, antimicrobial, and toxicologic characteristics. They are used to treat infections caused by gram-negative microorganisms such as *Pseudomonas* and *Proteus* species, *Escherichia coli*, and *Klebsiella, Enterobacter,* and *Serratia* species.

3. Aminoglycosides drugs are poorly absorbed from the gastrointestinal (GI) tract. When given orally, they exert local effects in the GI tract. They are well absorbed from intramuscular injection sites and reach peak effects in 30 to 90 minutes if circulatory status is good. After intravenous (IV) administration, peak effects occur within 30 to 60 minutes. Plasma half-life is 2 to 4 hours with normal renal function.

4. After parenteral administration, aminoglycosides are widely distributed in extracellular fluid and reach therapeutic levels in blood, urine, bone, inflamed joints, and pleural and ascitic fluids. They accumulate in high concentrations in the proximal renal tubules of the kidney leading to acute tubular necrosis. This damage to the kidney is termed *nephrotoxicity*. They also accumulate in high concentrations in the inner ear, damaging sensory cells in the cochlea (disrupting hearing) and the vestibular apparatus (disturbing balance). This damage to the inner ear is termed *ototoxicity*. They are poorly distributed to the central nervous system, intraocular fluids, and respiratory tract secretions.

5. Injected aminoglycosides are not metabolized; they are excreted unchanged in the urine, primarily by glomerular filtration. Oral aminoglycosides are excreted in feces.

SECTION III: APPLYING YOUR KNOWLEDGE

ACTIVITY D
CASE STUDIES
1. Infections involving the respiratory and genitourinary tracts, skin, wounds, bowel, and bloodstream are commonly due to gram-negative organisms, although gram-negative infections can occur anywhere. Any infection with gram-negative organisms may be serious and potentially life-threatening.

2. Radical surgery, such as in Ms. Bouchard's case, can lower a patient's resistance to infection. Nosocomial infections have become more common with control of other types of infections, widespread use of antimicrobial drugs, and diseases (e.g., acquired immunodeficiency syndrome [AIDS]) or treatments (e.g., radical surgery, therapy with antineoplastic or immunosuppressive drugs) that lower host resistance. Management is difficult, because the organisms are in general less susceptible to antibacterial drugs and drug-resistant strains develop rapidly.

3. The combination of an aminoglycoside and piperacillin has synergistic therapeutic effects. Management of nosocomial infection is difficult, because the organisms are in general less susceptible to antibacterial drugs and drug-resistant strains develop rapidly. In pseudomonal infections, an aminoglycoside is often given concurrently with an antipseudomonal penicillin (e.g., piperacillin). The penicillin-induced breakdown of the bacterial cell wall makes it easier for the aminoglycoside to reach its site of action inside the bacterial cell.

4. Decreased mortality has been demonstrated from combination antibiotic therapy in the treatment of infections due to *Pseudomonas aeruginosa* and other multidrug-resistant gram-negative bacilli. Routine use of combination antibiotic therapy containing an aminoglycoside has not been associated with decreased mortality in cases of other gram-negative infections.

SECTION IV: PRACTICING FOR NCLEX

1. a. *Rationale:* Fluoroquinolones are associated with hyperglycemia and hypoglycemia, and older patients may be more at risk for these glucose disturbances.

2. a and b. *Rationale:* Aminoglycosides reach higher concentrations in the kidneys and inner ears than in other body tissues; this is a major factor in nephrotoxicity and ototoxicity.

3. a. *Rationale:* Multiple-dose regimens (conventional dosing) of aminoglycosides must be carefully monitored with evaluation of peak and trough serum levels. Once-daily regimens are monitored with random level (12-hour) serum evaluation.

4. neomycin, kanamycin

5. aerobic

6. d. *Rationale:* The choice of aminoglycoside depends on local susceptibility patterns and specific organisms causing an infection.

7. b. *Rationale:* An increasing number of individuals with CAP are being treated at home for a number of reasons, including increased availability and cost considerations of oral antibiotics. Oral drugs have demonstrated effectiveness and are the preferred route for individuals and family members, but management with oral drugs has widely varied. The American College of Chest Physicians' position statement, cosponsored by the American Academy of Home Care Physicians, outlines recommendations for home care for patients with CAP and follow-up. Recommendations in the position statement take into consideration the best plan of care incorporating the best available evidence with clinician judgment and patient preferences.

8. c. *Rationale:* Fluoroquinolones are associated with hyperglycemia and hypoglycemia. Older patients may be more at risk for these glucose disturbances. Severe hypoglycemia has occurred in patients receiving concomitant glyburide and fluoroquinolones.

9. c. *Rationale:* Gatifloxacin has been associated with hypoglycemic and hyperglycemic events more commonly than other fluoroquinolones. The explanation for an increased association with gatifloxacin is not currently known.

10. d. *Rationale:* Fluoroquinolones are usually infused IV in critically ill patients. However, administration orally or by GI tube (e.g., nasogastric, gastrostomy, jejunostomy) may be feasible in some patients. Concomitant administration of antacids or enteral feedings decreases absorption.

11. b. *Rationale:* Because critically ill patients are at high risk for development of nephrotoxicity and ototoxicity with aminoglycosides, guidelines for safe drug use should be strictly followed. Renal function should be monitored to assess for needed dosage reductions in patients with renal dysfunction receiving who are aminoglycosides or fluoroquinolones. Because fluoroquinolones may be hepatotoxic, hepatic function should be monitored during therapy.

12. critically ill

13. trovafloxacin

14. c. *Rationale:* With aminoglycosides, hepatic impairment is not a significant factor, because the drugs are excreted through the kidneys.

15. b, c, and d. *Rationale:* With fluoroquinolones, reported renal effects include azotemia, crystalluria, hematuria, interstitial nephritis, nephropathy, and renal failure.

16. nephrotoxic

17. a. *Rationale:* Aminoglycosides must be used cautiously in children as with adults. Dosage must be accurately calculated according to weight and renal function.

18. b. *Rationale:* Guidelines to decrease the incidence and severity of adverse effects when administering aminoglycosides include the following: Keep patients well hydrated to decrease drug concentration in serum and body tissues.

19. reduced

20. Maintenance

Chapter 32: Tetracyclines, Sulfonamides, and Urinary Agents

SECTION II: ASSESSING YOUR UNDERSTANDING

ACTIVITY A
FILL IN THE BLANKS
1. antiseptics
2. renal tubules
3. passive
4. renal failure
5. time

ACTIVITY B
MATCHING
1. A   2. C   3. D   4. B   5. E

ACTIVITY C
SHORT ANSWERS
1. The tetracyclines are similar in pharmacologic properties and antimicrobial activity. They are effective against a wide range of gram-positive and gram-negative organisms, although they are usually not drugs of choice. Bacterial infections caused by *Brucella* or by *Vibrio cholerae* are still treated with tetracyclines. The drugs also remain effective against rickettsiae, chlamydiae, some protozoans, spirochetes, and others. Doxycycline (Vibramycin) is one of the drugs of choice for *Bacillus anthracis* (anthrax) and *Chlamydia trachomatis,* and it is used in respiratory tract infections caused by *Mycoplasma pneumoniae.*

2. Tetracyclines are widely distributed into most body tissues and fluids. The older tetracyclines are excreted mainly in urine; doxycycline is eliminated in urine and feces; and minocycline is eliminated mainly by the liver.

3. Sulfonamides may be active against *Streptococcus pyogenes*, some staphylococcal strains, *Haemophilus influenzae, Nocardia, Chlamydia trachomatis,* and toxoplasmosis.

4. Tetracyclines penetrate microbial cells by passive diffusion and via an active transport system. Inside the cell, they bind to 30S ribosomes, like the aminoglycosides, and inhibit microbial protein synthesis. Sulfonamides act as antimetabolites of para-aminobenzoic acid (PABA); microorganisms require PABA to produce folic acid, which they need for the production of bacterial intracellular proteins. Sulfonamides enter into the reaction instead of PABA, compete for the enzyme involved, and cause formation of nonfunctional derivatives of folic acid.

5. Sulfonamides are commonly used to treat UTIs (e.g., acute and chronic cystitis, asymptomatic bacteriuria) caused by *Escherichia coli* and *Proteus* or *Klebsiella* organisms. In acute pyelonephritis, other agents are preferred.

SECTION III: APPLYING YOUR KNOWLEDGE

ACTIVITY D
CASE STUDIES

1. If a urinary tract infection is suspected, it is necessary to obtain urine culture and susceptibility tests before prescription of medication because of wide variability in possible pathogens and their susceptibility to antibacterial drugs. The best results are obtained with drug therapy indicated by the microorganisms isolated from each patient.

2. With systemically absorbed sulfonamides, an initial loading dose may be given, which is usually twice the maintenance dose. The purpose is to achieve therapeutic blood levels more rapidly.

3. Urine pH is important in drug therapy with sulfonamides and urinary antiseptics. With sulfonamide therapy, alkaline urine increases drug solubility and helps prevent crystalluria. It also increases the rate of sulfonamide excretion and the concentration of sulfonamide in the urine. The urine can be alkalinized by giving sodium bicarbonate. Alkalinization is not needed with sulfisoxazole (because the drug is highly soluble) or with sulfonamides used to treat intestinal infections or burn wounds (because there is little systemic absorption).

SECTION IV: PRACTICING FOR NCLEX

1. a. *Rationale:* Urinary antiseptics may be bactericidal for sensitive organisms in the urinary tract because these drugs are concentrated in renal tubules and reach high levels in urine.

2. b. *Rationale:* Urinary antiseptics are not used in systemic infections because they do not attain therapeutic plasma levels.

3. a. *Rationale:* Sulfasalazine (Azulfidine) is contraindicated in people who are allergic to salicylates.

4. d. *Rationale:* Sulfonamides are bacteriostatic against a wide range of gram-positive and gram-negative bacteria, although increasing resistance is making them less useful.

5. c. *Rationale:* The tetracyclines are effective against a wide range of gram-positive and gram-negative organisms, although they are usually not drugs of choice.

6. d. *Rationale:* Sulfonamides are rarely used in critical care settings, except that topical silver sulfadiazine (Silvadene) is used to treat burn wounds.

7. a. *Rationale:* Trimethoprim-sulfamethoxazole used to treat *Pneumocystis jiroveci* pneumonia.

8. a, b, and d. *Rationale:* Tetracyclines may be used to treat sepsis caused by rickettsial, chlamydial, or mycoplasma infection and pulmonary infection caused by *M. pneumoniae* or *Legionella pneumophila.*

9. a and d. *Rationale:* Tetracyclines are generally contraindicated in pregnant women because they may cause fatal hepatic necrosis in the mother (as well as interfere with bone and tooth development in the fetus).

10. a. *Rationale:* Because tetracyclines are metabolized in the liver, hepatic impairment or biliary obstruction slows drug elimination.

11. b. *Rationale:* In patients with renal impairment, high IV doses of tetracycline (>2 g/day) have been associated with death from liver failure.

12. cholestatic

13. 2 liters

14. a and b. *Rationale:* With the combination of trimethoprim-sulfamethoxazole, older adults are at increased risk for severe adverse effects. Severe skin reactions and bone marrow depression are most often reported. Folic acid deficiency may also occur, because both of the drugs interfere with folic acid metabolism.

15. inhibit

16. a. *Rationale:* Tetracyclines should not be used in children younger than 8 years of age because of their effects on teeth and bones.

17. a and d. *Rationale:* If a fetus or young infant receives a sulfonamide by placental transfer, in breast milk, or by direct administration, the drug displaces bilirubin from binding sites on albumin. As a result, bilirubin may accumulate in the bloodstream (hyperbilirubinemia) and in the central nervous system (kernicterus) and may cause life-threatening toxicity.

18. crystalluria

19. c. *Rationale:* Sulfonamides are often used to treat UTI in children older than 2 months of age.

20. b and d. *Rationale:* Tetracyclines must be used cautiously in the presence of liver or kidney impairment.

Chapter 33: Macrolides and Miscellaneous Antibacterials

SECTION II: ASSESSING YOUR UNDERSTANDING

ACTIVITY A
FILL IN THE BLANKS

1. bacteriostatic
2. human immunodeficiency virus
3. azithromycin
4. liver
5. ribosomes

ACTIVITY B
MATCHING

1. C 2. A 3. B 4. E 5. D

ACTIVITY C
SHORT ANSWERS

1. Erythromycin is metabolized in the liver and excreted mainly in bile; approximately 20% is excreted in urine. Depending on the specific salt formulation used, food can have a variable effect on the absorption of oral erythromycin.

2. The macrolides and ketolides enter microbial cells and reversibly bind to the 50S subunits of ribosomes, thereby inhibiting microbial protein synthesis. Ketolides have a greater affinity for ribosomal RNA, expanding their antimicrobial spectrum compared to macrolides.

3. Macrolides and ketolides are contraindicated in people who have had hypersensitivity reactions. Telithromycin is contraindicated in people who have had hypersensitivity reactions to macrolides. All macrolides and telithromycin must be used with caution in patients with preexisting liver disease. A black box warning for erythromycin estolate and an FDA alert for telithromycin emphasize the liver toxicity associated with these drugs. Use of erythromycin and telithromycin concurrently with drugs highly dependent on CYP3A4 liver enzymes for metabolism (e.g., pimozide) is contraindicated. The FDA has issued a black box warning alerting health care professionals that telithromycin is contraindicated in patients with myasthenia gravis due to the potential for life-threatening or fatal respiratory failure.

4. Clinical indications for use of metronidazole include prevention or treatment of anaerobic bacterial infections (e.g., in colorectal surgery, intra-abdominal infections) and treatment of *Clostridium difficile* infections associated with pseudomembranous colitis. As part of a combination regimen, it is also useful in the treatment of infections due to *Helicobacter pylori*. It is contraindicated during the first trimester of pregnancy and must be used with caution in patients with CNS or blood disorders.

5. Quinupristin-dalfopristin is a strong inhibitor of cytochrome P450 3A4 enzymes and therefore interferes with the metabolism of drugs such as cyclosporine, antiretrovirals, carbamazepine, and many others. Toxicity may occur with the inhibited drugs.

SECTION III: APPLYING YOUR KNOWLEDGE

ACTIVITY D
CASE STUDIES

1. Vancomycin (Vancocin) is active only against gram-positive microorganisms. It acts by inhibiting cell wall synthesis.

2. Oral vancomycin is used only to treat staphylococcal enterocolitis and pseudomembranous colitis caused by *C. difficile*. In initial treatment for *C. difficile* colitis, metronidazole is preferred.

3. Partly because of the widespread use of vancomycin, vancomycin-resistant enterococci (VRE) are being encountered more often, especially in critical care units, and treatment options for infections caused by these organisms are limited. To decrease the spread of VRE, the Centers for Disease Control and Prevention (CDC) recommend limiting the use of vancomycin.

4. "Red man syndrome" is an adverse reaction characterized by hypotension, flushing, and skin rash. It is caused by giving an IV infusion too quickly and is attributed to histamine release. It is very important to give IV infusions slowly, over 1 to 2 hours, to avoid this reaction.

5. Vancomycin is excreted through the kidneys; dosage should be reduced in the presence of renal impairment.

SECTION IV: PRACTICING FOR NCLEX

1. d. *Rationale:* Metronidazole is effective against infections with anaerobic bacteria and some protozoa.

2. a. *Rationale:* Spectinomycin is an alternative treatment for gonococcal infection when patients are unable to comply with the preferred regimen.

3. b. *Rationale:* Rifaximin is prescribed for travelers' diarrhea caused by *Escherichia coli* infection.

4. positive

5. c. *Rationale:* Quinupristin-dalfopristin belongs to the streptogramin class of antibiotics. It is indicated for VREF and MSSA.

6. c. *Rationale:* Tigecycline belongs to the glycylcline class of antibiotics. It is similar to tetracycline in structure and properties and can be used to treat skin infections caused by MRSA.

7. a. *Rationale:* Daptomycin belongs to the lipopeptide class of antibiotics that kills gram-positive bacteria by inhibiting synthesis of bacterial proteins, DNA and RNA.

8. d. *Rationale:* Clindamycin belongs to the lincosamide class of antimicrobials, similar to macrolides in its mechanism of action and antimicrobial spectrum. A life-threatening adverse effect of clindamycin is the development of pseudomembranous colitis.

9. b. *Rationale:* Chloramphenicol (Chloromycetin) is rarely used due to the possible development of serious and fatal blood dyscrasias with its use. It is effective against some strains of VRE.

10. a. *Rationale:* Telithromycin is contraindicated in patients with myasthenia gravis because of the potential for life-threatening or fatal respiratory failure.

11. liver

12. d. *Rationale:* The ketolide, telithromycin, is approved only for community-acquired pneumonia. Its mechanism of action is inhibition of microbial protein synthesis.

13. b. *Rationale:* Erythromycin shares a similar antibacterial spectrum with penicillin, making it a good choice for patients with penicillin allergy.

14. d. *Rationale:* For acute bacterial sinusitis, azithromycin is approved for an abbreviated 3-day treatment duration.

15. b. *Rationale:* With the drug linezolid, myelosuppression (anemia, leukopenia, pancytopenia, and thrombocytopenia) is a serious adverse effect that may occur with prolonged therapy lasting longer than 2 weeks. The patient's complete blood count should be monitored; if myelosuppression occurs, linezolid should be discontinued. Myelosuppression usually improves with drug discontinuation.

16. a. *Rationale:* Patients receiving linezolid and selective serotonin reuptake inhibitors (SSRIs) may be at risk for serotonin syndrome, which is characterized by fever and cognitive dysfunction.

17. a, c, and d. *Rationale:* Because linezolid is a weak monoamine oxidase (MAO) inhibitor, patients should avoid foods high in tyramine content (aged cheeses, fermented or air-dried meats, sauerkraut, soy sauce, tap beers, red wine) while taking the drug.

18. a. *Rationale:* Erythromycin is generally considered safe. Because it is metabolized in the liver and excreted in bile, it may be an alternative in patients with impaired renal function.

19. increase

20. slow

Chapter 34: Drugs for Tuberculosis and *Mycobacterium avium* Complex (MAC) Disease

SECTION II: ASSESSING YOUR UNDERSTANDING

ACTIVITY A
FILL IN THE BLANKS

1. kidneys
2. *Mycobacterium tuberculosis*
3. phagocytosis
4. antitubercular
5. one-third

ACTIVITY B
MATCHING
1. D 2. A 3. B 4. E 5. C

ACTIVITY C
SHORT ANSWERS
1. Transmission of tuberculosis occurs when an uninfected person inhales infected airborne particles that are exhaled by an infected person. Major factors affecting transmission are the number of bacteria expelled by the infected person and the closeness and duration of the contact between the infected and the uninfected person.
2. It is estimated that 30% of persons exposed to tuberculosis bacilli become infected and develop a mild, pneumonia-like illness that is often undiagnosed; this is the *primary infection*. About 6 to 8 weeks after exposure, those infected have positive reactions to tuberculin skin tests. Within approximately 6 months after exposure, spontaneous healing occurs as the bacilli are encapsulated into calcified tubercles.
3. The immune system is able to stop bacterial growth in most people who become infected with TB bacteria. The bacteria become inactive, although they remain alive in the body and can become active later. People with inactive or latent TB infection have no symptoms, do not feel sick, do not spread TB to others, usually have a positive skin-test reaction, and can develop active TB disease years later if the latent infection is not effectively treated. In many people with LTBI, the infection remains inactive throughout their lives. In others, the TB bacteria become active and cause tuberculosis, usually when the person's immune system becomes weak as a result of disease, immunosuppressive drugs, or aging.
4. Active tuberculosis has long been thought to result almost exclusively from reactivation of latent infection, with only a few cases from new primary infections. However, more recent studies indicate that almost half of new TB cases may result from new infections or reinfections from exogenous sources.
5. Signs and symptoms of active disease (e.g., cough that is persistent and often productive of sputum, chest pain, chills, fever, hemoptysis, night sweats, weight loss, weakness, lack of appetite, positive skin test, abnormal chest radiograph, positive sputum smear or culture) are estimated to develop in 5% of people with LTBI within 2 years and in another 5% after 2 years.

SECTION III: APPLYING YOUR KNOWLEDGE

ACTIVITY D
CASE STUDIES
1. "The resistant bacteria may always have been present in your system." In addition to LTBI, a major concern among public health and infectious-disease authorities is an increase in drug-resistant infections. Drug-resistant mutants of *M. tuberculosis* microorganisms are present in any infected person. When infected people receive antitubercular drugs, drug-resistant mutants are not killed or weakened by the drugs. Instead, they are able to reproduce in the presence of the drugs and to transmit the property of drug resistance to newly produced bacteria. Eventually, the majority of TB bacilli in the body are drug resistant.
2. Once a drug-resistant strain of TB develops, it can be transmitted to other people just like a drug-susceptible strain.
3. Multidrug-resistant tuberculosis (MDR-TB) organisms are resistant to isoniazid (INH) and rifampin, the most effective drugs available. They may or may not be resistant to other

antitubercular drugs. Factors contributing to the development of drug-resistant disease, whether acquired or new infection, include delayed diagnosis and delayed determination of drug susceptibility, which may take several weeks.
4. Delay in effective treatment allows rapid disease progression and rapid transmission to others, especially to those with impaired immune systems.

SECTION IV: PRACTICING FOR NCLEX
1. c. *Rationale:* In drug-resistant TB, there is no standardized treatment regimen; treatment must be individualized for each patient according to drug susceptibility reports.
2. rifampin
3. c. *Rationale:* INH is the treatment of choice for LTBI.
4. b. *Rationale:* Directly observed therapy (DOT) is recommended to prevent inadequate drug therapy and the development of drug-resistant TB organisms.
5. extensively drug-resistant
6. d. *Rationale:* TB is a worldwide problem. Although TB is not as extensive in the United States as in many other countries, the public health infrastructure for diagnosing and treating TB needs to be maintained.
7. a, b, and d. *Rationale:* With individual patients receiving antitubercular drugs for latent or active infection, the home care nurse needs to assist the patient in taking the drugs as directed. Specific interventions vary widely and may include administering the drugs (DOT); teaching about the importance of taking the drugs and the possible consequences of not taking them (i.e., more severe disease, longer treatment regimens with more toxic drugs, spreading the disease to others); monitoring for adverse drug effects and assisting the patient to manage them or reporting them to the drug prescriber; and assisting the patient in obtaining the drugs and keeping follow-up appointments for blood tests and chest radiographs.
8. a, b, and d. *Rationale:* In relation to community needs, the nurse needs to be active in identifying cases, investigating contacts of newly diagnosed cases, and promoting efforts to manage tuberculosis effectively.
9. a. *Rationale:* For patients at risk of developing hepatotoxicity, serum ALT and AST should be measured before starting and periodically during drug therapy. If hepatitis occurs, these enzyme levels usually increase before other signs and symptoms develop.
10. b. *Rationale:* Rifampin is mainly eliminated by the liver. However, up to 30% of a dose is excreted by the kidneys, and dose reduction may be needed in patients with renal impairment.
11. c. *Rationale:* Although INH is the drug of choice for treatment of LTBI, its use is controversial in older adults. Because risks of drug-induced hepatotoxicity are higher in this population, some clinicians believe that those patients with positive skin tests should have additional risk factors (e.g., recent skin-test conversion, immunosuppression, previous gastrectomy) before receiving INH.
12. b. *Rationale:* For treatment of LTBI, only one of the four regimens currently recommended for adults (INH for 9 months) is recommended for those younger than 18 years of age.
13. a. *Rationale:* A major difficulty with treatment of TB in patients with HIV infection is that rifampin interacts with many PIs and NNRTIs. If the drugs are given concurrently, rifampin decreases blood levels and therapeutic effects of the anti-HIV drugs.

14. b. *Rationale:* Treatment of active TB disease in HIV-positive patients is similar to that in persons who do not have HIV infection. Those with HIV infection who adhere to standard treatment regimens do not have an increased risk of treatment failure.

15. d. *Rationale:* Pyrazinamide may decrease effects of allopurinol and cyclosporine.

16. c. *Rationale:* The rifamycins (rifampin, rifabutin, rifapentine) induce cytochrome P450 drug-metabolizing enzymes and therefore accelerate the metabolism and decrease the effectiveness of many drugs. Rifampin is the strongest inducer and may decrease the effects of angiotensin-converting enzyme (ACE) inhibitors, anticoagulants, antidysrhythmics, some antifungals (e.g., fluconazole), anti-HIV protease inhibitors (e.g., amprenavir, indinavir), anti-HIV NNRTIs (e.g., efavirenz, nevirapine), benzodiazepines, beta-blockers, corticosteroids, cyclosporine, digoxin, and diltiazem, as well as estrogens and oral contraceptives.

17. a. *Rationale:* Isoniazid (INH) increases risks of toxicity with several drugs by inhibiting their metabolism and increasing their blood levels. These drugs include carbamazepine, fluconazole, haloperidol, phenytoin (effects of rifampin are opposite to those of INH and tend to predominate if both drugs are given with phenytoin), and vincristine.

18. laboratory

19. c. *Rationale:* Individualizing treatment regimens is used, when possible, to increase patient convenience and minimize disruption of usual activities of daily living. Short-course regimens, intermittent dosing (e.g., 2 or 3 times weekly rather than daily), and fixed-dose combinations of drugs (e.g., Rifater, Rifamate) reduce the number of pills and the duration of therapy.

20. 6 to 8

Chapter 35: Antiviral Drugs

SECTION II: ASSESSING YOUR UNDERSTANDING

ACTIVITY A
FILL IN THE BLANKS
1. pneumonia
2. breaks
3. intracellular
4. numbers
5. human immunodeficiency virus (HIV)

ACTIVITY B
MATCHING
1. E   2. C   3. A   4. B   5. D

ACTIVITY C
SHORT ANSWERS
1. Inside host cells, viruses use cellular metabolic activities for their own survival and replication. Viral replication involves dissolution of the protein coating and exposure of the genetic material—deoxyribonucleic acid (DNA) or ribonucleic acid (RNA). With DNA viruses, the viral DNA enters the host cell's nucleus, where it becomes incorporated into the host cell's chromosomal DNA. Then, host cell genes are coded to produce new viruses. In addition, the viral DNA incorporated with host DNA is transmitted to the host's daughter cells during host cell mitosis and becomes part of the inherited genetic information of the host cell and its progeny. With RNA viruses (e.g., HIV), viral RNA must be converted to DNA by an enzyme called reverse transcriptase before replication can occur.

2. After new viruses are formed, they are released from the infected cell either by budding out and breaking off from the cell membrane (leaving the host cell intact) or by causing lysis of the cell. When the cell is destroyed, the viruses are released into the blood and surrounding tissues, from which they can transmit the viral infection to other host cells.

3. Symptoms usually associated with acute viral infections include fever, headache, cough, malaise, muscle pain, nausea and vomiting, diarrhea, insomnia, and photophobia. White blood cell counts usually remain normal. Other signs and symptoms vary with the type of virus and body organs involved.

4. Some viruses (e.g., herpesviruses) can survive in host cells for many years and cause a chronic, latent infection that periodically becomes reactivated.

5. Antibodies are proteins that defend against microbial or viral invasion. They are very specific (i.e., an antibody protects only against a specific virus or other antigen). The protein coat of the virus allows the immune system of the host to recognize the virus as a "foreign invader" and to produce antibodies against it. Antibodies against infecting viruses can prevent the viruses from reaching the bloodstream or, if they are already in the bloodstream, prevent their invasion of host cells. After the virus has penetrated the cell, it is protected from antibody action, and the host depends on cell-mediated immunity (lymphocytes and macrophages) to eradicate the virus along with the cell harboring it.

SECTION III: APPLYING YOUR KNOWLEDGE
ACTIVITY D
CASE STUDIES
1. Acyclovir, famciclovir, and valacyclovir penetrate virus-infected cells, become activated by an enzyme, and inhibit viral DNA reproduction. Acyclovir is used to treat genital herpes; it decreases viral shedding and the duration of skin lesions and pain. It does not eliminate inactive virus in the body and therefore does not prevent recurrence of the disease unless oral drug therapy is continued. Prolonged or repeated courses of acyclovir therapy may result in the emergence of acyclovir-resistant viral strains, especially in immunocompromised patients.

2. The disease will reoccur. Acyclovir does not prevent recurrence of the disease unless oral drug therapy is continued.

3. Acyclovir does not eliminate inactive virus in the body and therefore does not prevent recurrence of the disease unless oral drug therapy is continued.

4. Acyclovir may be given orally, intravenously (IV), or applied topically to lesions.

SECTION IV: PRACTICING FOR NCLEX
1. a. *Rationale:* Antiretroviral drugs are given in combination to increase effectiveness and decrease emergence of drug-resistant viruses.
2. a. *Rationale:* Because viruses are intracellular parasites, antiviral drugs are relatively toxic to human cells.
3. b, c, and d. *Rationale:* Viral infections for which drug therapy is available include genital herpes, hepatitis B and C, HIV infection, and influenza.
4. b. *Rationale:* Vaccinations, avoiding contact with people who have viral infections, and thorough hand hygiene are effective ways to prevent viral infections.
5. c. *Rationale:* Viral infections commonly occur in all age groups.

6. b, c, and d. *Rationale:* Home care of patients with HIV infection may include teaching patients and caregivers about the disease and its treatment, assisting with drug therapy for HIV or opportunistic infections, coordinating medical and social services, managing symptoms of infection or adverse drug effects, and preventing or minimizing opportunistic infections.

7. c. *Rationale:* When antiviral agents are prescribed, all patients with hepatic impairment should be monitored closely for abnormal liver function tests (LFTs) and drug-related toxicity.

8. a. *Rationale:* Nevirapine may cause abnormal LFTs, and a few cases of fatal hepatitis have been reported. If moderate or severe LFT abnormalities occur, nevirapine administration should be discontinued until LFTs return to baseline. If liver dysfunction recurs when the drug is resumed, nevirapine should be discontinued permanently.

9. d. *Rationale:* Zidovudine is eliminated slowly and has a longer half-life in patients with moderate to severe liver disease. Therefore, daily doses should be reduced by 50% in patients with hepatic impairment.

10. c. *Rationale:* Amantadine, emtricitabine, entecavir, famciclovir, ganciclovir, lamivudine, telbivudine, and valacyclovir are eliminated mainly through the kidneys. In patients with renal impairment, they may accumulate, produce higher blood levels, have longer half-lives, and cause toxicity. For all of these drugs except famciclovir and emtricitabine, dosage should be reduced with creatinine clearance (CrCl) rates lower than 50 mL/minute.

11. c. *Rationale:* Foscarnet may cause or worsen renal impairment and should be used with caution in all patients. Manifestations of renal impairment are most likely to occur during the second week of induction therapy, but they may occur any time during treatment.

12. a. *Rationale:* When foscarnet is administered, renal impairment may be minimized by monitoring renal function (e.g., at baseline; two or three times weekly during induction; at least every 1 or 2 weeks during maintenance therapy) and reducing dosage accordingly. The drug should be stopped if creatinine clearance drops to less than 0.4 mL/minute/kg. Adequate hydration should also be maintained throughout the course of drug therapy.

13. c. *Rationale:* Indinavir may cause nephrolithiasis, flank pain, and hematuria. Symptoms usually subside with increased hydration and drug discontinuation. To avoid nephrolithiasis, patients taking indinavir should consume 48 to 64 ounces of water or other fluid daily.

14. b. *Rationale:* When amantadine is given to prevent or treat influenza A, dosage should be reduced with renal impairment, and older adults should be closely monitored for CNS effects (e.g., hallucinations, depression, confusion) and cardiovascular effects (e.g., congestive heart failure, orthostatic hypotension).

15. b. *Rationale:* Oseltamivir may be used in children 1 year of age and older. However, some serious adverse effects have been reported in children 16 years and younger who were taking oseltamivir. The adverse effects include neurologic and psychiatric problems (e.g., delirium, hallucinations, confusion, abnormal behavior, seizures, encephalitis) and a few severe skin reactions.

16. d. *Rationale:* HIV-seropositive pregnant women should receive zidovudine to prevent perinatal transmission. At 14 to 34 weeks of gestation, zidovudine should be administered at a dose of 100 mg PO five times a day until delivery.

17. c. *Rationale:* Viral load is a measure of the number of HIV RNA particles within the blood; it does not measure viral levels in tissues, where viral reproduction may be continuing.

18. 3

19. a. *Rationale:* Viral vaccines are used to control epidemics of viral disease in a community or to produce active immunity in patients who have not yet been exposed.

20. b and d. *Rationale:* With sexually transmitted viral infections such as genital herpes, transmission can be prevented by avoiding sex when skin lesions are present and by using condoms.

Chapter 36: Antifungal Drugs

SECTION II: ASSESSING YOUR UNDERSTANDING
ACTIVITY A
FILL IN THE BLANKS
1. Fungi
2. multicellular
3. dermatophytes
4. Dimorphic
5. coccidioidomycosis

ACTIVITY B
MATCHING
1. C   2. A   3. D   4. B   5. E

ACTIVITY C
SHORT ANSWERS
1. *Candida albicans* organisms are part of the normal microbial flora of the skin, mouth, gastrointestinal tract, and vagina. Growth of *Candida* organisms is normally restrained by intact immune mechanisms and bacterial competition for nutrients.
2. When the body's natural restraining forces are altered, such as by suppression of the immune system or antibacterial drug therapy, fungal overgrowth and opportunistic infection can occur.
3. *Aspergillus* organisms produce protease, an enzyme that allows them to destroy structural proteins and penetrate body tissues.
4. *Cryptococcus neoformans* organisms can become encapsulated, which allows them to evade the normal immune defense mechanism of phagocytosis.

SECTION III: APPLYING YOUR KNOWLEDGE
ACTIVITY D
CASE STUDIES
1. Amphotericin B is active against most types of pathogenic fungi and is fungicidal or fungistatic, depending on the concentration in body fluids and the susceptibility of the causative fungus. Because of its toxicity, the drug is used only for serious fungal infections. It is usually given for 4 to 12 weeks.
2. Lipid formulations of amphotericin B (Abelcet, AmBisome, and Amphotec) reach higher concentrations in diseased tissues than in normal tissues, so that larger doses can be given to increase therapeutic effects. At the same time, they cause less damage to normal tissues and decrease adverse effects. These products are much more expensive than the deoxycholate formulation (Fungizone). They are most likely to be used for patients with preexisting renal impairment or conditions in which other nephrotoxic drugs are routinely given (e.g., bone marrow transplantation) and when high doses are needed for difficult-to-treat infections.

3. "The formulations cannot be interchanged." The lipid preparations differ in their characteristics and cannot be used interchangeably.
4. Amphotericin B drug concentrations in most body fluids are higher in the presence of inflammation. Amphotericin B must be given intravenously for systemic infections. After infusion, the drug is rapidly taken up by the liver and other organs. It is then slowly released back into the bloodstream. Despite its long-term use, little is known about its distribution and metabolic pathways.
5. Nephrotoxicity is the most common and the most serious long-term adverse effect of amphotericin B use. The drug constricts afferent renal arterioles and reduces blood flow to the kidneys. Several strategies may decrease nephrotoxicity, such as keeping the patient well hydrated, giving 0.9% sodium chloride IV prior to drug administration, and avoiding the concomitant administration of other nephrotoxic drugs (e.g., aminoglycoside antibiotics).
6. Peripheral lines can become phlebitic. Hypokalemia and hypomagnesemia also occur and may require oral or IV mineral replacement. Additional adverse effects include anorexia, nausea, vomiting, anemia, and phlebitis at peripheral infusion sites. A central vein is preferred for administration.

SECTION IV: PRACTICING FOR NCLEX

1. d. *Rationale:* Liver function should be monitored with all systemic antifungal drugs; both hepatic and renal function should be monitored with amphotericin B.
2. a. *Rationale:* Systemic antifungal drugs may cause serious adverse effects. Nephrotoxicity is associated with amphotericin B; hepatotoxicity is associated with azole drugs.
3. c. *Rationale:* Fungal infections often require long-term drug therapy.
4. d. *Rationale:* Patients whose immune systems are suppressed are at high risk of serious fungal infections.
5. non-*albicans*
6. a, c, and d. *Rationale:* With IV antifungal drugs for serious infections, the home care nurse may need to assist in managing the environment, administering the drug, and monitoring for adverse effects.
7. b. *Rationale:* Because the immune function of these patients is often severely suppressed, protective interventions are needed. These may include teaching about frequent and thorough hand hygiene by patients, all members of the household, and visitors; safe food preparation and storage; removal of potted plants and fresh flowers; and avoiding activities that generate dust in the patient's environment. In addition, air conditioning and air filtering systems should be kept meticulously clean, and any plans for renovations should be postponed or canceled.
8. a. *Rationale:* When itraconazole is used in critically ill patients, a loading dose of 200 mg three times daily may be given for the first 3 days.
9. c. *Rationale:* Amphotericin B penetrates tissues well, except for CSF, and only small amounts are excreted in urine. With prolonged administration, the half-life increases from 1 to 15 days. Hemodialysis does not remove the drug.
10. b. *Rationale:* Amphotericin B penetrates tissues well, except for CSF, and only small amounts are excreted in urine. Fluconazole penetrates tissues well, including CSF.
11. d. *Rationale:* The azole antifungals are relatively contraindicated in patients with increased liver enzymes, active liver disease, or a history of liver damage from other drugs. They should be given only if expected benefits outweigh risks of liver injury.
12. *Aspergillus*
13. a and b. *Rationale:* With the impaired renal and cardiovascular functions that usually accompany aging, older adults are especially vulnerable to serious adverse effects. They must be monitored closely to reduce the incidence and severity of nephrotoxicity, hypokalemia, and other adverse drug reactions.
14. a, c, and d. *Rationale:* Terbinafine is a strong inhibitor of cytochrome P450 2D6 enzymes and may increase the effects of propafenone, metoprolol, desipramine, and nortriptyline.
15. c. *Rationale:* There are several recommendations for reducing toxicity of IV amphotericin B, but most have not been tested in controlled studies. The treatment to decrease fever and chills includes premedication with acetaminophen, diphenhydramine, and a corticosteroid.
16. a, b, and d. *Rationale:* There are several recommendations for reducing toxicity of IV amphotericin B, but most have not been tested in controlled studies. Recommendations to decrease phlebitis at injection sites include administering on alternate days, adding 500 to 2000 units of heparin to the infusion, rotating infusion sites, administering through a central vein, removing the needle after infusion, and using a pediatric scalp vein needle.
17. a. *Rationale:* Maintenance doses of Fungizone may be doubled and infused on alternate days. However, a single daily dose of Fungizone should not exceed 1.5 mg/kg; overdoses can result in cardiorespiratory arrest.
18. d. *Rationale:* Itraconazole, for 3 to 6 months, is the drug of choice for localized lymphocutaneous infection.
19. a. *Rationale:* Use of antihistamines is a predisposing factor for fungal infections. In addition, some candidal infections respond to the removal of predisposing factors such as antibacterial drugs, corticosteroids or other immunosuppressant drugs, and indwelling IV or bladder catheters.
20. Terbinafine (Lamisil)

Chapter 37: Antiparasitics

SECTION II: ASSESSING YOUR UNDERSTANDING

ACTIVITY A
FILL IN THE BLANKS
1. parasite
2. *Entamoeba histolytica*
3. amebic cysts
4. Trophozoites
5. enzyme

ACTIVITY B
MATCHING
1. D   2. A   3. B   4. E   5. C

ACTIVITY C
SHORT ANSWERS
1. Amebiasis is a common disease in Africa, Asia, and Latin America, but it can occur in any geographic region. In the United States, it is most likely to occur among residents of institutions for the mentally challenged; among men who have sex with men; and among residents or travelers in countries with poor sanitation.

2. Toxoplasmosis is caused by *Toxoplasma gondii*, a parasite that is spread by ingestion of undercooked meat or other food containing encysted forms of the organism; by contact with feces from infected cats; and by congenital spread from mothers with acute infection.

3. The most common form of trichomoniasis is a vaginal infection caused by *Trichomonas vaginalis*. The disease is usually spread by sexual intercourse.

4. Scabies is caused by the "itch mite" (*Sarcoptes scabiei*), which burrows into the skin and lays eggs that hatch in 4 to 8 days. The burrows may produce visible skin lesions, most often between the fingers and on the wrists.

5. Pediculosis capitis (head lice) is the most common type of lice infestation in the United States. It is diagnosed by finding louse eggs (nits) attached to hair shafts close to the scalp.

SECTION III: APPLYING YOUR KNOWLEDGE

ACTIVITY D
CASE STUDIES

1. Eating locally grown food and drinking fruit juice reconstituted at a local restaurant are possible sources of the patient's infection. Giardiasis is caused by *Giardia lamblia*, a common intestinal parasite. It is spread by food or water contaminated with human feces containing encysted forms of the organism or by contact with infected people or animals.

2. Giardial infections usually occur 1 to 2 weeks after ingestion of the cysts, so symptoms often do not appear until travelers are back home. Giardial infections may be asymptomatic, or they may produce diarrhea, abdominal cramping, and abdominal distention.

3. If giardiasis is left untreated, it may resolve spontaneously, or it may progress to a chronic disease with anorexia, nausea, malaise, weight loss, and continued diarrhea with large, foul-smelling stools. Malaise and fatigue can develop, which are attributable to deficiencies of vitamin B_{12} and fat-soluble vitamins that are a consequence of untreated giardiasis.

4. Adults and children older than 8 years of age with symptomatic giardiasis are usually treated with oral metronidazole.

SECTION IV: PRACTICING FOR NCLEX

1. a. *Rationale:* Antiparasitic drugs are usually given for local effects in the GI tract or on the skin.

2. b. *Rationale:* Personal and public health hygienic practices can prevent many parasitic infections and should be followed diligently.

3. d. *Rationale:* Travelers to malarious regions should generally receive chloroquine to prevent malaria and take precautions to avoid or minimize exposure to the causative mosquito.

4. injure

5. b. *Rationale:* When children have parasitic infestations, the home care nurse may need to collaborate with daycare centers and schools to prevent or control outbreaks.

6. a, b, and d. *Rationale:* The home care nurse may need to examine close contacts of the infected person and assess their need for treatment; assist parents and patients so that drugs are used appropriately; and teach personal and environmental hygiene measures to prevent reinfection.

7. a. *Rationale:* Children often receive an antiparasitic drug for head lice or worm infestations. These products should be used exactly as directed and with appropriate precautions to prevent reinfection.

8. a. *Rationale:* Malaria is usually more severe in children than in adults, and children should be protected from exposure whenever possible. If chemoprophylaxis or treatment for malaria is indicated, the same drugs are used for children as for adults, with appropriate dosage adjustments. The tetracyclines are an exception and should not be given to children younger than 8 years of age.

9. personal

10. b. *Rationale:* Malathion (Ovide) is a pediculicide used in the treatment of resistant head lice infestations, and pyrethrin preparations (e.g., RID) are available over-the-counter for treatment of pediculosis. These preparations require two applications approximately 10 days apart.

11. lindane

12. Permethrin

13. b. *Rationale:* Mebendazole (Vermox) is a broad-spectrum anthelmintic that is usually the drug of choice for treatment of hookworm, pinworm, roundworm, and whipworm infestations. It is also useful in tapeworm infection. The drug kills helminths by preventing uptake of the glucose necessary for parasitic metabolism.

14. a. *Rationale:* Nitazoxanide (Alinia) is approved for treatment of diarrhea caused by giardiasis or cryptosporidiosis in children. It is the first drug approved for treatment of cryptosporidiosis, which may be life-threatening in immunocompromised hosts.

15. d. *Rationale:* Quinine also relaxes skeletal muscles and has been used for prevention and treatment of nocturnal leg cramps.

16. c. *Rationale:* When used to prevent initial occurrence of malaria (causal prophylaxis), primaquine is given concurrently with a suppressive agent (e.g., chloroquine, hydroxychloroquine) after the patient has returned from a malarious area.

17. d. *Rationale:* Chloroquine is a widely used antimalarial agent. It acts against erythrocytic forms of plasmodial parasites to prevent or treat malarial attacks.

18. a and c. *Rationale:* Tetracycline and doxycycline are antibacterial drugs that act against amebae in the intestinal lumen by altering the bacterial flora required for amebic viability. One of these drugs may be used with other amebicides in the treatment of all forms of amebiasis except asymptomatic intestinal amebiasis.

19. a. *Rationale:* Metronidazole is contraindicated during the first trimester of pregnancy and must be used with caution in patients with central nervous system (CNS) or blood disorders. Patients should also avoid all forms of ethanol while taking this medication.

20. helminthiasis

Chapter 38: Physiology of the Hematopoietic and Immune Systems

SECTION II: ASSESSING YOUR UNDERSTANDING

ACTIVITY A
FILL IN THE BLANKS

1. pluripotent
2. bone marrow
3. cytokines
4. hematopoiesis
5. receptors

ACTIVITY B
MATCHING
1. C   2. A   3. E   4. B   5. D

ACTIVITY C
SHORT ANSWERS
1. Immunity indicates protection from a disease, and the main function of the immune system is host protection. To this end, the immune system detects and eliminates foreign substances that may cause tissue injury or disease. It also regulates tissue homeostasis and repair as cells of the immune system identify and remove injured, damaged, dead, or malignant cells.
2. Non-self or foreign antigens are also recognized by distinctive molecules, called epitopes, on their surfaces. Epitopes vary widely in type, number, and ability to elicit an immune response.
3. When the system is hypoactive, immunodeficiency disorders develop, because the person is highly susceptible to infectious and neoplastic diseases.
4. When the system is hyperactive, it perceives ordinarily harmless environmental substances (e.g., foods, plant pollens) as harmful and induces allergic reactions.
5. When the system is inappropriately activated (i.e., loses its ability to distinguish between self and non-self, so that an immune response is aroused against the host's own body tissues), the result is autoimmune disorders such as rheumatoid arthritis and systemic lupus erythematosus (SLE).

SECTION III: APPLYING YOUR KNOWLEDGE

ACTIVITY D
CASE STUDIES
1. Adaptive immunity is divided into cellular immunity (mainly involving activated T lymphocytes in body tissues) and humoral immunity (mainly involving B lymphocytes and antibodies in the blood). The two types of adaptive immunity are closely connected: virtually all antigens elicit both cellular and humoral responses, and most humoral (B cell) responses require cellular (T cell) stimulation.
2. Although most humoral responses occur when antibodies or B cells encounter antigens in blood, some occur when antibodies or B cells encounter antigens in other body fluids (e.g., tears, sweat, saliva, mucus, breast milk). The antibodies in these body fluids other than blood are produced by a part of humoral immunity sometimes called the secretory or mucosal immune system. The B cells of the mucosal system migrate through lymphoid tissues of tear ducts, salivary glands, breasts, bronchi, intestines, and genitourinary structures. The antibodies (mostly immunoglobulin A) secreted at these sites act locally rather than systemically.
3. Local protection combats foreign substances, especially pathogenic microorganisms that are inhaled, swallowed, or otherwise come in contact with external body surfaces. When the foreign substances bind to local antibodies, they are unable to attach to and invade mucosal tissue.

SECTION IV: PRACTICING FOR NCLEX
1. b. *Rationale:* Autoimmune disorders occur when the body erroneously perceives its own tissues as antigens and initiates an immune response.
2. Immunoglobulins
3. d. *Rationale:* T lymphocytes are major regulators of both humoral and cellular immunity.
4. Interleukins
5. a, c, and d. *Rationale:* Interferons alfa, beta, and gamma have antiviral and immunomodulating effects.
6. a and b. *Rationale:* Hematopoietic growth factors include G-CSF, M-CSF, GM-CSF, erythropoietin, and thrombopoietin.
7. a. *Rationale:* All hematopoietic and immune blood cells are derived from stem cells in the bone marrow.
8. restrict
9. b. *Rationale:* The HIV paralyzes the immune system by targeting helper T cells, macrophages, and dendritic cells. More specifically, it decreases the numbers and almost all functions of T lymphocytes and several functions of B lymphocytes and monocytes.
10. c and d. *Rationale:* In autoimmune disorders, the body perceives its own tissues as antigens and elicits an immune response, usually chronic and inflammatory in nature. Hashimoto's thyroiditis, multiple sclerosis, myasthenia gravis, rheumatoid arthritis, systemic lupus erythematosus, and type 1 diabetes mellitus are considered autoimmune disorder.
11. b. *Rationale:* In allergic disorders, the body perceives normally harmless substances (e.g., foods, pollens) as antigens and mounts an immune response. More specifically, IgE binds to antigen on the surface of mast cells and causes the release of chemical mediators (e.g., histamine) that produce the allergic manifestations.
12. b. *Rationale:* There is evidence that stress depresses immune function and therefore increases risks for development of infection and cancer.
13. d. *Rationale:* Vitamin deficiencies may also depress T- and B-cell function because several vitamins (e.g., A, E, folic acid, pantothenic acid, pyridoxine) also are enzyme cofactors in lymphocytes.
14. a. *Rationale:* Older adults have impaired immune responses to antigens. Therefore, achieving protective antibody titers may require higher doses of immunizing antigens in older adults than in younger adults.
15. c. *Rationale:* At birth, the neonatal immune system is still immature, but IgG levels (from maternal blood) are at near-adult levels in umbilical cord blood.
16. a. *Rationale:* The source of maternal antibodies is severed at birth. Antibody titers in infants decrease over approximately 6 months as maternal antibodies are catabolized.
17. c. *Rationale:* Cytokines regulate the immune response by stimulating or inhibiting the activation, proliferation, and differentiation of various cells and by regulating the secretion of antibodies or other cytokines.
18. b. *Rationale:* IgM protects against bacteria, toxins, and viruses that gain access to the bloodstream. It acts only in the bloodstream, because its large molecular size prevents its movement through capillary walls. It activates complement to destroy microorganisms.
19. d. *Rationale:* IgG is the most abundant immunoglobulin. It protects against bacteria, toxins, and viruses as it circulates in the bloodstream. Molecules of IgG combine with molecules of antigen, and the antigen–antibody complex activates complement. Activated complement causes an inflammatory reaction, promotes phagocytosis, and inactivates or destroys the antigen.
20. T

Chapter 39: Immunizing Agents

SECTION II: ASSESSING YOUR UNDERSTANDING

ACTIVITY A
FILL IN THE BLANKS
1. Immunization
2. Vaccines
3. Attenuated
4. Toxoids
5. boosters

ACTIVITY B
MATCHING
1. C   2. E   3. A   4. B   5. D

ACTIVITY C
SHORT ANSWERS
1. Additional components of vaccines and toxoids may include aluminum phosphate, aluminum hydroxide, or calcium phosphate. Products containing aluminum should be given intramuscularly only, because they cannot be given intravenously and greater tissue irritation occurs with subcutaneous injections.
2. Additives are used to delay absorption and increase antigenicity.
3. Preparations used for immunization are biologic products prepared by pharmaceutical companies and regulated by the United States Food and Drug Administration (FDA). Widespread use of these products has dramatically decreased the incidence of many infectious diseases.
4. The single vaccines for measles, mumps and rubella has been largely replaced by the combination product containing all three vaccines (MMR).
5. Immunization of prepubertal girls or women of childbearing age against rubella is important because rubella during the first trimester of pregnancy is associated with a high incidence of birth defects in the newborn.

SECTION III: APPLYING YOUR KNOWLEDGE

ACTIVITY D
CASE STUDIES
1. The immune globulin will give temporary immunity to people exposed to a particular disease. Immune serums are the biologic products used for passive immunity. They act rapidly to provide temporary (1 to 3 months) immunity in people who have been exposed to or are experiencing a particular disease. You can explain to the patient that immune globulin products are made from the serum of individuals with high concentrations of the specific antibody or immunoglobulin (Ig) required and will not cause the disease.
2. The goal of therapy is to prevent or modify the disease process (i.e., decrease the incidence and severity of symptoms).
3. These products may consist of whole serum or of the immunoglobulin portion of serum in which the specific antibodies are concentrated. Immunoglobulin fractions are preferred over whole serum because they are more likely to be effective. Plasma used to prepare these products is negative for hepatitis B surface antigen (HbsAg).
4. Hyperimmune serums are available for cytomegalovirus, hepatitis B, rabies, rubella, tetanus, varicella zoster (shingles), and respiratory syncytial virus infections.

SECTION IV: PRACTICING FOR NCLEX
1. b. *Rationale:* Health care providers need to assess and inform patients about recommended immunizations.

2. b. *Rationale:* For patients with active malignant disease, live vaccines should not be given. Although killed vaccines and toxoids may be given, antibody production may be inadequate to provide immunity. If possible, patients should receive needed immunizations 2 weeks before or 3 months after immunosuppressive radiation or chemotherapy treatments.
3. c. *Rationale:* For children with HIV infection, most routine immunizations (DTaP, IPV, MMR, Hib, influenza) are recommended.
4. 2
5. c. *Rationale:* Patients with HIV infection have less-than-optimal responses to immunizing agents because the disease produces major defects in cell-mediated and humoral immunity. Live bacterial (BCG, oral typhoid) or viral (MMR, varicella) vaccines should not be given, because the bacteria or viruses may be able to reproduce and cause active infection.
6. d. *Rationale:* Persons with asymptomatic HIV infection should receive inactivated vaccines; those exposed to measles or varicella may be given immune globulin or varicella-zoster immune globulin for passive immunization.
7. 3 months
8. d. *Rationale:* Long-term alternate-day therapy with short-acting corticosteroids; maintenance physiologic doses; and the use of topical, aerosol, or intra-articular injections are not contraindications to immunization.
9. c. *Rationale:* Immunizations are not contraindicated with short-term use (less than 2 weeks) or low to moderate doses (less than 20 mg/day) of prednisone.
10. d. *Rationale:* Patients with active malignant disease may be given killed vaccines or toxoids but should not be given live vaccines. (An exception is persons with leukemia who have not received chemotherapy for at least 3 months.)
11. b. *Rationale:* When vaccines are used, they should be given at least 2 weeks before the start of chemotherapy or 3 months after chemotherapy is completed. Passive immunity with immunoglobulins may be used in place of active immunity.
12. a, b, and c. *Rationale:* Clients diagnosed with diabetes mellitus or chronic pulmonary, renal, or hepatic disorders who are not receiving immunosuppressant drugs may be given both live attenuated and killed vaccines and toxoids to induce active immunity
13. b. *Rationale:* Vaccine to prevent shingles is available for adults 60 years and older.
14. 64
15. varicella-zoster
16. a, c, and d. *Rationale:* Recommended immunizations for older adults have usually consisted of a tetanus-diphtheria (Td) booster every 10 years, annual influenza vaccine, and a one-time administration of pneumococcal vaccine at 65 years of age.
17. a. *Rationale:* A second dose of pneumococcal vaccine may be given at age 65 years if the first dose was given 5 years previously.
18. a and b. *Rationale:* Adolescents who received all primary immunizations as infants and young children should have a second dose of varicella (chickenpox) vaccine, hepatitis A and hepatitis B vaccines (if not received earlier); a tetanus-diphtheria-pertussis booster (Tdap) between 11 and 18 years if 5 years has passed since a tetanus-diphtheria (Td) booster was given; and meningococcal vaccine at 11 or 12 years of age.

19. b. *Rationale*: MMR is administered to adolescent females if they are not pregnant and their rubella titer is inadequate or proof of immunization is unavailable.
20. d. *Rationale*: Recommendations regarding immunizations change periodically as additional information and new immunizing agents become available. Consequently, health care providers need to update their knowledge at least annually. The best source of information for current recommendations is the Centers for Disease Control and Prevention (http://www.cdc.gov).

Chapter 40: Hematopoietic and Immunostimulant Drugs

SECTION II: ASSESSING YOUR UNDERSTANDING

ACTIVITY A
FILL IN THE BLANKS
1. hematopoiesis
2. immunocompetence
3. hematopoiesis
4. immunostimulants
5. immunorestoratives

ACTIVITY B
MATCHING
1. D   2. A   3. E   4. B   5. C

ACTIVITY C
SHORT ANSWERS
1. Exogenous drug preparations have the same mechanisms of action as the endogenous products. CSF binds to receptors on the cell surfaces of immature blood cells in the bone marrow and increases the number, maturity, and functional ability of the cells. Interferons, called alfa, beta, or gamma according to specific characteristics, also bind to specific cell-surface receptors and alter intracellular activities. In viral infections, they induce enzymes that inhibit protein synthesis and degrade viral ribonucleic acid. As a result, viruses are less able to enter uninfected cells, reproduce, and release new viruses.
2. In addition to their antiviral effects, interferons also have antiproliferative and immunoregulatory activities. They can increase expression of major histocompatibility complex (MHC) molecules; augment the activity of natural killer (NK) cells; increase the effectiveness of antigen-presenting cells in inducing the proliferation of cytotoxic T cells; aid the attachment of cytotoxic T cells to target cells; and inhibit angiogenesis (formation of blood vessels). Because of these characteristics, the interferons are used mainly to treat viral infections and cancers.
3. Exogenous cytokines are given by subcutaneous (Sub-Q) or intravenous (IV) injection because they are proteins that would be destroyed by digestive enzymes if given orally.
4. Erythropoietin is a hormone from the kidney that stimulates bone marrow production of red blood cells.
5. In AIDS, the human immunodeficiency virus (HIV) causes severe immune system dysfunction, so the antiviral drugs indirectly improve immunologic function.

SECTION III: APPLYING YOUR KNOWLEDGE

ACTIVITY D
CASE STUDIES
1. Epoetin alfa is a drug formulation of a hormone, erythropoiesis, from the kidneys that stimulates bone marrow production of red blood cells. Erythropoiesis-stimulating drugs have been used to raise the hemoglobin level and reduce the need for blood transfusions in many patients with anemia. Epoetin is prescribed at the lowest dose that is effective in raising hemoglobin levels just enough to avoid the need for blood transfusion. The hemoglobin levels must be regularly monitored until they stabilize.
2. Exogenous cytokines are given by subcutaneous (Sub-Q) or intravenous (IV) injection. Mrs. Cantos must be taught how to administer these injections for herself.
3. Studies indicated an increased risk of serious cardiovascular problems (e.g., hypertension, thromboembolic events) and death in patients with chronic renal failure and an increased risk of tumor progression and death in patients with cancer. These problems became evident when the drugs were used to achieve normal hemoglobin levels of 12 to 14 grams per deciliter (g/dL). A black box warning for this drug advises prescribers to avoid using Epogen in patients with hemoglobin values of 12 g/dL or greater.

SECTION IV: PRACTICING FOR NCLEX
1. pegylation
2. b. *Rationale*: Interferons are used mainly for viral hepatitis and certain types of cancer.
3. a. *Rationale*: Filgrastim is used to increase white blood cells and decrease risks of infection in patients who have or are at high risk for severe neutropenia.
4. c. *Rationale*: Adverse effects of epoetin and darbepoetin include increased risks of hypertension, myocardial infarction, and stroke, especially when used to increase hemoglobin above 12/dL.
5. b. *Rationale*: A drug formulation of erythropoietin is given to increase red blood cells in patients with anemia associated with chronic renal failure or bone marrow(damaging anticancer drug therapy.
6. a. *Rationale*: Epoetin is not effective unless sufficient iron is present, and most patients need an iron supplement. When an iron preparation is prescribed, the home care nurse may need to emphasize the importance of taking it.
7. d. *Rationale*: With filgrastim, the nurse may need to help the patient and family with techniques to reduce exposure to infection.
8. a. *Rationale*: With preexisting hepatic impairment, sargramostim increase serum bilirubin and liver enzymes. Values decline to baseline levels when the drug is stopped or its dosage is reduced. Liver function tests are recommended every 2 weeks for clients with preexisting impairment.
9. c. *Rationale*: Hepatitis B becomes chronic in 5% to 10% of patients. Interferon alfa and lamivudine or other antiviral drugs may be used for treatment. Drug resistance may develop, and active hepatitis may resume when the drugs are discontinued.
10. peginterferon
11. suppressed
12. b. *Rationale*: Bacillus Calmette-Guérin, when instilled into the urinary bladder of patients with superficial bladder cancer, causes remission in up to 82% of patients for an average of 4 years.
13. a. *Rationale*: Interferon alfa has demonstrated antitumor effects in multiple myeloma, renal cell carcinoma, and others.
14. b. *Rationale*: In hairy-cell leukemia, interferons normalize WBC counts in 70% to 90% of patients. Drug therapy must be continued indefinitely to avoid relapse, which usually develops rapidly after the drug is discontinued.
15. d. *Rationale*: When sargramostim is given to patients with cancer who have undergone bone marrow transplantation, the drug should be started 2 to 4 hours after the bone marrow infusion and at least 24 hours after the last dose of antineoplastic chemotherapy or 12 hours after the last radiotherapy treatment.

16. 24
17. b. *Rationale:* With darbepoetin and epoetin, iron stores (transferrin saturation and serum ferritin) should be measured before and periodically during treatment. Hemoglobin should be measured twice weekly until the level is stabilized and maintenance drug doses are established.
18. b. *Rationale:* With darbepoetin and epoetin, dosage is adjusted to achieve and maintain a hemoglobin value of no more than 12 g/dL (serous adverse effects may occur with values higher than 12 g/dL). Dosage should be reduced if the hemoglobin level approaches 12 g/dL or increases by more than 1 g/dL in any 2-week period.
19. 50%
20. platelet count

Chapter 41: Immunosuppressants

SECTION II: ASSESSING YOUR UNDERSTANDING

ACTIVITY A
FILL IN THE BLANKS
1. cytokines
2. antigens
3. proteins
4. immunosuppressant
5. immunosuppression

ACTIVITY B
MATCHING
1. D   2. A   3. C   4. B   5. E

ACTIVITY C
SHORT ANSWERS
1. An appropriate but undesirable immune response occurs when foreign tissue is transplanted into the body. If the immune response is not suppressed, the body reacts as with other antigens and attempts to destroy the foreign tissue (graft rejection reaction). Although numerous advances have been made in transplantation technology, the immune response remains a major factor in determining the success or failure of transplantation.
2. Tumor necrosis factor (TNF)–alpha is a cytokine that plays a major role in the response to infection. Functions of TNF include activation of monocytes, macrophages, and cytotoxic T cells; enhancement of natural killer (NK) cell functions; increased leukocyte movement into areas of tissue injury; increased phagocytosis by neutrophils; and stimulation of B and T lymphocytes. Despite the beneficial effects of a "normal" amount of TNF, however, an excessive TNF response has been associated with the pathogenesis of autoimmune disorders such as RA and Crohn's disease.
3. Several factors prevent the immune system from "turning off" the abnormal immune or inflammatory process. One of these factors may be an inadequate number of suppressor T cells, which are thought to be a subpopulation of helper or cytotoxic T cells. Another factor may be inadequate amounts of anti-inflammatory cytokines (e.g., interleukin-10).
4. A rejection reaction occurs when the host's immune system is stimulated to destroy the transplanted organ. The immune cells of the transplant recipient attach to the donor cells of the transplanted organ and react against the antigens of the donor organ. The rejection process involves T and B lymphocytes, antibodies, multiple cytokines, and inflammatory mediators. In general, T-cell activation and proliferation are more important in the rejection reaction than B-cell activation and formation of antibodies. Cytotoxic and helper T cells are activated; activated helper T cells stimulate B cells to produce antibodies, leading to a delayed hypersensitivity reaction. The antibodies injure the transplanted organ by activating complement, producing antigen–antibody complexes, or causing antibody-mediated tissue breakdown.
5. Acute reactions may occur from 10 days to a few months after transplantation and mainly involve cellular immunity and proliferation of T lymphocytes. Characteristics include signs of organ failure and vasculitis lesions that often lead to arterial narrowing or obliteration. Treatment with immunosuppressant drugs is usually effective in ensuring short-term survival of the transplant but does not prevent chronic rejection.

SECTION III: APPLYING YOUR KNOWLEDGE

ACTIVITY D
CASE STUDIES
1. With bone marrow/stem cell transplantation, the donor cells mount an immune response (mainly by stimulating T lymphocytes) against antigens on the host's tissues, producing GVHD. Tissue damage is produced directly by the action of cytotoxic T cells or indirectly through the release of inflammatory mediators (e.g., complement) and cytokines (e.g., TNF-alpha, interleukins).
2. Acute GVHD occurs in 30% to 50% of patients, usually within 6 weeks after transplant. Signs and symptoms include delayed recovery of blood cell production in the bone marrow, skin rash, liver dysfunction (indicated by increased alkaline phosphatase, aminotransferases, and bilirubin), and diarrhea. The skin reaction is usually a pruritic maculopapular rash that begins on the palms and soles and may extend over the entire body. Liver involvement can lead to bleeding disorders and coma. Chronic GVHD occurs when symptoms persist or occur 100 days or longer after transplantation. It is characterized by abnormal humoral and cellular immunity, severe skin disorders, and liver disease. Chronic GVHD appears to be an autoimmune disorder in which activated T cells perceive self-antigens as foreign antigens.
3. Methotrexate is used (with cyclosporine) to prevent GVHD after bone marrow transplantation. Lower doses are given for these conditions than for treatment of cancers, and adverse drug effects are fewer and less severe. When methotrexate is administered, CBC, platelet counts, and renal and liver function tests should be monitored.

SECTION IV: PRACTICING FOR NCLEX
1. a. *Rationale:* Newer immunosuppressants have more specific effects on the immune system and may cause fewer or less severe adverse effects than older drugs.
2. a. *Rationale:* Cyclosporine and tacrolimus are similar drugs that are effective immunosuppressants, are widely used in organ transplantation, cause nephrotoxicity, and are subject to numerous drug interactions (enzyme-inhibiting drugs increase blood levels and enzyme-inducing drugs decrease blood levels).
3. c. *Rationale:* Immunosuppressant drugs greatly increase risk of infection.
4. d. *Rationale:* With current treatments, most transplant patients must maintain on immunosuppressive drug therapy for the rest of their lives.
5. immune

6. b. *Rationale:* With patients who are taking immunosuppressant drugs, a major role of the home care nurse is to assess the environment for potential sources of infection, assist patients and other members of the household to understand the patient's susceptibility to infection, and teach ways to decrease risks of infection. Although infections often develop from the patient's own body flora, other potential sources include people with infections, caregivers, water or soil around live plants, and raw fruits and vegetables.

7. d. *Rationale:* Leflunomide may be hepatotoxic in patients with normal liver function and is not recommended for use in patients with liver impairment or in patients with positive serology tests for hepatitis B or C.

8. c. *Rationale:* Tacrolimus is metabolized in the liver by the cytochrome P450 enzyme system. Impaired liver function may decrease presystemic (first-pass) metabolism of oral tacrolimus and produce higher blood levels. Also, the elimination half-life is significantly longer. As a result, dosage must be decreased in patients with impaired liver function.

9. c. *Rationale:* Sirolimus is extensively metabolized in the liver and may accumulate in the presence of hepatic impairment. The maintenance dose should be reduced by 35%; it is not necessary to reduce the loading dose.

10. a. *Rationale:* Cyclosporine is nephrotoxic but is commonly used in patients with renal and other transplants. Nephrotoxicity usually subsides with decreased dosage or stopping the drug. In renal transplant recipients, when serum creatinine and blood urea nitrogen levels remain elevated, a complete evaluation of the patient must be done to differentiate cyclosporine-induced nephrotoxicity from a transplant rejection reaction.

11. b. *Rationale:* Immunosuppressants are used for the same purposes and produce similar therapeutic and adverse effects in older adults as in younger adults. Because older adults often have multiple disorders and organ impairments, it is especially important that drug choices, dosages, and monitoring tests be individualized. In addition, infections occur more commonly in older adults, and this tendency is increased with immunosuppressant therapy.

12. omalizumab

13. b. *Rationale:* Most immunosuppressants are used in children for the same disorders and with similar effects as in adults. Corticosteroids impair growth in children. As a result, some transplantation centers avoid prednisone therapy until a rejection episode occurs.

14. prednisone

15. a, b, and c. *Rationale:* Immunosuppressant drugs are relatively toxic, and adverse effects occur more often and are more severe with higher doses. Therefore, the general principle of using the smallest effective dose for the shortest period of time is especially important with immunosuppressant drug therapy. Dosage must be individualized according to the patient's serum drug levels and clinical response (i.e., improvement in signs and symptoms or occurrence of adverse effects).

16. T, B

17. b. *Rationale:* Rheumatoid arthritis is an abnormal immune response that leads to inflammation and damage of joint cartilage and bone. It is thought to involve the activation of T lymphocytes, release of inflammatory cytokines, and formation of antibodies.

18. d. *Rationale:* Psoriatic arthritis is a type of arthritis associated with psoriasis that is similar to RA. It may be characterized by extensive and disabling joint damage, especially in hand and finger joints. Etanercept (Enbrel) is a TNF-alpha inhibitor approved for treatment of psoriatic arthritis.

19. d. *Rationale:* Crohn's disease is a chronic, recurrent, inflammatory bowel disorder that can affect any area of the GI tract.

20. lymphomas

Chapter 42: Drugs Used in Oncologic Disorders

SECTION II: ASSESSING YOUR UNDERSTANDING
ACTIVITY A
FILL IN THE BLANKS
1. Oncology
2. Antineoplastic
3. cancer
4. Normal
5. cell cycle

ACTIVITY B
MATCHING
1. B   2. D   3. A   4. E   5. C

ACTIVITY C
SHORT ANSWERS
1. Antimetabolites are diverse drugs that are allowed to enter cancer cells because they are similar to metabolites or nutrients needed by the cells for reproduction. Inside the cell, the drugs replace normal metabolites or inhibit essential enzymes. These actions deprive the cell of substances needed for formation of DNA or cause formation of abnormal DNA.
2. Antimetabolites are cell cycle–specific because they exert their cytotoxic effects only during the S phase of the cell's reproductive cycle, when DNA is being synthesized.
3. Homocysteine is produced when proteins are broken down in the blood, and elevated blood levels are considered a risk factor for coronary artery disease and stroke. Treatment with folic acid and vitamin B_{12} supplements, which can reduce homocysteine blood levels, is required for all patients taking pemetrexed.
4. The toxic effects of folic acid antagonists include bone marrow depression, mucositis and ulceration of the GI tract, and hair loss.
5. Folic acid antagonists (e.g., methotrexate [prototype], pemetrexed), purine antagonists (e.g., mercaptopurine), and pyrimidine antagonists (e.g., fluorouracil) are most effective against rapidly growing tumors, and individual drugs vary in their effectiveness with different kinds of cancer.

SECTION III: APPLYING YOUR KNOWLEDGE
ACTIVITY D
CASE STUDIES
1. Most cytotoxic antineoplastic drugs kill malignant cells by interfering with cell replication, with the supply and use of nutrients (e.g., amino acids, purines, pyrimidines), or with the genetic materials in the cell nucleus (DNA or RNA). Each drug dose kills a specific percentage of cells. To achieve a cure, all malignant cells must be killed or reduced to a small number that can be killed by the person's immune system.

2. Doxorubicin and daunorubicin are available in conventional and liposomal preparations. The liposomal preparations increase drug concentration in malignant tissues and decrease concentration in normal tissues, thereby increasing effectiveness while decreasing toxicity (e.g., cardiotoxicity). With treatment of leukemias and lymphomas, a serious, life-threatening adverse effect called tumor lysis syndrome may occur. This syndrome occurs when large numbers of cancer cells are killed or damaged and release their contents into the bloodstream.

3. This patient needs more teaching, because he has not demonstrated accurate understanding of his condition. With tumor lysis syndrome, hyperkalemia, hyperphosphatemia, hyperuricemia, hypomagnesemia, hypocalcemia, and acidosis develop. Signs and symptoms depend on the severity of the metabolic imbalances but may include GI upset, fatigue, altered mental status, hypertension, muscle cramps, paresthesias (numbness and tingling), tetany, seizures, electrocardiographic changes (e.g., dysrhythmias), cardiac arrest, reduced urine output, and acute renal failure.

4. Tumor lysis syndrome can be prevented or minimized by aggressive hydration with IV normal saline, alkalinization with IV sodium bicarbonate, and administration of allopurinol (e.g., 300 mg daily for adults, 10 mg/kg/day for children) to reduce uric acid levels. Maintaining a urine pH of 7 or higher prevents renal failure from precipitation of uric acid crystals in the kidneys. Treatment of hyperkalemia may include IV dextrose and regular insulin (to drive potassium into cells) or Kayexalate to eliminate potassium in feces. Treatment of hyperphosphatemia may include administration of aluminum hydroxide or another phosphate-binding agent.

SECTION IV: PRACTICING FOR NCLEX

1. d. *Rationale:* Cancer in older adults presents a unique challenge, due in part to the presence of comorbidities and the physical, biologic, and physiologic changes that occur with normal aging. Until recently, older adults were excluded from participating in clinical trials.

2. c. *Rationale:* Hormonal therapies that block the effects of estrogen (in an estrogen-responsive tumor) and androgen (in an androgen-responsive tumor), respectively, are essential in the treatment of breast and prostate cancers.

3. cancer

4. a. *Rationale:* Traditional cytotoxic antineoplastic drugs are nonselective in their effect on proliferating cells; therefore, bone marrow toxicity is a common adverse effect of many cytotoxic drugs. These drugs kill the same fraction of cells with each cycle of chemotherapy treatment; repeated cycles of cytotoxic drugs potentially lower the number of cancer cells to a level where a person's immune responses are able to take over and destroy the remaining cancer cells.

5. a. *Rationale:* Patients may receive parenteral cytotoxic drugs as outpatients and return home, or these and other antineoplastic drugs may be administered at home by the patient or a caregiver. If a patient is receiving erythropoietin or oprelvekin subcutaneously, the patient or a caregiver may need to be taught injection technique.

6. c. *Rationale:* Some antineoplastic drugs are hepatotoxic, and many are metabolized in the liver. With impaired hepatic function, risks of further impairment or accumulation of toxic drug levels are increased. However, abnormal values for the usual liver function tests (e.g., aspartate aminotransferase [AST], alanine aminotransferase [ALT], bilirubin, alkaline phosphatase) may indicate liver injury but do not indicate decreased ability to metabolize drugs. Patients with metastatic cancer often have impaired liver function.

7. c. *Rationale:* L-Asparaginase is hepatotoxic in most patients; it may increase preexisting hepatic impairment and hepatotoxicity of other medications. Signs of liver impairment, which usually subsides when the drug is discontinued, include increased AST, ALT, alkaline phosphatase, and bilirubin and decreased serum albumin, cholesterol, and plasma fibrinogen.

8. d. *Rationale:* Capecitabine blood levels are significantly increased with hepatic impairment, and patients with liver metastases should be monitored closely.

9. d. *Rationale:* Some antineoplastic drugs are nephrotoxic (e.g., cisplatin, MTX), and many are excreted through the kidneys. In the presence of impaired renal function, risks of further impairment or accumulation of toxic drug levels are increased. Therefore, renal function should be monitored carefully during therapy, and drug dosages are often reduced based on CrCl levels.

10. renal failure

11. a, c, and d. *Rationale:* In addition to comorbidities, issues that affect treatment for older adults include access to care, financial and transportation issues, functional status, need for independence, and social support.

12. d. *Rationale:* Creatinine clearance (CrCl) should be monitored; serum creatinine level is not a reliable indicator of renal function in older adults because of their decreased muscle mass.

13. c. *Rationale:* In recent years, there have been rapid advances in cancer care for children and high cure rates for many pediatric malignancies. Many of these advances have resulted from the systematic enrollment of children in well-designed clinical trials.

14. oncologists

15. b. *Rationale:* Dosage of cytotoxic drugs for children should be based on body surface area, because this measurement takes size into account.

16. a. *Rationale:* Children who receive an anthracycline drug (e.g., doxorubicin) are at increased risk of developing cardiotoxic effects (e.g., heart failure) during treatment or after receiving the drug. Efforts to reduce cardiotoxicity include using alternative drugs when effective, giving smaller cumulative doses of anthracycline drug, and observing patients closely so that early manifestations can be recognized and treated before heart failure occurs.

17. a, b, and c. *Rationale:* Most cytotoxic antineoplastic drugs are carcinogenic, mutagenic, and teratogenic. Exposure during pregnancy increases risks of fetal abnormalities, ectopic pregnancy, and spontaneous abortion.

18. a. *Rationale:* When handling cytotoxic antineoplastic drugs, you should avoid direct contact with solutions for injection by wearing gloves, face shields, and protective clothing (e.g., disposable, liquid-impermeable gowns).

19. d. *Rationale:* When caring for clients receiving cytotoxic antineoplastic drugs; wear gloves when handling patients' clothing, bed linens, or excreta. Blood and body fluids are contaminated with drugs or metabolites for about 48 hours after a dose.

20. b. *Rationale:* When both hormone inhibitor and cytotoxic drug therapies are needed, they are not given concurrently, because hormone antagonists decrease malignant cell growth and cytotoxic agents are most effective when the cells are actively dividing.

Chapter 43: Physiology of the Respiratory System

SECTION II: ASSESSING YOUR UNDERSTANDING

ACTIVITY A
FILL IN THE BLANKS
1. cellular
2. anoxia
3. carbon dioxide (CO_2)
4. acidosis
5. alveolar–capillary

ACTIVITY B
MATCHING
1. B   2. E   3. A   4. D   5. C

ACTIVITY C
SHORT ANSWERS
1. Respiration is the process of gas exchange by which O_2 is obtained and CO_2 is eliminated. This gas exchange occurs between the lung and the blood across the alveolar–capillary membrane and between the blood and body cells.
2. Cilia are tiny, hair-like projections that sweep mucus toward the pharynx to be expectorated or swallowed.
3. Air passes from the nasal cavities to the pharynx (throat). Pharyngeal walls are composed of skeletal muscle, and their lining is composed of mucous membrane. The pharynx contains the palatine tonsils, which are large masses of lymphatic tissue. The pharynx is a passageway for food, fluids, and air. Food and fluids go from the pharynx to the esophagus, and air passes from the pharynx into the trachea.
4. The larynx is composed of nine cartilages joined by ligaments and controlled by skeletal muscles. It contains the vocal cords and forms the upper end of the trachea. It closes on swallowing to prevent aspiration of food and fluids into the lungs.
5. The alveoli are composed of two types of cells. Type I cells are flat, thin epithelial cells that fuse with capillaries to form the alveolar–capillary membrane across which gas exchange occurs. Oxygen enters the bloodstream to be transported to body cells; CO_2 enters the alveoli to be exhaled from the lungs. Type II cells produce *surfactant*, a lipoprotein substance that decreases the surface tension in the alveoli and aids lung inflation. The alveoli also contain macrophages that help to protect and defend the lungs.

SECTION III: APPLYING YOUR KNOWLEDGE

ACTIVITY D
CASE STUDIES
1. The pulmonary circulatory system transports O_2 and CO_2. After oxygen enters the bloodstream across the alveolar–capillary membrane, it combines with hemoglobin in red blood cells for transport to body cells, where it is released. Carbon dioxide combines with hemoglobin in the cells for return to the lungs and elimination from the body. The lungs receive the total cardiac output of blood and are supplied with blood from two sources, the pulmonary and bronchial circulations. The pulmonary circulation provides for gas exchange because the pulmonary arteries carry deoxygenated blood to the lungs and the pulmonary veins return oxygenated blood to the heart.
2. The bronchial circulation facilitates the development of collateral circulation. The bronchial arteries arise from the thoracic aorta and supply the air passages and supporting structures. The bronchial circulation also warms and humidifies incoming air and can form new vessels and develop collateral circulation when normal vessels are blocked (e.g., in pulmonary embolism). The latter ability helps to keep lung tissue alive until circulation can be restored.
3. Capillaries in the lungs are lined by a single layer of epithelial cells called endothelium. Once thought to be a passive conduit for blood, it is now known that the endothelium performs several important functions. It forms a barrier that prevents leakage of water and other substances into lung tissue. Capillary epithelial cells secrete vasodilating substances such as nitric oxide and prostacyclin. Nitric oxide also regulates smooth muscle tone in the bronchi, and prostacyclin also inhibits platelet aggregation.
4. Endotoxins or drugs such as bleomycin, an anticancer drug, can injure pulmonary endothelium. When pulmonary endothelium is injured, functions are impaired.

SECTION IV: PRACTICING FOR NCLEX
1. c. *Rationale:* Major drug groups used to treat respiratory symptoms are bronchodilating and anti-inflammatory agents, antihistamines, and nasal decongestants, antitussives, and cold remedies.
2. a, b, and c. *Rationale:* The respiratory system is subject to many disorders that interfere with respiration and other lung functions, including respiratory tract infections, allergic disorders, inflammatory disorders, and conditions that obstruct airflow.
3. a, b, and c. *Rationale:* The nervous system regulates the rate and depth of respiration by the respiratory center in the medulla oblongata, the pneumotaxic center in the pons, and the apneustic center in the reticular formation.
4. a, c, and d. *Rationale:* The efficiency of the respiratory system depends on the quality and quantity of air inhaled, the patency of air passages, the ability of the lungs to expand and contract, and the ability of O_2 and CO_2 to cross the alveolar–capillary membrane.
5. a. *Rationale:* When the oxygen supply is inadequate, cell function is impaired; when oxygen is absent, cells die.
6. c. *Rationale:* In general, drug therapy is more effective in relieving respiratory symptoms than in curing the underlying disorders that cause the symptoms.
7. c. *Rationale:* Common signs and symptoms of respiratory disorders include cough, increased secretions, mucosal congestion, and bronchospasm. Severe disorders or inadequate treatment may lead to cell necrosis or respiratory failure.
8. a. *Rationale:* Overall, normal respiration requires Atmospheric air containing at least 21% O_2.
9. a. *Rationale:* The musculoskeletal system participates in chest expansion and contraction. Normally, the diaphragm and external intercostal muscles expand the chest cavity and are called muscles of inspiration.
10. d. *Rationale:* The abdominal and internal intercostal muscles are the muscles of expiration.
11. b. *Rationale:* The nervous system also operates several reflexes important to respiration. The cough reflex is especially important because it helps protect the lungs from foreign particles, air pollutants, bacteria, and other potentially harmful substances. A cough occurs when nerve endings in the respiratory tract mucosa are stimulated by dryness, pressure, cold, irritant fumes, or excessive secretions.

12. b. *Rationale:* The respiratory center is stimulated primarily by increased CO_2 in the fluids of the center. (However, excessive CO_2 depresses the respiratory center.) When the center is stimulated, the rate and depth of breathing are increased, and excessive CO_2 is exhaled. A lesser stimulus to the respiratory center is decreased oxygen in arterial blood.
13. biologically
14. blood vessels
15. d. *Rationale:* Angiotensin-converting enzyme converts angiotensin I to angiotensin II, which is important in regulating blood pressure.
16. c. *Rationale:* The respiratory tract is a series of branching tubes with progressively smaller diameters. These tubes (nose, pharynx, larynx, trachea, bronchi, and bronchioles) function as air passageways and air "conditioners" that filter, warm, and humidify incoming air. Most of the conditioning is done by the ciliated mucous membrane that lines the entire respiratory tract, except the pharynx and alveoli.
17. alveoli
18. b. *Rationale:* The lungs are encased in a membrane called the pleura, which is composed of two layers. The inner layer, which adheres to the surface of the lung, is called the visceral pleura.
19. a. *Rationale:* The outer layer of the pleura, which lines the thoracic cavity, is called the parietal pleura. The potential space between the layers is called the pleural cavity. It contains fluid that allows the layers to glide over each other and minimizes friction.
20. compliance

Chapter 44: Drugs for Asthma and Other Bronchoconstrictive Disorders

SECTION II: ASSESSING YOUR UNDERSTANDING

ACTIVITY A
FILL IN THE BLANKS
1. Occupational asthma
2. hyperreactivity
3. Wheezing
4. bronchoconstriction
5. sulfites

ACTIVITY B
MATCHING
1. C   2. E   3. A   4. B   5. D

ACTIVITY C
SHORT ANSWERS
1. Asthma is an airway disorder that is characterized by bronchoconstriction, inflammation, and hyperreactivity to various stimuli. Resultant symptoms include dyspnea, wheezing, chest tightness, cough, and sputum production. Wheezing is a high-pitched, whistling sound caused by turbulent airflow through an obstructed airway.
2. Symptoms of asthma vary in incidence and severity, from occasional episodes of mild respiratory distress with normal functioning between "attacks" to persistent, daily, or continual respiratory distress if not adequately controlled. Inflammation and damaged airway mucosa are chronically present, even when clients appear symptom free.
3. Viral infections of the respiratory tract are often the causative agents of asthma, especially in infants and young children, whose airways are small and easily obstructed. Asthma symptoms may persist for days or weeks after the viral infection resolves.

4. Clients with severe asthma should be cautioned against ingesting food and drug products containing sulfites or metabisulfites.
5. Gastroesophageal reflux disease (GERD), a common disorder characterized by heartburn and esophagitis, is also associated with asthma. Asthma that worsens at night may be associated with nighttime acid reflux.

SECTION III: APPLYING YOUR KNOWLEDGE

ACTIVITY D
CASE STUDIES
1. The main xanthine used clinically is theophylline. Despite many years of use, the drug's mechanism of action is unknown. Various mechanisms have been proposed, such as inhibiting phosphodiesterase enzymes that metabolize cyclic AMP, increasing endogenous catecholamines, inhibiting calcium ion movement into smooth muscle, inhibiting prostaglandin synthesis and release, or inhibiting the release of bronchoconstrictive substances from mast cells and leukocytes.
2. Theophylline should be used cautiously in those with cardiovascular disorders that could be aggravated by drug-induced cardiac stimulation.
3. Theophylline increases the ability of the body to clear mucus from the airways. In addition to bronchodilation, other effects that may be beneficial in asthma and COPD include inhibiting pulmonary edema by decreasing vascular permeability, increasing the ability of cilia to clear mucus from the airways, strengthening contractions of the diaphragm, and decreasing inflammation.
4. Mrs. Livingston should be taught that it is important to keep all her appointments, because her serum drug levels need to be monitored. Theophylline increases cardiac output, causes peripheral vasodilation, exerts a mild diuretic effect, and stimulates the CNS. The cardiovascular and CNS effects are adverse effects. Serum drug levels should be monitored to help regulate dosage and avoid adverse effects.
5. Theophylline is metabolized in the liver; metabolites and some unchanged drug are excreted through the kidneys. In a patient with impaired liver function, metabolism of the drug can be compromised. Theophylline preparations are contraindicated in clients with acute gastritis or peptic ulcer disease.

SECTION IV: PRACTICING FOR NCLEX
1. c. *Rationale:* The FDA has issued a black box warning that initiating salmeterol in individuals with significantly worsening or acutely deteriorating asthma may be life-threatening.
2. anaphylaxis
3. a. *Rationale:* Cigarette smoking and drugs that stimulate drug-metabolizing enzymes in the liver (e.g., phenobarbital, phenytoin) increase the rate of metabolism and therefore the dosage requirements of aminophylline.
4. d. *Rationale:* Almost all over-the-counter aerosol products promoted for use in asthma contain epinephrine, which may produce hazardous cardiac stimulation and other adverse effects.
5. c. *Rationale:* Asthma may aggravate GERD, because antiasthma medications that dilate the airways also relax muscle tone in the gastroesophageal sphincter and may increase acid reflux
6. a, b, and c. *Rationale:* Because aerosol products act directly on the airways, drugs given by inhalation can usually be given in smaller doses and produce fewer adverse effects than oral or parenteral drugs

7. a. *Rationale:* A selective, short-acting, inhaled beta$_2$-adrenergic agonist (e.g., albuterol) is the initial rescue drug of choice for acute bronchospasm; subcutaneous epinephrine may also be considered.

8. anti-inflammatory

9. d. *Rationale:* Two general classifications of drugs are used for asthma management: long-term control medications to achieve and maintain control of persistent asthma and quick relief medications used during periods of acute symptoms and exacerbations.

10. c. *Rationale:* A specific monitoring plan for clients with asthma should be in place, whether through peak-flow or symptom monitoring.

11. a, b, and d. *Rationale:* With theophylline, the home care nurse needs to assess the client and the environment for substances that may affect metabolism of theophylline and decrease therapeutic effects or increase adverse effects

12. a. *Rationale:* The nurse needs to reinforce the importance of not exceeding the prescribed dose, not crushing long-acting formulations, reporting adverse effects, and keeping appointments for follow-up care.

13. b, c, and d. *Rationale:* In children, high doses of nebulized albuterol have been associated with tachycardia, hypokalemia, and hyperglycemia.

14. d. *Rationale:* Montelukast and zafirlukast produce higher blood levels and are eliminated more slowly in clients with hepatic impairment. However, no dosage adjustment is recommended for clients with mild to moderate hepatic impairment.

15. a. *Rationale:* Cromolyn is eliminated by renal and biliary excretion; the drug should be given in reduced doses, if at all, in clients with renal impairment.

16. a and d. *Rationale:* Older adults often have chronic pulmonary disorders for which bronchodilators and antiasthmatic medications are used. The main risks with adrenergic bronchodilators are excessive cardiac and CNS stimulation.

17. b. *Rationale:* If the client is obese, the dosage of theophylline should be based on lean or ideal body weight, because theophylline is not highly distributed in fatty tissue.

18. Cromolyn aerosol solution may be used in children 5 years of age and older, and nebulizer solution is used with children 2 years and older.

19. c. *Rationale:* Adrenal insufficiency is most likely to occur with systemic or high doses of inhaled corticosteroids.

20. b. *Rationale:* For theophylline overdose in clients without seizures, induce vomiting unless the level of consciousness is impaired. Precautions to prevent aspiration are needed, especially in children. If overdose is identified within 1 hour after drug ingestion, gastric lavage may be helpful if vomiting cannot be induced or is contraindicated. Administration of activated charcoal and a cathartic is also recommended, especially for overdoses of sustained-release formulations, if benefit exceeds risk.

Chapter 45: Antihistamines and Allergic Disorders

SECTION II: ASSESSING YOUR UNDERSTANDING

ACTIVITY A
FILL IN THE BLANKS
1. Antihistamines
2. Histamine
3. mast cells
4. Hypersensitivity
5. H$_1$

ACTIVITY B
MATCHING
1. C   2. E   3. A   4. B   5. D

ACTIVITY C
SHORT ANSWERS
1. Histamine is the first chemical mediator to be released in immune and inflammatory responses. It is synthesized and stored in most body tissues, with high concentrations in tissues exposed to environmental substances (such as the skin and mucosal surfaces of the eyes, nose, lungs, and gastrointestinal tract). It is also found in the central nervous system (CNS). In these tissues, histamine is located mainly in secretory granules of mast cells (tissue cells surrounding capillaries) and basophils (circulating blood cells).

2. When H$_2$ receptors are stimulated, the main effects are increased secretion of gastric acid and pepsin, increased rate and force of myocardial contraction, and decreased immunologic and proinflammatory reactions (e.g., decreased release of histamine from basophils, decreased movement of neutrophils and basophils into areas of injury, inhibited T- and B-lymphocyte function). Stimulation of both H$_1$ and H$_2$ receptors causes peripheral vasodilation (with hypotension, headache, and skin flushing) and increased bronchial, intestinal, and salivary secretion of mucus.

3. Hypersensitivity or allergic reactions are exaggerated responses by the immune system that produce tissue injury and may cause serious disease. The mechanisms that eliminate pathogens in adaptive immune responses are essentially identical to those of natural immunity. Allergic reactions may result from specific antibodies, sensitized T lymphocytes, or both, formed during exposure to an antigen.

4. Type I immune response (also called immediate hypersensitivity because it occurs within minutes after exposure to the antigen) is an immunoglobulin E (IgE)-induced response triggered by the interaction of antigen with antigen-specific IgE bound on mast cells, causing mast cell activation. Histamine and other mediators are released immediately, and cytokines, chemokines, and leukotrienes are synthesized after activation.

5. Type II responses are mediated by IgG or IgM generating direct damage to the cell surface. These cytotoxic reactions include blood transfusion reactions, hemolytic disease of newborns, autoimmune hemolytic anemia, and some drug reactions. Hemolytic anemia (caused by destruction of erythrocytes) and thrombocytopenia (caused by destruction of platelets), both type II hypersensitivity responses, are adverse effects of certain drugs (e.g., penicillin, methyldopa, heparin).

SECTION III: APPLYING YOUR KNOWLEDGE

ACTIVITY D
CASE STUDIES
1. Allergic rhinitis is inflammation of nasal mucosa caused by a type I hypersensitivity reaction to inhaled allergens.

2. There are two types of allergic rhinitis. Seasonal disease (often called hay fever) produces acute symptoms in response to the protein components of airborne pollens from trees, grasses and weeds, mainly in the spring or fall.

3. Allergic rhinitis is an immune response in which normal nasal breathing and filtering of air brings inhaled antigens into contact with mast cells and basophils in nasal mucosa, blood vessels, and submucosal tissues. With initial exposure, the inhaled antigens are processed by lymphocytes that produce IgE, an antigen-specific antibody that binds to mast cells. With later exposures, the IgE interacts with inhaled antigens and triggers the breakdown of the mast cell.

4. In people with allergies, mast cells and basophils are increased in both number and reactivity. Therefore, these cells may be capable of releasing large amounts of histamine and other mediators.

5. Allergic rhinitis that is not effectively treated may lead to chronic fatigue, impaired ability to perform usual activities of daily living, difficulty sleeping, sinus infections, postnasal drip, cough, and headache. In addition, this condition is a strong risk factor for asthma.

SECTION IV: PRACTICING FOR NCLEX

1. b. *Rationale:* For children with allergies, provide all family members, daycare, and school personnel with an emergency plan.
2. medical alert
3. a. *Rationale:* Azelastine (Astelin) is the only antihistamine formulated as a nasal spray for topical use.
4. d. *Rationale:* Second-generation H_1 antagonists cause less CNS depression because they are selective for peripheral H_1 receptors and do not cross the blood–brain barrier.
5. c. *Rationale:* First-generation antihistamines have substantial anticholinergic effects; therefore, they may cause dry mouth, urinary retention, constipation, and blurred vision.
6. c. *Rationale:* First-generation antihistamines (e.g., diphenhydramine) may cause drowsiness and decreased mental alertness in children as in adults.
7. a, b, and c. *Rationale:* Some food allergens such as shellfish, egg, milk, peanut, and tree nuts have a higher inherent risk for triggering anaphylaxis than others.
8. d. *Rationale:* Allergic rhinitis is inflammation of nasal mucosa caused by a type I hypersensitivity reaction to inhaled allergens.
9. tissue
10. a. *Rationale:* A first-generation antihistamine may cause drowsiness and safety hazards in the environment (e.g., operating a car or other potentially hazardous machinery). In most people, tolerance develops to the sedative effects within a few days if they are not taking other sedative-type drugs or alcoholic beverages.
11. d. *Rationale:* Diphenhydramine may be given by injection, usually as a single dose, to a patient who is having a blood transfusion or a diagnostic test, to prevent allergic reactions. Hydroxyzine or promethazine may be given by injection for nausea and vomiting or to provide sedation, but they are not usually the first drugs of choice for these indications.
12. c. *Rationale:* Clients with hepatic impairment who take promethazine should be aware that cholestatic jaundice has been reported and the drug should be used with caution.
13. a. *Rationale:* The dosing interval of diphenhydramine should be extended to 12 to 18 hours in patients with severe kidney failure.

14. a. *Rationale:* Second-generation antihistamines should be used for older adults. They are much safer because they do not impair consciousness, thinking, or ability to perform activities of daily living (e.g., driving a car or operating various machines).
15. a and c. *Rationale:* First-generation antihistamines (e.g., diphenhydramine) may cause confusion (with impaired thinking, judgment, and memory), dizziness, hypotension, sedation, syncope, unsteady gait, and paradoxical CNS stimulation in older adults.
16. a and d. *Rationale:* First-generation antihistamines (e.g., diphenhydramine) may cause drowsiness and decreased mental alertness in children as in adults. Young children may experience paradoxical excitement. These reactions may occur with therapeutic dosages. In overdosage, hallucinations, convulsions, and death may occur. Close supervision and appropriate dosages are required for safe drug usage in children.
17. b. *Rationale:* For treatment of the common cold, studies have demonstrated that antihistamines do not relieve symptoms and are not recommended. However, an antihistamine is often included in prescription and OTC combination products for the common cold.
18. c. *Rationale:* For chronic allergic symptoms (e.g., allergic rhinitis), long-acting preparations provide more consistent relief. A patient may respond better to one antihistamine than to another. Therefore, if one antihistamine does not relieve symptoms or produces excessive sedation, another may be effective.
19. short
20. second

Chapter 46: Nasal Decongestants, Antitussives, and Cold Remedies

SECTION II: ASSESSING YOUR UNDERSTANDING

ACTIVITY A
FILL IN THE BLANKS
1. common cold
2. rhinoviruses
3. Sinusitis
4. Rhinitis
5. Nasal congestion

ACTIVITY B
MATCHING
1. E   2. D   3. A   4. C   5. B

ACTIVITY C
SHORT ANSWERS
1. Colds can be caused by many types of virus, most often the rhinoviruses. Shedding of these viruses by infected people, mainly from nasal mucosa, can result in rapid spread to other people. The viruses can enter the body through mucous membranes. Cold viruses can survive for several hours on the skin and on hard surfaces such as wood or plastic. There may also be airborne spread from sneezing and coughing, but this source is considered secondary. After the viruses gain entry, the incubation period is usually 5 days, the most contagious period is about 3 days after symptoms begin, and the cold usually lasts about 7 days.
2. Sinusitis is inflammation of the paranasal sinuses, air cells that connect with the nasal cavity and are lined by similar mucosa. As in other parts of the respiratory tract, ciliated

mucous membranes help move fluid and microorganisms out of the sinuses and into the nasal cavity. This movement becomes impaired when sinus openings are blocked by nasal swelling, and the impairment is considered a major cause of sinus infections. Another contributing factor is a lower oxygen content in the sinuses, which aids the growth of microorganisms and impairs local defense mechanisms.

3. Rhinorrhea is defined as the secretions discharged from the nose.

4. Rhinitis is defined as inflammation of nasal mucosa and is usually accompanied by nasal congestion, rhinorrhea, and sneezing.

5. Cough is a forceful expulsion of air from the lungs. It is normally a protective reflex for removing foreign bodies, environmental irritants, or accumulated secretions from the respiratory tract.

SECTION III: APPLYING YOUR KNOWLEDGE

ACTIVITY D

CASE STUDIES

1. Many combination products are available for treating symptoms of the common cold. Many of the products contain an antihistamine, a nasal decongestant, and an analgesic. Some contain antitussives, expectorants, and other agents as well. Many cold remedies are over-the-counter (OTC) formulations. Commonly used ingredients include chlorpheniramine (antihistamine), pseudoephedrine (adrenergic nasal decongestant), acetaminophen (analgesic and antipyretic), dextromethorphan (antitussive), and guaifenesin (expectorant).

2. Although antihistamines are popular OTC drugs because they dry nasal secretions, they are not recommended because they can also dry lower respiratory secretions and worsen secretion retention and cough. Allergy remedies contain an antihistamine; "nondrowsy" or "daytime" formulas contain a nasal decongestant but do not contain an antihistamine; "PM" or "night" formulas contain a sedating antihistamine to promote sleep. Pain, fever, and multisymptom formulas usually contain acetaminophen; the term "maximum strength" usually refers only to the amount of acetaminophen per dose, usually 1000 milligrams for adults.

3. The use of OTC products containing pseudoephedrine to manufacture methamphetamine has increased at an alarming rate. Most states have passed laws placing these products behind pharmacy counters to restrict sales. Mrs. Hoyer would have to ask the pharmacist for the drug.

4. Many products come in several formulations, with different ingredients, and are advertised for different purposes (e.g., allergy, sinus disorders, multisymptom cold and flu remedies). In addition, labels on OTC combination products list ingredients by generic name, without identifying the type of drug. As a result of these bewildering products, consumers, including nurses and other health care providers, may not know what medications they are taking or whether some drugs increase or block the effects of other drugs.

5. The use of antivirals agents for cold treatment has increased in popularity. Oseltamivir (Tamiflu) limits spread of virus within the respiratory tract and may also prevent virus penetration of respiratory secretions to initiate replication. Oseltamivir has activity against influenza A and B. Although the drug was effective in treating community-acquired colds caused by rhinoviruses in two placebo-controlled trials, there is not sufficient evidence to support its use in viral upper respiratory tract infections.

SECTION IV: PRACTICING FOR NCLEX

1. b. *Rationale:* Several OTC cough and cold medicines for use in infants have been recalled voluntarily due to concerns about possible misuse that could result in overdoses.

2. d. *Rationale:* There is limited or no support for the use of dietary or herbal supplements to prevent or treat symptoms of the common cold.

3. a, b, and c. *Rationale:* First-generation antihistamines (e.g., chlorpheniramine, diphenhydramine) have anticholinergic effects that may reduce sneezing, rhinorrhea, and cough.

4. c. *Rationale:* Rebound nasal swelling can occur with excessive or extended use of nasal sprays.

5. b, c, and d. *Rationale:* An adequate fluid intake, humidification of the environment, and sucking on hard candy or throat lozenges can help relieve mouth dryness and cough.

6. d. *Rationale:* Nonrespiratory conditions that predispose to secretion retention include immobility, debilitation, cigarette smoking, and postoperative status.

7. c. *Rationale:* Retention of secretions commonly occurs with influenza, pneumonia, upper respiratory infections, acute and chronic bronchitis, emphysema, and acute attacks of asthma.

8. a. *Rationale:* Most upper respiratory infections are viral in origin, and antibiotics are not generally recommended.

9. b. *Rationale:* Before recommending a particular product, the nurse needs to assess the intended recipient for conditions or other medications that contraindicate the product's use.

10. b and c. *Rationale:* A major consideration is that older adults are at high risk of adverse effects from oral nasal decongestants (e.g., hypertension, cardiac dysrhythmias, nervousness, insomnia).

11. b. *Rationale:* Parents often administer a medication (e.g., acetaminophen, ibuprofen) for pain and fever when a child has cold symptoms, whether the child has pain and fever or not. Some pediatricians suggest treating fevers higher than 101 degrees if the child seems uncomfortable but not to treat them otherwise. Parents may need to be counseled that fever is part of the body's defense mechanism and may help the child recover from an infection.

12. c. *Rationale:* Nasal congestion may interfere with an infant's ability to nurse. Phenylephrine nasal solution, applied just before feeding time, is usually effective.

13. a. *Rationale:* Excessive amounts or too-frequent administration of topical agents (i.e. phenylephrine) may result in rebound nasal congestion and systemic effects of cardiac and central nervous system stimulation. Therefore, the drug should be given to infants only when recommended by a pediatric specialist.

14. d. *Rationale:* For sore throat, a throat culture for streptococcal organisms should be performed and the results obtained before an antibiotic is prescribed.

15. b. *Rationale:* Single-drug formulations allow flexibility and individualization of dosage, whereas combination products may contain unneeded ingredients and are more expensive. However, many people find combination products more convenient to use.

16. c. *Rationale:* With nasal decongestants, topical preparations (i.e., nasal solutions or sprays) are often preferred for short-term use. They are rapidly effective because they come into direct contact with nasal mucosa.

17. a. *Rationale:* Antihistamines are clearly useful in allergic conditions, but their use to relieve cold symptoms is controversial. First-generation antihistamines (e.g., chlorpheniramine, diphenhydramine) have anticholinergic effects that may reduce sneezing, rhinorrhea, and cough. Also, their sedative effects may aid sleep. Many multi-ingredient cold remedies contain an antihistamine.
18. postnasal drainage
19. c. *Rationale:* Cough syrups serve as vehicles for antitussive drugs and may exert antitussive effects of their own by soothing irritated pharyngeal mucosa.
20. Cromolyn

Chapter 47: Physiology of the Cardiovascular System

SECTION II: ASSESSING YOUR UNDERSTANDING

ACTIVITY A
FILL IN THE BLANKS
1. blood
2. antibodies
3. patency
4. two-sided
5. atria

ACTIVITY B
MATCHING
1. B 2. D 3. A 4. E 5. C

ACTIVITY C
SHORT ANSWERS
1. The heart has four chambers: two atria and two ventricles. The *atria* are receiving chambers. The right atrium receives deoxygenated blood from the upper part of the body by way of the superior vena cava; from the lower part of the body by way of the inferior vena cava; and from veins and sinuses within the heart itself. The left atrium receives oxygenated blood from the lungs through the pulmonary veins.
2. The *ventricles* are distributing chambers. The right ventricle sends deoxygenated blood through the pulmonary circulation. It is small and thin walled because it contracts against minimal pressure. The left ventricle pumps oxygenated blood through the systemic circuit. It is much more muscular and thick walled because it contracts against relatively high pressure.
3. The right atrium and right ventricle form one pump, and the left atrium and left ventricle form another. A muscular wall called the *septum* separates the right and left sides of the heart.
4. The myocardium is the strong muscular layer of the heart that provides the pumping power for circulation of blood.
5. The epicardium is the outer, serous layer of the heart. The heart is enclosed in a fibroserous sac called the *pericardium*.

SECTION III: APPLYING YOUR KNOWLEDGE

ACTIVITY D
CASE STUDIES
1. The heart contains special cells that can carry electrical impulses much more rapidly than ordinary muscle fibers. This special conduction system consists of the sinoatrial (SA) node, the atrioventricular node, bundle of His, the right and left bundle branches, and the Purkinje fibers.
2. The SA node, the normal pacemaker of the heart, generates a burst of electrical energy approximately 60 to 100 times each minute under normal circumstances. The electrical current flows over the heart in an orderly way to produce contraction of both atria, then both ventricles. A unique characteristic of the heart is that any cell in any chamber can generate its own electrical impulse to contract.
3. The ventricles can beat independently, but at a rate of less than 40 beats per minute. This provides a backup mechanism should the SA node fail to fire, with an inherent rate that does not compete with SA node firing.
4. The autonomic nervous system does influence heart rate. Sympathetic nerves increase heart rate (through the release of epinephrine and norepinephrine); parasympathetic nerves (by way of the vagus nerve) decrease heart rate.

SECTION IV: PRACTICING FOR NCLEX
1. a. *Rationale:* The goal of drug therapy in cardiovascular disorders is to restore homeostasis or physiologic balance between opposing factors.
2. a, b, and c. *Rationale:* Cardiovascular drugs may be given to increase or decrease cardiac output, blood pressure, and heart rate; to alter heart rhythm; to increase or decrease blood clotting; to alter the quality of blood; and to decrease chest pain of cardiac origin.
3. c and d. *Rationale:* Cardiovascular disorders usually managed with drug therapy include atherosclerosis, heart failure, cardiac dysrhythmias, ischemia, myocardial infarction, hypertension, hypotension, and shock. Peripheral vascular disease and valvular disease are usually managed surgically.
4. circulatory
5. endothelial cells
6. b. *Rationale:* Dysfunctional endothelium is considered a major factor in atherosclerosis, acute coronary syndromes (symptomatic myocardial ischemia, asymptomatic myocardial infarction [MI], and MI with or without ST-segment elevation), hypertension, and thromboembolic disorders.
7. a. *Rationale:* Pathologic changes in the structure of the capillary and venular endothelium also result in the accumulation of excess fluid in interstitial space (edema), a common symptom of cardiovascular and other disorders.
8. b. *Rationale:* Platelets are essential for blood coagulation.
9. nucleus
10. d. *Rationale:* The main cause of endothelial dysfunction is injury to the blood vessel wall from trauma or disease processes.
11. hemoglobin
12. c. *Rationale:* Serum albumin, which helps maintain blood volume by exerting colloid osmotic pressure.
13. b and c. *Rationale:* Blood functions to nourish and oxygenate body cells, protect the body from invading microorganisms, and initiate hemostasis when a blood vessel is injured.
14. b. *Rationale:* Blood transports absorbed food products from the gastrointestinal tract to tissues; at the same time, it carries metabolic wastes from tissues to the kidneys, skin, and lungs for excretion.
15. d. *Rationale:* Blood transports leukocytes and antibodies to sites of injury, infection, and inflammation.
16. b. *Rationale:* Blood vessel walls are composed of two types of cells, smooth muscle cells and endothelial cells.
17. a. *Rationale:* The intima, or inner lining, is composed of a layer of endothelial cells next to the blood (to provide a smooth surface for blood circulation) and an elastic layer that joins the media.
18. b. *Rationale:* Coronary arteries originate at the base of the aorta in the aortic cusps and fill during diastole, the resting or filling phase of the cardiac cycle
19. pulmonic
20. aortic

Chapter 48: Drug Therapy for Heart Failure

SECTION II: ASSESSING YOUR UNDERSTANDING

ACTIVITY A
FILL IN THE BLANKS
1. Heart failure
2. systolic dysfunction
3. diastolic dysfunction
4. fluid accumulation
5. heart failure

ACTIVITY B
MATCHING
1. D   2. A   3. B   4. E   5. C

ACTIVITY C
SHORT ANSWERS
1. At the cellular level, HF stems from dysfunction of contractile myocardial cells and the endothelial cells that line the heart and blood vessels (see Chapter 47). Vital functions of the endothelium include maintaining equilibrium between vasodilation and vasoconstriction, coagulation and anticoagulation, and cellular growth promotion and inhibition. Endothelial dysfunction allows processes that narrow the blood vessel lumen (e.g., buildup of atherosclerotic plaque, growth of cells, inflammation, activation of platelets) and leads to blood-clot formation and vasoconstriction that further narrow the blood vessel lumen. These are major factors in coronary artery disease and hypertension, the most common conditions leading to HF.
2. As the heart fails, the low cardiac output and inadequately filled arteries activate the neurohormonal system by several feedback mechanisms. One mechanism is increased sympathetic activity and circulating *catecholamines* (neurohormones), which increases the force of myocardial contraction, increases heart rate, and causes vasoconstriction. The effects of the baroreceptors in the aortic arch and carotid sinus that normally inhibit undue sympathetic stimulation are blunted in patients with HF, and the effects of the high levels of circulating catecholamines are intensified. Endothelin, a neurohormone secreted primarily by endothelial cells, is the most potent endogenous vasoconstrictor and may exert direct toxic effects on the heart and result in myocardial cell proliferation.
3. Cardinal manifestations of HF are dyspnea and fatigue, which can lead to exercise intolerance and fluid retention resulting in pulmonary congestion and peripheral edema. Patients with compensated (asymptomatic) HF usually have no symptoms at rest and no edema; dyspnea and fatigue occur only with activities involving moderate or higher levels of exertion. Symptoms that occur with minimal exertion or at rest and are accompanied by ankle edema and distention of the jugular vein (from congestion of veins and leakage of fluid into tissues) reflect decompensation (symptomatic HF). Acute, severe cardiac decompensation is manifested by pulmonary edema, a medical emergency that requires immediate treatment. Two models currently exist for classification of HF. The New York Heart Association (NYHA) classifies HF based on functional limitations. A newer system of staging HF, proposed by the American College of Cardiology (ACC) and the American Heart Association (AHA), is based on the progression of HF.

4. Renin is an enzyme produced in the kidneys in response to impaired blood flow and tissue perfusion. When released into the bloodstream, renin stimulates the production of angiotensin II, a powerful vasoconstrictor. Arterial vasoconstriction impairs cardiac function by increasing the resistance (afterload) against which the ventricle ejects blood. This raises filling pressures inside the heart, increases stretch and stress on the myocardial wall, and predisposes to subendocardial ischemia. In addition, patients with severe HF have constricted arterioles in cerebral, myocardial, renal, hepatic, and mesenteric vascular beds. This results in increased organ hypoperfusion and dysfunction. Venous vasoconstriction limits venous capacitance, resulting in venous congestion and increased diastolic ventricular filling pressures (preload). Angiotensin II also promotes sodium and water retention by stimulating aldosterone release from the adrenal cortex and the release of vasopressin (antidiuretic hormone) from the posterior pituitary gland.
5. Increased blood volume and pressure in the heart chambers; stretching of muscle fibers; and dilation, hypertrophy, and changes in the shape of the heart (a process called *cardiac or ventricular remodeling*) make it contract less efficiently.

SECTION III: APPLYING YOUR KNOWLEDGE

ACTIVITY D
CASE STUDIES
1. Food may decrease digoxin absorption, so she should take it on an empty stomach. In addition to drug dosage forms, other factors that may decrease digoxin absorption include the presence of food in the GI tract, delayed gastric emptying, malabsorption syndromes, and concurrent administration of some drugs (e.g., antacids, cholestyramine).
2. When digoxin is given orally, absorption varies among available preparations. Lanoxicaps, which are liquid-filled capsules, and the elixir used for children are better absorbed than tablets. With tablets, the most frequently used formulation, differences in bioavailability are also important, because a person who is stabilized on one formulation may be underdosed or overdosed if another formulation is taken. Differences are attributed to the rate and extent of tablet dissolution rather than amounts of digoxin.
3. The physician will decrease the digoxin dose. Therapeutic serum levels of digoxin are 0.5 to 2 nanograms per milliliter (ng/mL); serum levels greater than 2 ng/mL are toxic. In elderly patients and in the presence of renal failure, therapeutic serum levels are 0.5 to 1.3 ng/mL. Research in the past decade has suggested that serum levels of 1.0 ng/mL or less are more appropriate in those with HF (see "Bridging the Gap with EBP"). However, toxicity may occur at virtually any serum level. Dosage must be reduced in the presence of renal failure to prevent drug accumulation and toxicity, because most of the digoxin (60% to 70%) is excreted unchanged by the kidneys. The remainder is metabolized or excreted by nonrenal routes.
4. In patients with atrial dysrhythmias, digoxin slows the rate of ventricular contraction (negative chronotropic effect). With IV digoxin, the onset of action occurs within 10 to 30 minutes, and peak effects occur in 1 to 5 hours. Digoxin is given orally or intravenously. Although it can be given intramuscularly, this route is not recommended, because pain and muscle necrosis may occur at injection sites. When digoxin is given orally, the onset of action occurs in 30 minutes to 2 hours, and peak effects occur in approximately 6 hours.

SECTION IV: PRACTICING FOR NCLEX

1. d. *Rationale:* The normal digoxin level is 0.5 to 2.0 ng/mL. Serum levels greater than 2 ng/mL are toxic; however, toxicity may occur at any serum level.
2. Digitalis
3. b. *Rationale:* For acute HF, the first drugs of choice may include an IV loop diuretic, a cardiotonic–inotropic agent (e.g., digoxin, dobutamine, milrinone), and vasodilators (e.g., nitroglycerin and hydralazine or nitroprusside).
4. c. *Rationale:* Beta-blockers are not recommended for patients in acute HF because of the potential for an initial decrease in myocardial contractility.
5. c. *Rationale:* Cardinal manifestations of HF are dyspnea and fatigue, which can lead to exercise intolerance and fluid retention resulting in pulmonary congestion and peripheral edema.
6. hypertension
7. a, b, and c. *Rationale:* Heart failure may result from impaired myocardial contraction during systole (systolic dysfunction), impaired relaxation and filling of ventricles during diastole (diastolic dysfunction), or a combination of systolic and diastolic dysfunction.
8. a. *Rationale:* Natural licorice blocks the effects of spironolactone and causes sodium retention and potassium loss, effects that may worsen HF and potentiate the effects of digoxin.
9. a. *Rationale:* When patients are receiving a combination of drugs for management of HF, the nurse needs to assist them in understanding that the different types of drugs have different actions and produce different responses. As a result, they work together to be more effective and maintain a more balanced state of cardiovascular function. Changing drugs or dosages can upset the balance and lead to acute and severe symptoms that may require hospitalization or may even cause death from HF. Therefore, it is extremely important that patients take all their medications as prescribed. If they are unable to take the medications for any reason, patients or caregivers should notify the prescribing health care provider. They should be instructed not to wait until symptoms become severe before seeking care.
10. d. *Rationale:* Hepatic impairment has little effect on digoxin clearance, and no dosage adjustments are needed
11. c. *Rationale:* Digoxin should be used cautiously, in reduced dosages, because renal impairment delays its excretion. Both loading and maintenance doses should be reduced. Patients with advanced renal impairment can achieve therapeutic serum concentrations with a dosage of 0.125 mg three to five times per week.
12. b. *Rationale:* Digoxin is commonly used in children for the same indications as for adults and should be prescribed or supervised by a pediatric cardiologist when possible. The response to a given dose varies with age, size, and renal and hepatic function. There may be little difference between a therapeutic dose and a toxic dose. Very small amounts are often given to children. These factors increase the risks of dosage errors in children. In a hospital setting, institutional policies may require that each dose be verified by another nurse before it is administered. Liquid digoxin must be precisely measured in a syringe, and the dose should not be rounded. ECG monitoring is desirable when digoxin therapy is started.
13. Digoxin immune Fab
14. a. *Rationale:* Atropine or isoproterenol, used in the management of bradycardia or conduction defects, may be administered to clients with digoxin toxicity.

15. c. *Rationale:* Digoxin dosages must be interpreted with consideration of specific patient characteristics, including age, weight, gender, renal function, general health state, and concurrent drug therapy. Loading or digitalizing doses are necessary for initiating therapy, because digoxin's long half-life make therapeutic serum levels difficult to obtain without loading. Loading doses should be used cautiously in patients who have taken digoxin within the previous 2 or 3 weeks.
16. b. *Rationale:* In chronic HF, hypokalemia may be less likely to occur because lower doses of potassium-losing diuretics are usually being given. In addition, there may be more extensive use of potassium-sparing diuretics (e.g., amiloride, triamterene) and the aldosterone antagonist, spironolactone.
17. diuretic
18. vasodilators
19. b. *Rationale:* For patients who are obese, weight loss is desirable to decrease systemic vascular resistance and myocardial oxygen demand.
20. a, c, and d. *Rationale:* Administer oxygen, if needed, to relieve dyspnea, improve oxygen delivery, reduce the work of breathing, and decrease constriction of pulmonary blood vessels (which is a compensatory measure in patients with hypoxemia).

Chapter 49: Antidysrhythmic Drugs

SECTION II: ASSESSING YOUR UNDERSTANDING

ACTIVITY A
FILL IN THE BLANKS
1. Dysrhythmias
2. contractile
3. Automaticity
4. calcium
5. excitability

ACTIVITY B
MATCHING
1. D   2. A   3. E   4. B   5. C

ACTIVITY C
SHORT ANSWERS
1. The heart is an electrical pump. Its "electrical" activity resides primarily in the specialized tissues that can generate and conduct an electrical impulse. Although impulses are also conducted through muscle cells, the rate is much slower. The mechanical or "pump" activity resides in contractile tissue. Normally, these activities result in effective cardiac contraction and distribution of blood throughout the body. Heart beats occur at regular intervals and consist of four events: *stimulation* from an electrical impulse, *transmission* of the electrical impulse to adjacent conductive or contractile tissue, *contraction* of atria and then ventricles, and *relaxation* of atria and then ventricles.
2. Automaticity is the heart's ability to generate an electrical impulse. Any part of the conduction system can spontaneously start an impulse, but the sinoatrial (SA) node normally has the fastest rate of automaticity and therefore the fastest rate of spontaneous impulse formation. Because it has a faster rate of electrical discharge or depolarization than other parts of the conduction system, the SA node serves as the pacemaker site.

3. The ability of a cardiac muscle cell to respond to an electrical stimulus is called *excitability*. The stimulus must reach a certain threshold to cause contraction. After contraction, sodium and calcium ions return to the extracellular space, potassium ions return to the intracellular space, muscle relaxation occurs, and the cell prepares for the next electrical stimulus followed by contraction.
4. After a contraction, there is also a period of decreased excitability (called the *absolute refractory period*) during which the cell cannot respond to a new stimulus. Before the resting membrane potential is reached, a stimulus greater than normal can evoke a response in the cell. This period is called the *relative refractory period*.
5. Conductivity is the ability of cardiac tissue to transmit electrical impulses. The orderly, rhythmic transmission of impulses to all cells is needed for effective myocardial contraction.

SECTION III: APPLYING YOUR KNOWLEDGE

ACTIVITY D
CASE STUDIES
1. Lidocaine decreases myocardial irritability (automaticity) in the ventricles. Lidocaine has little effect on atrial tissue and therefore is not useful in treating atrial dysrhythmias.
2. A bolus dose has a rapid onset and a short duration of action. After intravenous (IV) administration of a bolus dose of lidocaine, therapeutic effects occur within 1 to 2 minutes and last approximately 10 to 20 minutes. This characteristic is advantageous in emergency management but limits lidocaine use to intensive care settings.
3. The physician would decrease the dosage of the lidocaine in an alcoholic patient or in a patient with liver damage. Lidocaine is metabolized in the liver, so the dosage must be reduced in patients with hepatic insufficiency or right-sided heart failure to avoid drug accumulation and toxicity. Hives, as well as shortness of breath, are signs of an allergic reaction. Lidocaine is contraindicated for such a patient.
4. With a lidocaine serum level of 0.75 mcg/mL, the patient has achieved a subtherapeutic level of the drug. Therapeutic serum levels of lidocaine are 1.5 to 6 mcg/mL. Toxic serum levels are those greater than 6 mcg/mL.

SECTION IV: PRACTICING FOR NCLEX
1. d. *Rationale:* The FDA has issued a black box warning for amiodarone recommending that it be used only in patients with life-threatening dysrhythmias due to the risk of developing potentially fatal pulmonary toxicity.
2. a and d. *Rationale:* Amiodarone is a potassium channel blocker that prolongs conduction in all cardiac tissues and decreases heart rate; it also decreases contractility of the left ventricle.
3. prodysrhythmic
4. a and d. *Rationale:* As Class IV drugs, diltiazem and verapamil are the only calcium channel blockers approved for management of dysrhythmias.
5. a. *Rationale:* Class II beta-adrenergic blockers are being used more extensively because of their effectiveness in reducing mortality after myocardial infarction and in patients with heart failure.
6. d. *Rationale:* Flecainide, propafenone, and moricizine are class 1C drugs that have no effect on the repolarization phase but greatly decrease conduction in the ventricles.

7. a, b, and c. *Rationale:* Lidocaine is the prototype of class IB antidysrhythmics used for treating serious ventricular dysrhythmias associated with acute myocardial infarction, cardiac catheterization, or cardiac surgery and digitalis-induced ventricular dysrhythmias.
8. a and c. *Rationale:* Quinidine, the prototype of class IA antidysrhythmics, reduces automaticity, slows conduction, and prolongs the refractory period. Phenytoin may be used to treat dysrhythmias produced by digoxin intoxication.
9. sodium, calcium
10. Atrial fibrillation
11. c. *Rationale:* Patients receiving chronic antidysrhythmic drug therapy are likely to have significant cardiovascular disease. With each visit, the home care nurse needs to assess the patient's physical, mental, and functional status and evaluate pulse and blood pressure. In addition, patients and caregivers should be taught to report symptoms (e.g., dizziness or fainting, chest pain) and to avoid over-the-counter agents unless discussed with a healthcare provider.
12. c. *Rationale:* Because serious problems may stem from either dysrhythmias or their treatment, healthcare providers should be adept in preventing, recognizing, and treating conditions that predispose to the development of serious dysrhythmias (e.g., electrolyte imbalances, hypoxia). If dysrhythmias cannot be prevented, early recognition and treatment are needed.
13. c. *Rationale:* Dosages of digoxin, disopyramide, propafenone, and quinidine should be reduced in patients with impairment of hepatic function.
14. a, b, and c. *Rationale:* Antidysrhythmic drug therapy in patients with renal impairment should be very cautious, with close monitoring of drug effects (e.g., plasma drug levels, ECG changes, symptoms that may indicate drug toxicity).
15. a. *Rationale:* Cardiac dysrhythmias are common in older adults, but in general only those causing symptoms of circulatory impairment should be treated with antidysrhythmic drugs.
16. Prodysrhythmia
17. Propranolol
18. d. *Rationale:* Adenosine is administered like the adult dosing for children over 50 kg. For children weighing less than 50 kg, initially 0.1 mg/kg IV push is given, with a maximum dose administration of 6 mg. If this initial dose if ineffective, a repeat dose of 0.2 mg/kg up to the maximum of 12 mg, may be administered by IV push.
19. c. *Rationale:* Low-dose amiodarone is a pharmacologic choice for preventing recurrent A-Fib after electrical or pharmacologic conversion. The low doses cause fewer adverse effects than the higher ones used for life-threatening ventricular dysrhythmias.
20. a and b. *Rationale:* Nonpharmacologic management is preferred, at least initially, for several dysrhythmias. For example, sinus tachycardia usually results from such disorders as dehydration, fever, infection, or hypotension, and intervention and management should attempt to relieve the underlying cause. For PSVT with mild or moderate symptoms, Valsalva's maneuver, carotid sinus massage, or other measures to increase vagal tone are preferred.

Chapter 50: Antianginal Drugs

SECTION II: ASSESSING YOUR UNDERSTANDING

ACTIVITY A
FILL IN THE BLANKS
1. Angina pectoris
2. myocardial
3. vasospasm
4. coronary artery disease (CAD)
5. variant

ACTIVITY B
MATCHING
1. C   2. A   3. E   4. B   5. D

ACTIVITY C
SHORT ANSWERS
1. Classic anginal pain is usually described as substernal chest pain of a constricting, squeezing, or suffocating nature. It may radiate to the jaw, neck, or shoulder; down the left or both arms; or to the back. The discomfort is sometimes mistaken for arthritis or for indigestion, because the pain may be associated with nausea, vomiting, dizziness, diaphoresis, shortness of breath, or fear of impending doom. The discomfort is usually brief, typically lasting 5 minutes or less until the balance of oxygen supply and demand is restored.
2. Current research indicates that gender differences exist in the type and quality of cardiac symptoms, with women reporting epigastric or back discomfort.
3. Older adults may have atypical symptoms of CAD and may experience "silent" ischemia that may delay them from seeking professional help.
4. Atherosclerosis begins with accumulation of lipid-filled macrophages (i.e., foam cells) on the inner lining of coronary arteries. Foam cells, which promote growth of atherosclerotic plaque, develop in response to elevated blood cholesterol levels. These early lesions progress to fibrous plaques containing foam cells covered by smooth muscle cells and connective tissue. Advanced lesions also contain hemorrhages, ulcerations, and scar tissue. Factors contributing to plaque development and growth include endothelial injury, lipid infiltration (i.e., cholesterol), recruitment of inflammatory cells (mainly monocytes and T lymphocytes), and smooth muscle cell proliferation. Endothelial injury may be the initiating factor in plaque formation, because it allows monocytes, platelets, cholesterol, and other blood components to come in contact with and stimulate abnormal growth of smooth muscle cells and connective tissue in the arterial wall.
5. Myocardial ischemia occurs when the coronary arteries are unable to provide sufficient blood and oxygen for normal cardiac functions. Also known as *ischemic heart disease, CAD,* or *coronary heart disease,* myocardial ischemia may manifest as an acute coronary syndrome with three main consequences. One consequence is unstable angina, with the occurrence of pain (symptomatic myocardial ischemia).

SECTION III: APPLYING YOUR KNOWLEDGE

ACTIVITY D
CASE STUDIES
CASE STUDY 1
1. Mrs. Smith is at risk for metabolic syndrome. *The Third Report of the National Cholesterol Education Program Expert Panel on Detection, Evaluation, and Treatment of High Blood Cholesterol in Adults* (NCEP III) defines metabolic syndrome as a cluster several cardiovascular risk factors linked with obesity: elevated waist circumference, elevated triglycerides, reduced high-density lipoprotein cholesterol, elevated blood pressure, and elevated fasting glucose.
2. Smoking cessation is a good place for this patient to start. Patients should avoid circumstances known to precipitate acute attacks, and those who smoke should stop.

CASE STUDY 2
1. Organic nitrates relax smooth muscle in blood vessel walls. This action produces vasodilation, which relieves anginal pain by several mechanisms. First, dilation of veins reduces venous pressure and venous return to the heart. This decreases blood volume and pressure within the heart (preload), which in turn decreases cardiac workload and oxygen demand. Second, nitrates dilate coronary arteries at higher doses and can increase blood flow to ischemic areas of the myocardium. Third, nitrates dilate the arterioles, which lowers peripheral vascular resistance (afterload). This results in lower systolic blood pressure and, consequently, reduced cardiac workload.
2. When given sublingually, nitroglycerin is absorbed directly into the systemic circulation. It acts within 1 to 3 minutes, and its effects last for 30 to 60 minutes. Contraindications include hypersensitivity reactions, severe anemia, hypotension, and hypovolemia. The drugs should be used cautiously in the presence of head injury or cerebral hemorrhage because they may increase intracranial pressure.
3. Males taking nitroglycerin or any other nitrate should not take phosphodiesterase enzyme type 5 inhibitors such as sildenafil (Viagra) and vardenafil (Levitra) for erectile dysfunction. Nitrates and phosphodiesterase enzyme type 5 inhibitors decrease blood pressure, and the combined effect can produce profound, life-threatening hypotension.

SECTION IV: PRACTICING FOR NCLEX
1. b. *Rationale:* Starting with relatively small doses of antianginal drugs and increasing them at appropriate intervals as necessary should achieve optimal benefit and minimal adverse effects.
2. c. *Rationale:* Aspirin, antilipemics, and antihypertensives are used in conjunction with antianginal drugs to prevent progression of myocardial ischemia to MI.
3. c. *Rationale:* In angina pectoris, calcium channel blockers improve blood supply to the myocardium by dilating coronary arteries and decrease the workload of the heart by dilating peripheral arteries; in variant angina, the drugs reduce coronary artery vasospasm.
4. b. *Rationale:* Patients who take long-acting dosage forms of nitrates on a regular schedule develop tolerance to the vasodilating (antianginal) effects of the drug.
5. a. *Rationale:* Traditional antianginal drugs that act via hemodynamic mechanisms (e.g., beta-blockers, calcium antagonists, nitrates) can pose a problem in older adults because of the associated higher risk of drug interactions and greater incidence of adverse drug effects.
6. d. *Rationale:* Beta-blockers are more effective than nitrates or calcium channel blockers in decreasing the likelihood of silent ischemia and improving the mortality rate after transmural MI.
7. nitrates
8. b, c, and d *Rationale:* Because oral nitroglycerin is rapidly metabolized in the liver, relatively small proportions reach systemic circulation; transmucosal, transdermal, and IV preparations are more effective.

9. a, c, and d. *Rationale:* The goals of antianginal drug therapy are to relieve acute anginal pain, to reduce the number and severity of acute anginal attacks, to improve exercise tolerance and quality of life, to delay progression of CAD, to prevent MI, and to prevent sudden cardiac death.

10. a. *Rationale:* Angina pectoris results from deficit in myocardial oxygen supply (myocardial ischemia) in relation to myocardial oxygen demand, most often caused by atherosclerotic plaque in the coronary arteries.

11. a, b, and d. *Rationale:* The home care nurse's responsibilities may include monitoring the patient's response to antianginal medications; teaching patients and caregivers how to use, store, and replace medications to ensure a constant supply; and discussing circumstances in which the patient should seek emergency care.

12. a. *Rationale:* In addition to reduced effectiveness, absorption of oral drugs or topical forms of nitroglycerin may be impaired in patients with extensive edema, heart failure, hypotension, or other conditions that impair blood flow to the gastrointestinal tract or skin.

13. a, b, and d. *Rationale:* Antianginal drugs have multiple cardiovascular effects and may be used alone or in combination with other cardiovascular drugs in patients with critical illness. They are probably used most often to manage severe angina, severe hypertension, or serious cardiac dysrhythmias.

14. contraindicated

15. a. *Rationale:* Nitroglycerin has been given IV for heart failure and intraoperative control of blood pressure, with the initial dose adjusted for weight and later doses titrated to response.

16. a. *Rationale:* For relief of acute angina and for prophylaxis before events that cause acute angina, nitroglycerin (sublingual tablets or translingual spray) is usually the primary drug of choice.

17. a. *Rationale:* Ranolazine (Ranexa) represents a new classification of antianginal medication, metabolic modulators, used in individuals with chronic angina. The drug is labeled for use in combination with amlodipine, beta-blockers, or nitrates. After oral administration, peak plasma concentrations are reached within 2 to 5 hours. The drug is rapidly and extensively metabolized in the liver. Because of a risk of dose-dependent QT prolongation on electrocardiogram, ranolazine is reserved for the treatment of patients with chronic angina who have not achieved a satisfactory antianginal response with traditional drugs.

18. c. *Rationale:* Propranolol, the prototype beta-blocker, is used to reduce the frequency and severity of acute attacks of angina. It is usually added to the antianginal drug regimen when nitrates do not prevent anginal episodes. It is especially useful in preventing exercise-induced tachycardia, which can precipitate anginal attacks.

19. isosorbide dinitrate

20. a. *Rationale:* Isosorbide dinitrate (Isordil) is used to reduce the frequency and severity of acute anginal episodes. When given sublingually or in chewable tablets, it acts in about 2 minutes, and its effects last 2 to 3 hours. When higher doses are given orally, more drug escapes metabolism in the liver and produces systemic effects in approximately 30 minutes. Therapeutic effects last about 4 hours after oral administration. The effective oral dose is usually determined by increasing the dose until headache occurs, indicating the maximum tolerable dose. Sustained-release capsules also are available.

Chapter 51: Drugs Used in Hypotension and Shock

SECTION II: ASSESSING YOUR UNDERSTANDING
ACTIVITY A
FILL IN THE BLANKS
1. Shock
2. Hypovolemic
3. Cardiogenic
4. Distributive
5. neurogenic

ACTIVITY B
MATCHING
1. E   2. C   3. A   4. B   5. D

ACTIVITY C
SHORT ANSWERS
1. Shock is a clinical condition of insufficient perfusion of cells and vital organs causing tissue hypoxia. Clinical symptoms depend on the degree of impaired perfusion of vital organs (e.g., brain, heart, kidneys). Common signs and symptoms include oliguria, heart failure, mental confusion, cool extremities, and coma. Most, but not all, people in shock are hypotensive.
2. An additional consequence of inadequate blood flow to tissues is that cells change from aerobic (oxygen-based) to anaerobic metabolism. Lactic acid produced by anaerobic metabolism leads to generalized metabolic acidosis and eventually to organ failure and death if blood flow is not promptly restored.
3. Anaphylactic shock is due to massive vasodilation caused by release of histamine in response to a severe allergic reaction.
4. Septic shock is due to massive vasodilation caused by release of mediators of the inflammatory process in response to overwhelming infection.
5. Neurogenic shock is due to massive vasodilation caused by a suppression of the sympathetic nervous system.

SECTION III: APPLYING YOUR KNOWLEDGE
ACTIVITY D
CASE STUDIES
1. Epinephrine is a naturally occurring catecholamine produced by the adrenal glands. At low doses, epinephrine stimulates beta receptors, which increases cardiac output by increasing the rate and force of myocardial contractility. Epinephrine causes bronchodilation. Larger doses act on alpha receptors to increase blood pressure.
2. Epinephrine is the drug of choice for management of anaphylactic shock because of its rapid onset of action and antiallergic effects. It prevents the release of histamine and other mediators that cause symptoms of anaphylaxis, thereby reversing vasodilation and bronchoconstriction. In early management of anaphylaxis, it is given subcutaneously to produce therapeutic effects within 5 to 10 minutes, with peak activity in approximately 20 minutes.
3. Epinephrine is also used to manage other kinds of shock and is usually given by continuous IV infusion. However, bolus doses may be given in emergencies, such as cardiac arrest.
4. Epinephrine may produce excessive cardiac stimulation, ventricular dysrhythmias, and reduced renal blood flow. Epinephrine has an elimination half-life of about 2 minutes and is rapidly inactivated to metabolites, which are then excreted by the kidneys.

SECTION IV: PRACTICING FOR NCLEX

1. a, b, and c. *Rationale:* The adrenergic catecholamines (dobutamine, dopamine, epinephrine, and norepinephrine) are widely used in patients with a low cardiac output that persists despite adequate fluid replacement and correction of electrolyte imbalance. Dobutamine is usually the cardiotonic agent of choice in critically ill patients.

2. a. *Rationale:* In hypotension and shock, drugs with alpha-adrenergic activity (e.g., norepinephrine, phenylephrine) are used to increase peripheral vascular resistance and raise blood pressure.

3. b. *Rationale:* For all drugs used to manage shock, blood pressure should be monitored frequently during infusion.

4. b and c. *Rationale:* The overall goal in the treatment of hypotension and shock is to maximize oxygen delivery to the tissues by maintaining vascular volume and optimal hemoglobin levels.

5. b. *Rationale:* Shock is a clinical condition of insufficient perfusion of cells and vital organs causing tissue hypoxia.

6. d. *Rationale:* Continuous invasive hemodynamic monitoring using a mixed venous oxygen pulmonary artery catheter and an arterial catheter is indicated to titrate drug dosage and monitor response to drug therapy. Close monitoring of critically ill patients is essential, because they often have multiple organ impairments and are clinically unstable.

7. c. *Rationale:* Patients should be monitored closely and drug dosage should be adjusted as symptoms warrant. However, the half-life of most adrenergic drugs are very brief, and this decreases the chance of drug accumulation in hepatically impaired patients.

8. a. *Rationale:* Older adults often have disorders such as atherosclerosis, peripheral vascular disease, and diabetes mellitus and may not demonstrate common symptoms of volume depletion (e.g., thirst, skin turgor changes). Also, when adrenergic drugs are given, the vasoconstricting effects may decrease blood flow and increase risks of tissue ischemia and thrombosis.

9. d. *Rationale:* Little information is available about adrenergic drugs for the management of hypotension and shock in children. Children who lose up to one fourth of their circulating blood volume may exhibit minimal changes in arterial blood pressure and a relatively low heart rate. In general, management is the same as for adults, with drug dosages adjusted for weight.

10. nonadrenergic

11. b and d. *Rationale:* Cardiogenic shock may be complicated by pulmonary congestion, for which diuretic drugs are indicated and IV fluids are contraindicated (except to maintain a patent IV line).

12. b. *Rationale:* Clients diagnosed with hypovolemic shock may require volume replacement to optimize the SVO_2 yet avoid hypothermia.

13. vasopressor

14. a. *Rationale:* The choice of drug depends primarily on the pathophysiology involved. For cardiogenic shock and decreased cardiac output, dobutamine is given.

15. a. *Rationale:* With severe heart failure characterized by decreased cardiac output and high peripheral vascular resistance, vasodilator drugs (e.g., nitroprusside, nitroglycerin) may be given along with the cardiotonic drugs.

16. c. *Rationale:* Norepinephrine (Levophed) is a pharmaceutical preparation of the naturally occurring catecholamine norepinephrine. It stimulates alpha-adrenergic receptors and thus increases blood pressure primarily by vasoconstriction.

17. cardiogenic

18. d. *Rationale:* Dobutamine is a synthetic catecholamine developed to provide less vascular activity than dopamine. It acts mainly on $beta_1$ receptors in the heart to increase the force of myocardial contraction with a minimal increase in heart rate.

19. increase

20. c. *Rationale:* Dobutamine has a short plasma half-life and therefore must be administered by continuous intravenous (IV) infusion. A loading dose is not required, because the drug has a rapid onset of action and reaches steady state within approximately 10 minutes.

Chapter 52: Antihypertensive Drugs

SECTION II: ASSESSING YOUR UNDERSTANDING

ACTIVITY A

FILL IN THE BLANKS

1. Arterial
2. homeostatic
3. cardiac output
4. Cardiac output
5. Stroke volume

ACTIVITY B

MATCHING

1. D   2. A   3. E   4. B   5. C

ACTIVITY C

SHORT ANSWERS

1. Autoregulation is the ability of body tissues to regulate their own blood flow. Local blood flow is regulated primarily by nutritional needs of the tissue, such as lack of oxygen or accumulation of products of cellular metabolism (e.g., carbon dioxide, lactic acid). Local tissues produce vasodilating and vasoconstricting substances to regulate local blood flow. Important tissue factors include histamine, bradykinin, serotonin, and prostaglandins.

2. Histamine is found mainly in mast cells surrounding blood vessels and is released when these tissues are injured. In some tissues, such as skeletal muscle, mast cell activity is mediated by the sympathetic nervous system (SNS) and histamine is released when SNS stimulation is blocked or withdrawn.

3. Bradykinin is released from a protein in body fluids. Kinins dilate arterioles, increase capillary permeability, and constrict venules.

4. Serotonin is released from aggregating platelets during the blood clotting process. It causes vasoconstriction and plays a major role in control of bleeding.

5. Prostaglandins are formed in response to tissue injury and include vasodilators (e.g., prostacyclin) and vasoconstrictors (e.g., thromboxane A_2).

SECTION III: APPLYING YOUR KNOWLEDGE

ACTIVITY D

CASE STUDIES

CASE STUDY 1

1. Hypertension is persistently high blood pressure that results from abnormalities in regulatory mechanisms. Hypertension is usually defined as a systolic pressure greater than 140 mm Hg or a diastolic pressure greater than 90 mm Hg on multiple blood pressure measurements.

2. Secondary hypertension may result from renal, endocrine, or central nervous system disorders or from drugs that stimulate the SNS or cause retention of sodium and water.

CASE STUDY 2
1. A systolic pressure of 140 mm Hg or greater, with a diastolic pressure lower than 90 mm Hg, is called *isolated systolic hypertension* and is more common in the elderly.
2. Hypertension profoundly alters cardiovascular function by increasing the workload of the heart and causing thickening and sclerosis of arterial walls.

SECTION IV: PRACTICING FOR NCLEX
1. a. *Rationale:* The FDA has issued a black box warning for minoxidil, because the drug can exacerbate angina and precipitate effusion (which can progress to cardiac tamponade).
2. a *Rationale:* The FDA has issued a black box warning for ACE inhibitors and ARBs during pregnancy, because their use can cause injury and even death to a developing fetus.
3. c. *Rationale:* The FDA has issued a black box warning for patients with CAD who are withdrawing from oral forms of atenolol, metoprolol, nadolol, propranolol, and timolol; abrupt withdrawal has resulted in exacerbation of angina, increased incidence of ventricular dysrhythmias, and the occurrence of MIs.
4. a, b, and c. *Rationale:* African Americans are more likely to have severe hypertension and to require multiple drugs as a result of having low circulating renin, increased salt sensitivity, and a higher incidence of obesity.
5. d. *Rationale:* In general, individuals of Asian descent with hypertension require much smaller doses of beta blockers, because they metabolize and excrete the drugs slowly.
6. b. *Rationale:* Beta-adrenergic blockers are the drugs of first choice for patients younger than 50 years of age who have high-renin hypertension, tachycardia, angina pectoris, myocardial infarction, or left ventricular hypertrophy.
7. ARBs
8. b. *Rationale:* Alpha$_1$-adrenergic receptor blocking agents should be administered at bedtime to minimize the first-dose phenomenon.
9. b. *Rationale:* Key behavioral determinants of blood pressure are related to dietary consumption of calories and salt; the prevalence of hypertension rises proportionally to average body mass index.
10. b. *Rationale:* Yohimbe, used to treat erectile dysfunction, is a central nervous system stimulant and can affect blood pressure.
11. b, c, and d. *Rationale:* Whether the patient or another member of the household is taking antihypertensive medications, the home care nurse may be helpful in teaching about the drugs, monitoring for drug effects, and promoting compliance with the prescribed regimen (pharmacologic and lifestyle modifications).
12. d. *Rationale:* There are risks with severe hypertension, there are also risks associated with lowering blood pressure excessively or too rapidly, including stroke, myocardial infarction, and acute renal failure. Therefore, the goal of management is usually to lower blood pressure over several minutes to several hours, with careful titration of drug dosage to avoid precipitous drops.
13. c. *Rationale:* Nitroglycerin is especially beneficial in patients with both severe hypertension and myocardial ischemia. The dose is titrated according to blood pressure response and may range from 5 to 100 micrograms per minute. Tolerance develops to IV nitroglycerin over 24 to 48 hours.

14. a. *Rationale:* Urgencies can be treated with oral antihypertensive agents such as captopril 25 to 50 mg every 1 to 2 hours, or clonidine 0.2 mg initially and then 0.1 mg hourly until the diastolic blood pressure falls to less than 110 mm Hg or 0.7 mg has been given.
15. c. *Rationale:* Patients who have jaundice or marked elevations of hepatic enzymes while taking an ACE inhibitor should have the drug discontinued, because these drugs have been associated with cholestatic jaundice which can progress to hepatic necrosis and possibly death.
16. d. *Rationale:* Approximately 25% of patients taking an ACE inhibitor for heart failure experience an increase in BUN and serum creatinine levels. These patients usually do not require drug discontinuation unless they have severe, preexisting renal impairment.
17. 140
18. a, b, and c. *Rationale:* Nonpharmacologic management of hypertension should be tried alone or with drug therapy. For example, weight reduction, limited alcohol intake, moderate sodium restriction, and smoking cessation may be the initial treatment of choice if the patient is hypertensive and overweight.
19. b. *Rationale:* The National High Blood Pressure Education Program Working Group on High Blood Pressure in Children and Adolescents produced the fourth report on the diagnosis, evaluation, and treatment of high blood pressure in children and adolescents in 2004. These guidelines established parameters for blood pressure in children and adolescents of comparable age, body size (height and weight), and sex. Normal blood pressure is defined as systolic and diastolic values less than the 90th percentile; prehypertension is defined as an average of systolic or diastolic pressures within the 90th to 95th percentiles; hypertension is defined as pressures beyond the 95th percentile.
20. 60

Chapter 53: Diuretics

SECTION II: ASSESSING YOUR UNDERSTANDING
ACTIVITY A
FILL IN THE BLANKS
1. output
2. composition
3. glomerulus
4. capillaries
5. Bowman's capsule

ACTIVITY B
MATCHING
1. C 2. E 3. A 4. B 5. D

ACTIVITY C
SHORT ANSWERS
1. The tubules are often called *convoluted tubules* because of their many twists and turns. The convolutions provide a large surface area that brings the blood flowing through the peritubular capillaries and the glomerular filtrate flowing through the tubular lumen into close proximity. Consequently, substances can be readily exchanged through the walls of the tubules.
2. The nephron functions by three processes: glomerular filtration, tubular reabsorption, and tubular secretion. These processes normally maintain the fluid volume, electrolyte concentration, and pH of body fluids within a relatively narrow range. They also remove waste products

of cellular metabolism. A minimum daily urine output of approximately 400 milliliters is required to remove normal amounts of metabolic end products.

3. Arterial blood enters the glomerulus via the afferent arteriole at the relatively high pressure of approximately 70 mm Hg. This pressure pushes water, electrolytes, and other solutes out of the capillaries into Bowman's capsule and then to the proximal tubule. This fluid, called glomerular filtrate, contains the same components as blood except for blood cells, fats, and proteins that are too large to be filtered.

4. The glomerular filtration rate (GFR) is about 180 liters per day, or 125 milliliters per minute. Most of this fluid is reabsorbed as the glomerular filtrate travels through the tubules. The end product is about 2 liters of urine daily. Because filtration is a nonselective process, the reabsorption and secretion processes determine the composition of the urine. After it is formed, urine flows into collecting tubules, which carry it to the renal pelvis, then through the ureters, bladder, and urethra for elimination from the body.

5. Blood that does not become part of the glomerular filtrate leaves the glomerulus through the efferent arteriole. The efferent arteriole branches into the peritubular capillaries that eventually empty into veins, which return the blood to systemic circulation.

SECTION III: APPLYING YOUR KNOWLEDGE

ACTIVITY D
CASE STUDIES

1. The term *reabsorption*, in relation to renal function, indicates movement of substances from the tubule (glomerular filtrate) to the blood in the peritubular capillaries. Most reabsorption occurs in the proximal tubule. Almost all glucose and amino acids are reabsorbed; about 80% of water, sodium, potassium, chloride, and most other substances is reabsorbed.

2. About 20% of the glomerular filtrate enters the loop of Henle. In the descending limb of the loop of Henle, water is reabsorbed; in the ascending limb, sodium is reabsorbed. A large fraction of the total amount of sodium (up to 30%) filtered by the glomeruli is reabsorbed in the loop of Henle.

3. Antidiuretic hormone (ADH) from the posterior pituitary gland promotes reabsorption of water from the distal tubules and the collecting ducts of the kidneys. This conserves water needed by the body and produces more concentrated urine. Aldosterone, a hormone from the adrenal cortex, promotes sodium–potassium exchange mainly in the distal tubule and collecting ducts. Thus, aldosterone promotes sodium reabsorption and potassium loss.

4. The term *secretion*, in relation to renal function, indicates movement of substances from blood in the peritubular capillaries to glomerular filtrate flowing through the renal tubules. Secretion occurs in the proximal and distal tubules, across the epithelial cells that line the tubules. In the proximal tubule, uric acid, creatinine, hydrogen ions, and ammonia are secreted; in the distal tubule, potassium ions, hydrogen ions, and ammonia are secreted. Secretion of hydrogen ions is important in maintaining acid–base balance in body fluids.

SECTION IV: PRACTICING FOR NCLEX

1. c. *Rationale:* When digoxin and diuretics are given concomitantly, the risk of digoxin toxicity is increased due to diuretic-induced hypokalemia.

2. a. *Rationale:* High-dose furosemide continuous IV infusions should be given at a rate of 4 mg/minute or less

to decrease or avoid risks of adverse effects, including ototoxicity.

3. c. *Rationale:* Thiazides and related diuretics are the drugs of choice for most patients who require diuretic therapy, especially for long-term management of heart failure and hypertension.

4. a. *Rationale:* There is a known cross-sensitivity of some sulfonamide-allergic patients to sulfonamide nonantibiotics, such as thiazides.

5. b. *Rationale:* Potassium-sparing diuretics are contraindicated in patients with renal impairment because of the high risk of hyperkalemia.

6. d. *Rationale:* Loop diuretics have a sodium-losing effect up to 10 times greater than that of thiazide diuretics.

7. b. *Rationale:* Excessive table salt and salty foods (e.g., ham, packaged sandwich meats, potato chips, dill pickles, most canned soups) may aggravate edema or hypertension.

8. 2.2 lb (1 kg)

9. reabsorption

10. a and b. *Rationale:* Diuretics are often taken in the home setting. The home care nurse may need to assist patients and caregivers in using the drugs safely and effectively; monitor patient responses (e.g., with each home visit, assess nutritional status, blood pressure, weight, use of over-the-counter medications that may aggravate edema or hypertension); and provide information as indicated.

11. a and d. *Rationale:* Fast-acting, potent diuretics such as furosemide and bumetanide are the most likely diuretics to be used in critically ill patients (e.g., those with pulmonary edema).

12. b. *Rationale:* Although IV bolus doses of the drugs are often given to critically ill clients, continuous IV infusions may be more effective and less likely to produce adverse effects in critically ill patients.

13. c. *Rationale:* Diuretics are often used to manage edema and ascites in patients with hepatic impairment. These drugs must be used with caution, because diuretic-induced fluid and electrolyte imbalances may precipitate or worsen hepatic encephalopathy and coma.

14. a. *Rationale:* patients with cirrhosis, diuretic therapy should be initiated in a hospital setting, with small doses and careful monitoring. To prevent hypokalemia and metabolic alkalosis, supplemental potassium or spironolactone may be needed.

15. b. *Rationale:* Potassium-sparing diuretics are contraindicated in patients with renal impairment because of the high risk of hyperkalemia. If they are used at all, frequent monitoring of serum electrolytes, creatinine, and BUN is needed.

16. c. *Rationale:* For continuous infusion, furosemide should be mixed with normal saline or lactated Ringer's solution, because D5W may accelerate degradation of furosemide.

17. c. *Rationale:* With loop diuretics, older adults are at greater risk of excessive diuresis, hypotension, fluid volume deficit, and possibly thrombosis or embolism.

18. d. *Rationale:* The smallest effective dose to treat elder adults in need of diuresis is recommended, usually a daily dose of 12.5 to 25 milligrams of hydrochlorothiazide or equivalent doses of other thiazides and related drugs.

19. a. *Rationale:* Thiazides may be useful in managing edema caused by renal disorders such as nephrotic syndrome and acute glomerulonephritis. However, their effectiveness decreases as the GFR decreases, and the drugs become ineffective when the GFR is less than 30 mL/minute.

20. b. *Rationale:* Furosemide is the loop diuretic used most often in children. Oral therapy is preferred when feasible, and doses greater than 6 milligrams per kilogram of body weight per day are not recommended.

Chapter 54: Drugs That Affect Blood Coagulation

SECTION II: ASSESSING YOUR UNDERSTANDING

ACTIVITY A
FILL IN THE BLANKS
1. thrombus
2. Blood clotting
3. embolus
4. macrophages
5. foam cells

ACTIVITY B
MATCHING
1. D   2. E   3. A   4. B   5. C

ACTIVITY C
SHORT ANSWERS
1. Hemostasis is prevention or stoppage of blood loss from an injured blood vessel and is the process that maintains the integrity of the vascular compartment. It involves activation of several mechanisms, including vasoconstriction, formation of a platelet plug (a cluster of aggregated platelets), sequential activation of clotting factors in the blood, and growth of fibrous tissue (fibrin) into the blood clot to make it more stable and to repair the tear (opening) in the damaged blood vessel.
2. When a blood clot is being formed, plasminogen (an inactive protein found in many body tissues and fluids) is bound to fibrin and becomes a component of the clot. After the outward blood flow is stopped and the tear in the blood vessel is repaired, plasminogen is activated by plasminogen activator (produced by endothelial cells or the coagulation cascade) to produce plasmin. Plasmin is an enzyme that breaks down the fibrin meshwork that stabilizes the clot; this fibrinolytic or thrombolytic action dissolves the clot.
3. Arterial thrombosis is usually associated with atherosclerotic plaque, hypertension, and turbulent blood flow. These conditions damage arterial endothelium and activate platelets to initiate the coagulation process. Arterial thrombi cause disease by obstructing blood flow. If the obstruction is incomplete or temporary, local tissue ischemia (deficient blood supply) occurs. If the obstruction is complete or prolonged, local tissue death (infarction) occurs.
4. Venous thrombosis is usually associated with venous stasis. When blood flows slowly, thrombin and other procoagulant substances present in the blood become concentrated in local areas and initiate the clotting process. With a normal rate of blood flow, these substances are rapidly removed from the blood, primarily by Kupffer's cells in the liver. A venous thrombus is less cohesive than an arterial thrombus, and an embolus can easily become detached and travel to other parts of the body.
5. Venous thrombi cause disease by two mechanisms. First, thrombosis causes local congestion, edema, and perhaps inflammation by impairing normal outflow of venous blood (e.g., thrombophlebitis, deep vein thrombosis). Second, embolization obstructs the blood supply when the embolus becomes lodged. The pulmonary arteries are common sites of embolization.

SECTION III: APPLYING YOUR KNOWLEDGE

ACTIVITY D
CASE STUDIES
1. Heparin combines with antithrombin III (a natural anticoagulant in the blood) to inactivate clotting factors IX, X, XI, and XII; inhibit the conversion of prothrombin to thrombin; and prevent thrombus formation. After thrombosis has developed, heparin can inhibit additional coagulation by inactivating thrombin, preventing the conversion of fibrinogen to fibrin, and inhibiting factor XIII (the fibrin-stabilizing factor). Other effects include inhibiting factors V and VIII and platelet aggregation.
2. Heparin acts immediately after intravenous (IV) injection and within 20 to 30 minutes after subcutaneous (Sub-Q) injection.
3. Heparin does not cross the placental barrier and is not secreted in breast milk, making it the anticoagulant of choice for use during pregnancy and lactation.
4. Heparin is prescribed for patients who are expected to be on bedrest or to have limited activity for longer than 5 days.
5. DIC is disseminated intravascular coagulation, a life-threatening condition characterized by widespread clotting, which depletes the blood of coagulation factors. Heparin is prescribed for DIC also. The goal of heparin therapy in DIC is to prevent blood coagulation long enough for clotting factors to be replenished and thus be able to control hemorrhage.

SECTION IV: PRACTICING FOR NCLEX

1. b. *Rationale:* When the thrombolytic agents are used in acute myocardial infarction, cardiac dysrhythmias may occur when blood flow is re-established; antidysrhythmic drugs should be readily available.
2. a, b, and d. *Rationale:* The FDA has issued a black box warning for the use of protamine sulfate due to the risk of severe hypotension, cardiovascular collapse, noncardiogenic pulmonary edema, catastrophic pulmonary vasoconstriction, and pulmonary hypertension.
3. Protamine sulfate
4. c. *Rationale:* Monitoring of aPTT is not necessary with low-dose standard heparin given Sub-Q for prophylaxis of thromboembolism or with the LMWHs.
5. c. *Rationale:* Currently available LMWHs (dalteparin, enoxaparin) differ from standard heparin and each other and are not interchangeable.
6. d. *Rationale:* The FDA has issued a black box warning for warfarin due to its risk of causing major or fatal bleeding.
7. Vitamin K
8. a. *Rationale:* Herbs commonly used that may increase the effects of warfarin include alfalfa, celery, clove, feverfew, garlic, ginger, ginkgo biloba, ginseng, and licorice.
9. c. *Rationale:* Warfarin dosage is regulated according to the INR (derived from the prothrombin [PT] time), for which a therapeutic value is between 2.0 to 3.0 in most conditions. A therapeutic PT value is approximately 1.5 times the control, or 18 seconds.
10. b. *Rationale:* No antidote exists for the effects of aspirin or the adenosine diphosphate receptor antagonists, because both produce irreversible platelet effects; platelet transfusion may be required.
11. a and b. *Rationale:* Thrombolytic agents are used to dissolve thrombi and limit tissue damage in selected thromboembolic disorders.

12. arterial
13. d. *Rationale:* Anticoagulant drugs are given to prevent formation of new clots and extension of clots already present.
14. d. *Rationale:* Many commonly used herbs and supplements have a profound effect on drugs used for anticoagulation. Multivitamin supplements may contain 25 to 28 micrograms of vitamin K and should be taken consistently to avoid fluctuating vitamin K levels.
15. c. *Rationale:* Daily visits by a home care nurse may be needed if the patient or a family member is unable or unwilling to inject the medication. Platelet counts should be obtained before therapy and every 2 to 3 days during heparin therapy. Heparin should be discontinued if the platelet count falls to less than 100,000 or to less than half the baseline value.
16. a. *Rationale:* Warfarin is more likely to cause bleeding in patients with liver disease because of decreased synthesis of vitamin K. In addition, warfarin is eliminated only by hepatic metabolism and may accumulate with liver impairment.
17. a. *Rationale:* Most anticoagulant, antiplatelet, and thrombolytic drugs may be used in patients with impaired renal function. For example, heparin and warfarin may be used in usual dosages, and thrombolytic agents (e.g., streptokinase, urokinase) may be used to dissolve clots in IV catheters or vascular access sites for hemodialysis.
18. c. *Rationale:* NSAIDs, which are commonly used by older adults, also have antiplatelet effects. Patients who take an NSAID daily may not need low-dose aspirin for antithrombotic effects.
19. benzyl alcohol
20. b. *Rationale:* When warfarin is started, PT and INR should be assessed daily until a stable daily dose is reached (the dose that maintains PT and INR within therapeutic ranges and does not cause bleeding).

Chapter 55: Drugs for Dyslipidemia

SECTION II: ASSESSING YOUR UNDERSTANDING

ACTIVITY A
FILL IN THE BLANKS
1. Dyslipidemic
2. intestine
3. cell membranes
4. steroid
5. cholic acid

ACTIVITY B
MATCHING
1. E   2. B   3. A   4. C   5. D

ACTIVITY C
SHORT ANSWERS
1. Blood lipids are transported in plasma by specific proteins called lipoproteins. Each lipoprotein contains cholesterol, phospholipid, and triglyceride bound to protein.
2. The lipoproteins vary in density and in their amounts of lipid and protein. Density is determined mainly by the amount of protein, which is more dense than fat. Therefore, density increases as the proportion of protein increases.
3. Metabolic syndrome is a group of cardiovascular risk factors linked with obesity. *The Third Report of the National Cholesterol Education Program Expert Panel on Detection, Evaluation, and Treatment of High Blood Cholesterol in Adults* (NCEP III) clustered several elements of the metabolic syndrome: elevated waist circumference

(central adiposity), elevated triglycerides, reduced high-density lipoprotein cholesterol, elevated blood pressure, and elevated fasting glucose.
4. These risk factors frequently produce an additive effect on cardiovascular, cerebrovascular, and peripheral vascular disease and are principal contributors to the significant morbidity and mortality of these conditions.
5. Improvements in insulin resistance and lipid profiles are essential lifestyle modifications and constitute first-line treatment of metabolic syndrome.

SECTION III: APPLYING YOUR KNOWLEDGE
ACTIVITY D
CASE STUDIES
1. Elevated total and LDL cholesterol and reduced HDL cholesterol are the abnormalities that are major risk factors for coronary artery disease. Triglycerides also play a role in cardiovascular disease. For example, high blood levels of triglycerides reflect excessive caloric intake (excessive dietary fats are stored in adipose tissue; excessive proteins and carbohydrates are converted to triglycerides and also stored in adipose tissue) and obesity.
2. For accurate interpretation of a patient's lipid profile, blood samples for laboratory testing of triglycerides should be drawn after the patient has fasted for 12 hours. Fasting is not required for cholesterol testing.
3. NCEP III recommends treatment of patients according to their blood levels of total and LDL cholesterol and their risk factors for cardiovascular disease. Therapeutic lifestyle changes (TLC), including exercise, smoking cessation, changes in diet, and drug therapy, are recommended at lower serum cholesterol levels in patients who already have cardiovascular disease or diabetes mellitus. Also, the target LDL serum level is lower in these patients. The so-called Mediterranean diet, which includes moderate amounts of monounsaturated fats (e.g., canola, olive oils) and polyunsaturated fats (e.g., safflower, corn, cottonseed, sesame, soybean, sunflower oils), also decreases risks of cardiovascular disease. Further, the patient should be encouraged to increase dietary intake of soluble fiber (e.g., psyllium preparations, oat bran, pectin, fruits and vegetables). This diet lowers serum LDL cholesterol by 5% to 10%.

SECTION IV: PRACTICING FOR NCLEX
1. a. *Rationale:* Fibrates are the most effective drugs for reducing serum triglyceride levels.
2. c. *Rationale:* Skin flushing may occur with niacin.
3. c. *Rationale:* Lovastatin should be taken with food; fluvastatin, pravastatin, or simvastatin should be taken in the evening, with or without food; atorvastatin may be taken with or without food and without regard to time of day.
4. a. *Rationale:* Lifestyle changes that can help improve cholesterol levels include a low fat diet, regular aerobic exercise, losing weight, and not smoking.
5. a, b, and c. *Rationale:* Metabolic syndrome is a group of cardiovascular risk factors that are linked with obesity and include elevated waist circumference (central adiposity), elevated triglycerides, reduced high-density lipoprotein cholesterol, elevated blood pressure, and elevated fasting glucose.
6. d. *Rationale:* For accurate interpretation of a patient's lipid profile, blood samples for laboratory testing of triglycerides should be drawn after the patient has fasted for 12 hours. Fasting is not required for cholesterol testing.
7. a. *Rationale:* Unless a person has a genetic disorder of lipid metabolism, the amount of cholesterol in the blood is strongly related to dietary intake of saturated fat.

8. b. *Rationale:* Flax or flax seed is used internally as a laxative and a dyslipidemic agent. Absorption of all medications may be decreased when taken with flax, resulting in a less than therapeutic effect.

9. a *Rationale:* Niacin may cause hepatotoxicity, especially with doses greater than 2 grams daily, with timed-release preparations, and if given in combination with a statin or a fibrate.

10. c. *Rationale:* Cholesterol absorption inhibitors as monotherapy (without statins) do not require dosage reduction in mild hepatic insufficiency.

11. b. *Rationale:* Statins are metabolized in the liver and may accumulate in patients with impaired hepatic function. They are contraindicated in patients with active liver disease or unexplained elevations of serum aspartate or alanine aminotransferase.

12. b. *Rationale:* Fluvastatin is cleared hepatically, and less than 6% of the dose is excreted in urine; therefore, dosage reduction for mild to moderate renal impairment is unnecessary. Use caution with severe impairment. Recent randomized, controlled clinical trials have demonstrated the drug's safety in kidney transplant recipients.

13. d. *Rationale:* In postmenopausal women, estrogen replacement therapy increases HDL cholesterol.

14. a. *Rationale:* Dyslipidemic drugs are not recommended for children younger than 10 years of age, except for pravastatin, which has dosing recommendations for children as young as 8 years.

15. c. *Rationale:* Despite an increased prevalence of diabetes and obesity, American Indians appear to have lower cholesterol levels than the United States population as a whole. This suggests that diet and exercise may be more useful than lipid-lowering drugs for this group.

16. a, b, and c. *Rationale:* To lower cholesterol and triglycerides, a statin, a cholesterol absorption inhibitor, gemfibrozil, or niacin may be used.

17. a. *Rationale:* A fibrate–statin combination should be avoided because of increased risks of severe myopathy. A niacin–statin combination increases the risks of hepatotoxicity.

18. c. *Rationale:* The cholesterol absorption inhibitors (e.g., ezetimibe), the newest class of dyslipidemic drugs, act in the small intestine to inhibit absorption of cholesterol and decrease the delivery of intestinal cholesterol to the liver, resulting in reduced hepatic cholesterol stores and increased clearance of cholesterol from the blood. This distinct mechanism is complementary to that of HMG-CoA reductase inhibitors.

19. d. *Rationale:* Niacin (nicotinic acid) decreases both cholesterol and triglycerides. It inhibits mobilization of free fatty acids from peripheral tissues, thereby reducing hepatic synthesis of triglycerides and secretion of VLDL, which leads to decreased production of LDL cholesterol.

20. intestinal

Chapter 56: Physiology of the Digestive System

SECTION II: ASSESSING YOUR UNDERSTANDING

ACTIVITY A
FILL IN THE BLANKS
1. anus
2. liver
3. cellular
4. elimination
5. alimentary

ACTIVITY B
MATCHING
1. A   2. C   3. E   4. B   5. D

ACTIVITY C
SHORT ANSWERS
1. The pancreas secretes enzymes required for the digestion of carbohydrates, proteins, and fats. It also secretes insulin, glucagon, and somatostatin, hormones that regulate glucose metabolism and blood sugar levels.
2. The gallbladder is a small pouch attached to the underside of the liver that stores and concentrates *bile*. It has a capacity of 50 to 60 milliliters. The gallbladder releases bile when fats are present in the duodenum.
3. Mucus is secreted by mucous glands in every part of the gastrointestinal (GI) tract. The functions of mucus are to protect the lining of the tract from digestive juices, lubricate the food bolus for easier passage, promote adherence of the fecal mass, and neutralize acids and bases.
4. Saliva consists of mucus, ptyalin, and salivary amylase. It is produced by the salivary glands and totals about 1000 milliliters daily. Saliva has a slightly acidic to neutral pH (6 to 7); it lubricates the food bolus and begins starch digestion.
5. Hydrochloric acid provides the acid medium to promote pepsin activity.

SECTION III: APPLYING YOUR KNOWLEDGE

ACTIVITY D
CASE STUDIES
1. The hepatic artery carries blood to the connective tissue of the liver and bile ducts, then empties into the hepatic sinuses. Arterial blood mixes with blood from the portal circulation. Venous blood from the liver flows into the inferior vena cava for return to the systemic circulation. The ample blood flow facilitates the many functions of the liver. The liver serves as a blood reservoir for the body. The liver can eject 500 to 1000 mL of blood into the general circulation in response to stress, decreased blood volume, or sympathetic nervous system stimulation (e.g., hemorrhagic or hypovolemic shock).
2. The liver serves as a blood filter and detoxifier. Kupffer cells in the liver phagocytize bacteria carried from the intestines by the portal vein. They also break down worn-out erythrocytes, saving iron for reuse in hemoglobin synthesis, and form bilirubin, a waste product excreted in bile.
3. The liver metabolizes many body secretions and most drugs to prevent accumulation and harmful effects on body tissues. Most drugs are active as the parent compound and are metabolized in the liver to an inactive metabolite, which is then excreted by the kidneys. However, some drugs become active only after formation of a metabolite in the liver. The liver detoxifies or alters substances by oxidation, hydrolysis, or conjugation.

SECTION IV: PRACTICING FOR NCLEX
1. a, b, and c. *Rationale:* The liver plays numerous roles in digestion, including metabolism of carbohydrates, fats, and proteins; storage of fat-soluble vitamins, vitamin B_{12}, iron, phospholipids, cholesterol, and a small amount of protein and fat; and synthesis of bile.
2. fats
3. a. *Rationale:* Pancreatic juices are rich in bicarbonate and digestive enzymes.
4. d. *Rationale:* Most nutrients and drugs are absorbed in the small intestine.
5. prostaglandins

6. acetylcholine
7. c. *Rationale:* Pepsin requires an acidic pH in order to effectively digest proteins.
8. a and b. *Rationale:* Food is mixed in the stomach with *gastric juices* containing mucus, digestive enzymes such as pepsin, and hydrochloric acid.
9. d. *Rationale:* Failure of the lower esophageal sphincter results in reflux of gastric contents into the esophagus.
10. sphincters
11. a. *Rationale:* Digestion begins in the oral cavity with mastication and digestion of starches.
12. Sympathetic
13. b. *Rationale:* Peristalsis propels food through the digestive tract and mixes the food bolus with digestive juices.
14. a and b. *Rationale:* The main functions of the digestive system are to provide the body with useable nutrition and dispose of waste products that result from the digestive process.
15. d. *Rationale:* The digestive system and drug therapy have a reciprocal relationship. Many common symptoms (i.e., nausea, vomiting, constipation, diarrhea, abdominal pain) relate to GI dysfunction.
16. cholecystokinin
17. b. *Rationale:* The major digestive enzyme in gastric juice is pepsin, a proteolytic enzyme (named before the "ase" system of naming enzymes) that functions best at a pH of 2 to 3.
18. c. *Rationale:* One function of the liver is production of body heat by continuous cellular metabolism. The liver is the body organ with the highest rate of chemical activity during basal conditions, and it produces about 20% of total body heat.
19. ammonia
20. glycogen

Chapter 57: Nutritional Support Products, Vitamins, and Mineral–Electrolytes

SECTION II: ASSESSING YOUR UNDERSTANDING

ACTIVITY A
FILL IN THE BLANKS
1. Proteins
2. Carbohydrates
3. kilocalories
4. proteins
5. Vitamins

ACTIVITY B
MATCHING
1. D   2. E   3. A   4. B   5. C

ACTIVITY C
SHORT ANSWERS
1. Nurses encounter many patients who are unable to ingest, digest, absorb, or use sufficient nutrients to improve or maintain health. Debilitating illnesses such as cancer; acquired immunodeficiency syndrome; and chronic lung, kidney, or cardiovascular disorders often interfere with appetite and gastrointestinal (GI) function. Therapeutic drugs often cause anorexia, nausea, vomiting, diarrhea, or constipation. Nutritional deficiencies may impair the function of essentially every body organ. Signs and symptoms include unintended weight loss, increased susceptibility to infection, weakness and fatigability, impaired wound healing, impaired growth and development in children, edema, and decreased hemoglobin.

2. Numerous liquid enteral formulas are available over-the-counter or in healthcare settings for oral or tube feedings. Many are nutritionally complete, except for water, when given in sufficient amounts (e.g., Ensure, Isocal, Sustacal, Resource). Additional water must be given to meet fluid needs. Most oral products are available in a variety of flavors and contain 1 kcal per milliliter. Additional products are formulated for patients with special conditions (e.g., renal or hepatic failure, malabsorption syndromes) or special needs (e.g., high protein, increased calories).

3. Intravenous fluids are used when oral or tube feedings are contraindicated. Most are nutritionally incomplete and are used in the short term to supply fluids, electrolytes, and a few calories. Dextrose or dextrose and sodium chloride solutions are often used. When nutrients must be provided intravenously for more than a few days, a special parenteral nutritional formula can be designed to meet all nutritional needs or to supplement other feeding methods.

4. Pancreatic enzymes (amylase, protease, lipase) are required for absorption of carbohydrates, proteins, and fats. Pancrelipase and others are commercial preparations used as replacement therapy in deficiency states, including cystic fibrosis, chronic pancreatitis, pancreatectomy, and pancreatic obstruction. Dosage is 1 to 3 capsules or tablets with each meal or snack.

5. Vitamins are obtained from foods or supplements. Although foods are considered the best source, studies indicate that most adults and children do not consume enough fruits, vegetables, cereal grains, dairy products, and other foods to consistently meet their vitamin requirements. In addition, some conditions increase requirements above the usual recommended amounts (e.g., pregnancy, lactation, various illnesses).

SECTION III: APPLYING YOUR KNOWLEDGE

ACTIVITY D
CASE STUDIES
1. Iron preparations are used to prevent or treat iron deficiency anemia. For prevention, they are often given during periods of increased need, such as childhood or pregnancy.

2. The drug is well absorbed. Oral ferrous salts (sulfate, gluconate, fumarate) are preferred because of their absorption. Action starts in about 4 days, peaks in 7 to 10 days, and lasts 2 to 4 months. The drugs are not metabolized; a portion of a dose is lost daily in feces. Otherwise, the iron content is recycled and its half-life is unknown. Sustained-release or enteric-coated formulations are not as well absorbed as other preparations. Available ferrous salts differ in the amount of elemental iron they contain.

3. Adverse effects include nausea and other symptoms of GI irritation. Oral preparations also discolor feces, producing a black-green color that may be mistaken for blood in the stool. A guaiac test can tell whether the discoloration is from blood or from the iron preparation. Iron preparations are contraindicated in patients with peptic ulcer disease, inflammatory intestinal disorders, anemias other than iron deficiency anemia, multiple blood transfusions, hemochromatosis, or hemosiderosis. Ferrous gluconate (Fergon) may be less irritating to GI mucosa and therefore better tolerated than ferrous sulfate. It contains 12% elemental iron (i.e., 36 mg per 325 mg tablet).

SECTION IV: PRACTICING FOR NCLEX
1. b. *Rationale:* Although most adults and children probably benefit from a daily multivitamin, large doses of single vitamins do not prevent cancer or cardiovascular disease and should be avoided.

2. d. *Rationale:* Nutrients are best obtained from foods; when they cannot be obtained from foods, they can be provided by oral, enteral (via GI tubes), or parenteral (IV) feedings to meet a patient's nutritional needs.

3. a, b, and c. *Rationale:* Fat-soluble vitamins are A, D, E, and K.

4. a and c. *Rationale:* Water-soluble vitamins are B complex and C.

5. c. *Rationale:* Health promotion may involve assessing the nutritional status of all members of the household, especially children, older adults, and those with obvious deficiencies, and providing assistance to improve nutritional status.

6. a, b, and d. *Rationale:* For patients receiving tube feedings at home, the home care nurse may teach about the goals of treatment, administration, preparation or storage of solutions, equipment (e.g., obtaining, cleaning), and monitoring of responses (e.g., weight, urine output).

7. b. *Rationale:* Electrolyte and acid–base imbalances often occur in critically ill patients and are usually treated, as in other patients, with very close monitoring of serum electrolyte levels and avoidance of excessive amounts of replacement products.

8. d. *Rationale:* With parenteral nutrition, adequate types and amounts of nutrients are needed. When IV fat emulsions are given, they should be infused slowly, over 24 hours.

9. a. *Rationale:* The Nutrition Advisory Group of the American Medical Association (NAG-AMA) has established guidelines for daily intake of vitamins, and parenteral multivitamin formulations are available for adults and children. Those for adults do not contain vitamin K, which is usually injected weekly. The usual dose is 2 to 4 mg. Vitamin K is included in pediatric parenteral nutrition solutions.

10. b. *Rationale:* Patients with respiratory impairment may need an enteral formula that contains less carbohydrate and more fat than other products and produces less carbon dioxide (e.g., Pulmocare).

11. concentrated

12. d. *Rationale:* Protein restriction is usually needed in patients with cirrhosis to prevent or treat hepatic encephalopathy, which is caused by excessive protein or excessive production of ammonia (from protein breakdown in the GI tract).

13. Amin-Aid

14. b. *Rationale:* IV fat emulsions should not be given to patients with ARF if serum triglyceride levels exceed 300 mg/dL.

15. a. *Rationale:* With the high incidence of atherosclerosis, cardiovascular disease, and diabetes mellitus in older adults, it is especially important that intake of animal fats and high-calorie sweets be reduced.

16. b. *Rationale:* Accidental ingestion of iron-containing medications and dietary supplements is a common cause of poisoning death in children younger than 6 years of age. To help prevent poisoning, products containing iron must be labeled with a warning, and products with 30 mg or more of iron (e.g., prenatal products) must be packaged as individual doses. All iron-containing preparations should be stored in places that are inaccessible to young children.

17. candy

18. b. *Rationale:* Preterm infants need proportionately more vitamins than term infants, because their growth rate is faster and their absorption of vitamins from the intestine is less complete. A multivitamin product containing the equivalent of DRIs for term infants is recommended.

19. b. *Rationale:* Folic acid decreases effects of phenytoin and may decrease absorption and effects of zinc.

20. rhabdomyolysis

Chapter 58: Drugs Used to Aid Weight Management

SECTION II: ASSESSING YOUR UNDERSTANDING

ACTIVITY A
FILL IN THE BLANKS
1. Overweight
2. Obese
3. BMI
4. BMI
5. obesity

ACTIVITY B
MATCHING
1. B 2. A 3. C 4. E 5. D

ACTIVITY C
SHORT ANSWERS
1. Obesity may occur in anyone but is more likely to occur in women, members of minority groups, and poor people. It results from consistent ingestion of more calories than are used for energy, and it substantially increases risks for development of numerous health problems.

2. Most obesity-related disorders are attributed mainly to the multiple metabolic abnormalities associated with obesity. Abdominal fat out of proportion to total body fat (also called central or visceral obesity), which often occurs in men and postmenopausal women, is considered a greater risk factor for disease and death than lower-body obesity. In addition to the many health problems associated with obesity, obesity is increasingly being considered a chronic disease in its own right.

3. The prevalence of overweight people and obesity has dramatically increased during the past 25 years. Some authorities estimate that 60% of American adults are overweight or obese. There are differences in prevalence by gender, ethnicity, and socioeconomic status. In general, more women than men are obese, whereas more men than women are overweight; African American women and Mexican Americans of both sexes have the highest rates of overweight and obesity in the United States; and women in lower socioeconomic classes are more likely to be obese than those in higher socioeconomic classes.

4. The etiology of excessive weight is thought to involve complex and often overlapping interactions among physiologic, genetic, environmental, psychosocial, and other factors.

5. In general, increased weight is related to an energy imbalance in which energy intake (food/calorie consumption) exceeds energy expenditure. Total energy expenditure represents the energy expended at rest (i.e., the basal or resting metabolic rate), during physical activity, and during food consumption.

SECTION III: APPLYING YOUR KNOWLEDGE

ACTIVITY D
CASE STUDIES
1. "The drug decreases absorption of dietary fat from the intestine." Orlistat (Xenical, Alli) differs from phentermine and sibutramine because it decreases absorption of dietary fat from the intestine by binding to gastric and pancreatic lipases in the gastrointestinal tract lumen and making them unavailable to break down dietary fats into absorbable free fatty acids and monoglycerides.

2. The drug blocks absorption of approximately 30% of the fat ingested in a meal; increasing the dosage does not increase this percentage. Decreased fat absorption leads to decreased caloric intake, resulting in weight loss and improved serum cholesterol values (e.g., decreased total and low-density lipoprotein cholesterol levels). The improvement in cholesterol levels is thought to be independent of weight-loss effects.

3. Orlistat is not absorbed systemically, and its action occurs in the GI tract. Consequently, it does not cause systemic adverse effects or drug interactions as phentermine and sibutramine do. Orlistat's main disadvantages are the requirement for frequent administration (three times daily) and gastrointestinal symptoms (abdominal pain, oily spotting, fecal urgency, flatulence with discharge, fatty stools, fecal incontinence, and increased defecation). Adverse gastrointestinal effects occur in almost all orlistat users but usually subside after a few weeks of continued drug usage.

4. The patient should consult with her physician about other supplements to take with orlistat. The drug prevents absorption of the fat-soluble vitamins, A, D, E, and K, so people taking orlistat should also take a multivitamin containing these vitamins daily. The multivitamin should be taken 2 hours before or after the orlistat dose. If it is taken at the same time, the orlistat will prevent absorption of the fat-soluble vitamins. High-fat foods need to be decreased, because total caloric intake is a major determinant of weight, and adverse effects (e.g., diarrhea, fatty and malodorous stools) worsen with high fat consumption.

SECTION IV: PRACTICING FOR NCLEX

1. a, b, and d. *Rationale:* Many people lose weight but regain it within a few months if they do not change their lifestyle habits toward eating more healthfully and exercising more.

2. b. *Rationale:* Weight-loss drugs are generally recommended only for people who are seriously overweight or have health problems associated with or aggravated by obesity.

3. caloric intake

4. d. *Rationale:* Ingesting 500 calories more per day than those used in exercise and physical activity leads to a weight gain of 1 lb in 1 week; decreasing caloric intake or increasing caloric output of 500 calories per day for 1 week leads to a weight loss of 1 lb.

5. a and b. *Rationale:* Overweight and obesity are major concerns because of their association with numerous health problems, including diabetes, hypertension, other cardiovascular disorders, and muscle and joint disorders.

6. c. *Rationale:* The home care nurse should be able to provide accurate information about realistic and successful techniques for losing weight and keeping it off; the health benefits of even modest weight loss; and reasons to avoid "fad" diets, weight-loss herbal and dietary supplements, and programs that promise rapid and easy weight loss with little effort.

7. d. *Rationale:* In relation to drugs for obesity, little information is available about their use in patients with hepatic impairment. Because sibutramine is metabolized in the liver, it is contraindicated in patients with severe hepatic impairment.

8. d. *Rationale:* With sibutramine, dosage reductions are not recommended with mild to moderate impairment, because the drug and its active metabolites are eliminated by the liver. However, some inactive metabolites are also formed, and these are excreted renally. The drug is contraindicated in patients with severe renal impairment.

9. a, b, and c. *Rationale:* With orlistat, the manufacturer recommends conservative use and dosage because older adults often have decreased renal, cardiac, and hepatic function.

10. c. *Rationale:* Treatment of childhood obesity should focus on healthy eating and increasing physical activity. In general, children should not be put on "diets." For a child who is overweight, the recommended goal is to maintain weight or slow the rate of weight gain so that weight-for-height and BMI gradually decline as the child grows in height.

11. a. *Rationale:* If the child already exceeds the optimal adult weight, the goal of treatment should be a slow weight loss of 10 to 12 pounds per year until the optimal adult weight is reached.

12. b. *Rationale:* Although drug therapy has not been generally recommended for treatment of childhood obesity, orlistat is approved for use in children aged 12 to 16 years and is considered safe and effective for weight reduction in overweight adolescents. As with adults, common adverse effects in clinical trials were gastrointestinal effects(e.g., diarrhea, flatulence) and reduced concentrations of fat-soluble vitamins.

13. c. *Rationale:* For any patients following a weight-loss regimen, provide psychological support and positive reinforcement for efforts toward weight management. Programs or support groups involving supervision or regular participation within a social group appear to be more successful over time. However, a systematic review that evaluated major commercial weight-loss programs found few high-quality studies. In general, there was more evidence of success with the Weight Watchers program than with Health Management Resources, OPTIFAST, Jenny Craig, or L.A. Weight Loss.

14. d. *Rationale:* The National Institutes of Health do not recommend combining weight-loss medications except in the context of clinical trials. Thus far, studies indicate that combining sibutramine and orlistat has no additional benefit over using one of the drugs alone.

15. b. *Rationale:* For people who already have type 2 diabetes, weight loss reduces blood levels of glucose and glycosylated (A_{1c}) hemoglobin. These effects make the diabetes easier to manage, reduce complications of diabetes, and may allow smaller doses of antidiabetic medications.

16. a, c, and d. *Rationale:* Emphasize health benefits of weight reduction. There is strong evidence that weight loss reduces risk factors for cardiovascular disease, including blood pressure, serum triglycerides, and total and LDL cholesterol. It also increases HDL cholesterol.

17. b. *Rationale:* Drug therapy and bariatric surgery are recommended only for seriously overweight people with major medical problems that can be improved by weight loss. In addition, neither of these treatments is a substitute for the necessary changes in eating and physical activity patterns.

18. a. *Rationale:* Laxative and diuretic herbs (e.g., aloe, rhubarb root, buckthorn, cascara, senna, parsley, juniper, dandelion leaves) are found in several products such as Super Dieter's Tea, Trim-Maxx Tea, and Water Pill. These products cause a significant loss of body fluids and electrolytes, not fat. Adverse effects may include low serum potassium levels, with subsequent cardiac dysrhythmias and other heart problems.

19. c. *Rationale:* Guar gum is a dietary fiber that is included in weight-loss products because it is bulk-forming and produces feelings of fullness. Several small studies indicated it is no more effective than placebo for weight loss. It may cause esophageal or intestinal obstruction if not taken with an adequate amount of water and may interfere with the absorption of other drugs if taken at the same time. Adverse effects include nausea, diarrhea, flatulence, and abdominal discomfort.

20. diabetes.

Chapter 59: Drugs Used for Peptic Ulcer and Acid Reflux Disease

SECTION II: ASSESSING YOUR UNDERSTANDING

ACTIVITY A
FILL IN THE BLANKS
1. Peptic ulcer disease
2. duodenal
3. protective
4. pepsin
5. Gastric acid

ACTIVITY B
MATCHING
1. E   2. C   3. D   4. A   5. B

ACTIVITY C
SHORT ANSWERS
1. Antacids are alkaline substances that neutralize acids. They react with hydrochloric acid in the stomach to produce neutral, less acidic, or poorly absorbed salts and to raise the pH (alkalinity) of gastric secretions. Raising the pH to approximately 3.5 neutralizes more than 90% of gastric acid and inhibits conversion of pepsinogen to pepsin. Commonly used antacids are aluminum, magnesium, and calcium compounds.
2. Histamine is a substance that is found in almost every body tissue and is released in response to certain stimuli (e.g., allergic reactions, tissue injury). After it is released, histamine causes contraction of smooth muscle in the bronchi, GI tract, and uterus; dilation and increased permeability of capillaries; dilation of cerebral blood vessels; and stimulation of sensory nerve endings to produce pain and itching. Histamine also causes strong stimulation of gastric acid secretion. Vagal stimulation causes release of histamine from cells in the gastric mucosa. The histamine then acts on receptors located on the parietal cells to increase production of hydrochloric acid. These receptors are called the histamine$_2$ (H$_2$) receptors.
3. PPIs are strong inhibitors of gastric acid secretion. These drugs bind irreversibly to the gastric proton pump (e.g., the enzyme H$^+$,K$^+$-ATPase) to prevent the "pumping" or release of gastric acid from parietal cells into the stomach lumen, thereby blocking the final step of acid production. Inhibition of the proton pump suppresses gastric acid secretion in response to all primary stimuli including histamine, gastrin, and acetylcholine. Therefore, the drugs inhibit both daytime (including meal-stimulated) and nocturnal (unstimulated) acid secretion.
4. Naturally occurring prostaglandin E, which is produced in mucosal cells of the stomach and duodenum, inhibits gastric acid secretion and increases mucus and bicarbonate secretion, mucosal blood flow, and perhaps mucosal repair. It also inhibits the mucosal damage produced by gastric acid, aspirin, and NSAIDs.

5. Sucralfate is a preparation of sulfated sucrose and aluminum hydroxide that binds to normal and ulcerated mucosa. It is used to prevent and treat peptic ulcer disease. It is effective even though it does not inhibit secretion of gastric acid or pepsin and has little neutralizing effect on gastric acid. Its mechanism of action is unclear, but it is thought to act locally on the gastric and duodenal mucosa. Possible mechanisms include binding to the ulcer and forming a protective barrier between the mucosa and gastric acid, pepsin, and bile salts; neutralizing pepsin; stimulating prostaglandin synthesis in the mucosa; and exerting healing effects through the aluminum component. Sucralfate is effective in healing duodenal ulcers and in maintenance therapy to prevent ulcer recurrence. In general, the rates of ulcer healing with sucralfate are similar to the rates with H2RAs.

SECTION III: APPLYING YOUR KNOWLEDGE

ACTIVITY D
CASE STUDIES
1. Misoprostol is a synthetic form of prostaglandin E that is approved for concurrent use with NSAIDs to protect gastric mucosa from NSAID-induced erosion and ulceration. Prostaglandin E, which is produced in mucosal cells of the stomach and duodenum, inhibits gastric acid secretion and increases mucus and bicarbonate secretion, mucosal blood flow, and perhaps mucosal repair. It also inhibits the mucosal damage produced by gastric acid, aspirin, and NSAIDs. When synthesis of prostaglandin E is inhibited, erosion and ulceration of gastric mucosa may occur.
2. You should know more about Mrs. Dinwiddie before advising her husband. The FDA has issued a black box warning to alert health care professionals that misoprostol is contraindicated in women of childbearing potential (unless effective contraceptive methods are being used) and during pregnancy, because it may induce abortion, premature birth, or birth defects.
3. The most common adverse effects of misoprostol use are diarrhea (in 10% to 40% of recipients) and abdominal cramping. It is indicated for patients at who are at high risk of GI ulceration and bleeding, such as those taking high doses of NSAIDs.

SECTION IV: PRACTICING FOR NCLEX
1. a. *Rationale:* Sucralfate forms a protective barrier over mucosal ulcerations, protecting them from exposure to gastric juices. It requires an acid pH to be effective.
2. parietal
3. a, c, and d. *Rationale:* PPIs are considered drugs of choice for treatment of heartburn, gastric and duodenal ulcers, GERD, esophagitis, and hypersecretory syndromes such as Zollinger-Ellison syndrome.
4. gastric juices
5. a. *Rationale:* The treatment of choice for *Helicobacter pylori* infection is a PPI and clarithromycin plus either amoxicillin or metronidazole.
6. b. *Rationale:* Calcium antacids have high neutralizing capacity and rapid onset. They may cause rebound acidity and hypercalcemia.
7. c. *Rationale:* Magnesium antacids have high neutralizing capacity and may cause diarrhea and hypermagnesemia.
8. constipation
9. d. *Rationale:* Gastroesophageal reflux disease (GERD) is characterized by regurgitation of acidic gastric contents into the esophagus resulting in esophagitis or esophageal ulceration.

10. c. *Rationale:* Cell-protective effects include secretion of mucus and bicarbonate, dilution of hydrochloric acid by food and secretions, prevention of diffusion of hydrochloric acid from the stomach back into the gastric mucosal lining, the presence of prostaglandin E, and alkalinization of gastric secretions by pancreatic juices and bile.

11. a. *Rationale:* Cell-destructive effects include secretion of gastric acid (hydrochloric acid) and pepsin, *Helicobacter pylori* infection, and ingestion of NSAIDs.

12. duodenum

13. b. *Rationale:* The home care nurse can assist patients by providing information about taking the drugs correctly and monitoring responses. If cimetidine is being taken, the home care nurse needs to assess for potential drug–drug interactions.

14. b. *Rationale:* PPIs are metabolized in the liver and may cause transient elevations in liver function tests.

15. b. *Rationale:* Antacids containing magnesium are contraindicated in patients with impaired renal function.

16. c. *Rationale:* Sucralfate is well tolerated by older adults. PPIs are also well tolerated, but long-term use (greater than 1 year) is associated with increased risk of hip fractures in adults older than 50 years of age. The risk of fractures increases the longer the medications are taken. The risk of hip fractures is also greater in those taking higher dosages of PPIs.

17. a. *Rationale:* With H2RAs, older adults are more likely to experience adverse effects, especially confusion, agitation, and disorientation, with cimetidine. In addition, older adults often have decreased renal function, and doses need to be reduced.

18. a. *Rationale:* Smaller doses of antacids may be effective in older adults, because they usually secrete less gastric acid than younger adults do.

19. b. *Rationale:* When a patient has a nasogastric tube in place, antacid dosage may be titrated by aspirating stomach contents, determining pH, and then basing the dose on the pH. (Most gastric acid is neutralized and most pepsin activity is eliminated at a pH greater than 3.5.)

20. c. *Rationale:* Recommended doses of PPIs heal most gastric and duodenal ulcers in about 4 weeks. Large gastric ulcers may require 8 weeks.

Chapter 60: Laxatives and Cathartics

SECTION II: ASSESSING YOUR UNDERSTANDING

ACTIVITY A
FILL IN THE BLANKS
1. elimination
2. soft, formed
3. cathartic
4. Defecation
5. duodenocolic

ACTIVITY B
MATCHING
1. A   2. C   3. E   4. B   5. D

ACTIVITY C
SHORT ANSWERS
1. Defecation is normally stimulated by movements and reflexes in the gastrointestinal (GI) tract. When the stomach and duodenum are distended with food or fluids, gastrocolic and duodenocolic reflexes cause propulsive movements in the colon, which move feces into the rectum and arouse the urge to defecate. When sensory nerve fibers in the rectum are stimulated by the fecal mass, the defecation reflex causes strong peristalsis, deep breathing, closure of the glottis, contraction of abdominal muscles, contraction of the rectum, relaxation of anal sphincters, and expulsion of the fecal mass.

2. Constipation is the infrequent and painful expulsion of hard, dry stools. Although there is no "normal" number of stools because of variations in diet and other factors, most people report more than three bowel movements per week. Normal bowel elimination should produce a soft, formed stool without pain.

3. Cathartics and laxatives are used to relieve constipation in pregnant women, in elderly patients whose abdominal and perineal muscles have become weak and atrophied, in children with megacolon, and in patients who are receiving drugs that decrease intestinal motility (e.g., opioid analgesics, drugs with anticholinergic effects).

4. Cathartics and laxatives are used to prevent straining at stool in patients with coronary artery disease (e.g., post–myocardial infarction), hypertension, cerebrovascular disease, and hemorrhoids and other rectal conditions.

5. Cathartics and laxatives are used to prevent absorption of intestinal ammonia in patients with hepatic encephalopathy.

SECTION III: APPLYING YOUR KNOWLEDGE

ACTIVITY D
CASE STUDIES
1. Saline laxatives (e.g., magnesium citrate, milk of magnesia) are not well absorbed from the intestine. Consequently, they increase osmotic pressure in the intestinal lumen and cause water to be retained. Distention of the bowel leads to increased peristalsis and decreased intestinal transit time for the fecal mass. The resultant stool is semifluid.

2. Saline laxatives, including milk of magnesia, are used when rapid bowel evacuation is needed. With oral magnesium preparations, effects occur within 0.5 to 6 hours; with sodium phosphate–containing rectal enemas, effects occur within 15 minutes.

3. The patient is most likely experiencing a fluid and electrolyte imbalance. Saline laxatives are generally useful and safe for short-term treatment of constipation, for cleansing of the bowel before endoscopic examinations, and for treating fecal impaction. However, they are not safe for frequent or prolonged usage or for certain patients because they may produce fluid and electrolyte imbalances.

4. The patient must stay at home for the preparation, because the medication may cause rapid evacuation of the bowel. Polyethylene glycol–electrolyte solution (e.g., NuLYTELY) is a nonabsorbable oral solution that induces diarrhea within 30 to 60 minutes and rapidly evacuates the bowel, usually within 4 hours. It is a prescription drug used for bowel cleansing before GI examination (e.g., colonoscopy) and is contraindicated in patients with GI obstruction, gastric retention, colitis, or bowel perforation.

5. Polyethylene glycol solution (MiraLax) is an oral laxative that may be used to treat occasional constipation. Effects may require 2 to 4 days. It is a prescription drug and should not be taken for longer than 2 weeks.

SECTION IV: PRACTICING FOR NCLEX
1. a. *Rationale:* Lubiprostone (Amitiza) aids in treating chronic idiopathic constipation by increasing intestinal fluid secretion and thereby stimulating intestinal motility and defecation.

2. c. *Rationale:* Sorbitol is often given with sodium polystyrene sulfonate (Kayexalate) in the treatment of hyperkalemia to aid in the expulsion of the potassium–resin complex.

3. d. *Rationale:* Lactulose exerts an osmotic effect, pulling water into the colon and stimulating peristalsis. It is also useful in treating hepatic encephalopathy by decreasing the production of the waste product ammonia.

4. b. *Rationale:* Lubricant laxatives lubricate the fecal mass and slow colonic absorption of water from the fecal mass. These medications may interfere with the absorption of fat-soluble vitamins and, if aspirated, may result in a lipid aspiration pneumonia.

5. c. *Rationale:* Stimulant cathartics are the strongest and most abused laxative products. They irritate the GI mucosa, pull water into the colon, and stimulate peristalsis. They produce a watery stool and may lead to fluid, electrolyte, and acid–base imbalances

6. 4

7. a. *Rationale:* Saline laxatives increase the osmotic pressure in the intestinal lumen, resulting in the retention of water, which distends the bowel and stimulates peristalsis. They produce a semifluid stool and may lead to fluid and electrolyte imbalances.

8. c. *Rationale:* Surfactant laxatives decrease the surface tension of the fecal mass to allow water and fat to penetrate into the stool, making it softer and easier to expel. They have little true laxative effect.

9. d. *Rationale:* Bulk-forming laxatives add mass to the feces, stimulating peristalsis and defecation. They must be taken with water to avoid obstruction. In general, bulk-forming drugs are the most desirable laxative for long-term use.

10. a. *Rationale:* Laxatives and cathartics should not be used in the presence of undiagnosed abdominal pain or other signs of intestinal obstruction because of the risks of perforation and peritonitis.

11. a, b, and c. *Rationale:* Common reasons for abuse of laxatives and cathartics include eating disorders, desire for strict weight control, and the belief that a daily bowel movement is necessary for health.

12. Laxatives, cathartics

13. c. *Rationale:* Lifestyle modifications such as increased fluid and fiber intake and increased exercise are preferred to medications in the treatment of constipation.

14. Constipation

15. a. *Rationale:* Individuals with upper motor neuron injuries usually follow a bowel program that includes taking a daily stool softener such as docusate sodium and stimulating bowel movements at the desired time using digital stimulation and rectal suppositories such as bisacodyl or glycerin.

16. b. *Rationale:* Many patients with cancer require moderate to large amounts of opioid analgesics for pain control. The analgesics slow GI motility and cause constipation. These patients often need a bowel-management program that includes routine laxative administration.

17. once per week

18. a. *Rationale:* Constipation is responsible for 3% of visits to pediatric clinics and up to 30% of visits to pediatric gastroenterologists. As in adults, increasing fluids, high-fiber foods, and exercise is preferred when possible.

19. b. *Rationale:* Saline cathartics containing sodium salts are contraindicated in patients with edema or congestive heart failure, because enough sodium may be absorbed to cause further fluid retention and edema.

20. a, b, and d. *Rationale:* Oral use of mineral oil may cause potentially serious adverse effects (e.g., decreased absorption of fat-soluble vitamins and some drugs, lipid pneumonia if aspirated into the lungs).

Chapter 61: Antidiarrheals

SECTION II: ASSESSING YOUR UNDERSTANDING

ACTIVITY A
FILL IN THE BLANKS
1. Diarrhea
2. ground beef
3. hemolytic uremic
4. enterotoxigenic
5. *Campylobacter jejuni*

ACTIVITY B
MATCHING
1. C   2. D   3. E   4. B   5. A

ACTIVITY C
SHORT ANSWERS
1. *Salmonella* infections may occur when contaminated poultry and other meats, eggs, and dairy products are ingested. Elderly clients are especially susceptible to *Salmonella*-associated colitis.

2. Several strains of *Shigella* may produce diarrhea. Infection most often results from direct person-to-person contact, but it may also occur via food or water contamination. Hand washing is especially important in preventing the spread of *Shigella* from person to person.

3. Deficiency of pancreatic enzymes inhibits digestion and absorption of carbohydrates, proteins, and fats. Deficiency of lactase, which breaks down lactose to simple sugars (i.e., glucose and galactose) that can be absorbed by GI mucosa, inhibits digestion of milk and milk products. Lactase deficiency commonly occurs among people of African or Asian descent.

4. In inflammatory bowel disorders, such as gastroenteritis, diverticulitis, ulcerative colitis, and Crohn's disease, the inflamed mucous membrane secretes large amounts of fluids into the intestinal lumen, along with mucus, proteins, and blood, and absorption of water and electrolytes is impaired. In addition, when the ileum is diseased or a portion is surgically excised, large amounts of bile salts reach the colon, where they act as cathartics and cause diarrhea. Bile salts are normally reabsorbed from the ileum.

5. IBS is a functional disorder of intestinal motility with no evidence of inflammation or tissue changes. A change in bowel pattern (constipation, diarrhea, or a combination of both) accompanied by abdominal pain, bloating, and distention is the presenting symptom. The cause is unknown; however, activation of 5-HT3 (serotonin) receptors, which affect the regulation of visceral pain, colonic motility, and GI secretions, is thought to be involved in the pathophysiology of IBS.

SECTION III: APPLYING YOUR KNOWLEDGE

ACTIVITY D
CASE STUDIES
1. "Your physician belongs to a drug manufacturer prescribing program." To ensure safe and appropriate use of alosetron, the drug manufacturer has established a prescribing program, and only qualified health care providers enrolled in the program can prescribe this medication. Alosetron (Lotronex) is a selective 5-HT3 receptor antagonist that is indicated for treating women

with chronic severe diarrhea-predominant irritable bowel syndrome (IBS) that has not responded to conventional therapy.

2. The patient is likely to show signs of alosetron toxicity. Alosetron is extensively metabolized by the cytochrome P450 enzyme system (CYP2C9, CYP3A4, and CYP1A2) with multiple metabolites produced that are excreted primarily in the urine. Caution must be used with concurrent administration of CYP1A2 and CYP3A4 inhibitors. Concurrent administration with fluvoxamine is contraindicated. The physician will consult the psychiatrist and reduce the dose of the fluvoxamine. Alosetron should not be given to patients with a history of GI disorders, including chronic or severe constipation or sequelae of constipation, intestinal obstruction, stricture, toxic megacolon, GI perforation and/or adhesions, ischemic colitis, impaired intestinal circulation, thrombophlebitis or hypercoagulable state, Crohn's disease, ulcerative colitis, or diverticulitis.

3. Reduced dosages may be needed in some women older than 65 years of age to prevent drug accumulation and toxicity. Each patient must sign a patient–physician agreement indicting that she: understands the risks of taking alosetron and agrees to take the medication, will discontinue taking alosetron and immediately notify the physician if constipation or signs of ischemic colitis occur, and will stop taking alosetron and contact the physician after 4 weeks of therapy with alosetron if the symptoms of IBS are not controlled. The medication guide and patient–physician agreement are available at http://www.lotronex.com.

SECTION IV: PRACTICING FOR NCLEX

1. b. *Rationale:* In bacterial gastroenteritis or diarrhea, the choice of antibacterial drug depends on the causative organism and susceptibility tests.
2. a, b, and d. *Rationale:* Specific therapy for diarrhea is directed at the cause of the symptom and may include enzymatic replacement therapy, bile salt–binding drugs, antibacterial agents, and 5-HT3 receptor antagonists.
3. decreasing
4. d. *Rationale:* Bismuth subsalicylate has antisecretory, antimicrobial, and possibly anti-inflammatory effects. It is used in the control of travelers' diarrhea and relief of abdominal cramping.
5. b. *Rationale:* Octreotide, a synthetic form of somatostatin, decreases GI secretion and motility. It is used for diarrhea associated with carcinoid syndrome, intestinal tumors, or HIV/AIDS and diarrhea that does not respond to other antidiarrheal drugs.
6. opiates
7. Diarrhea
8. d. *Rationale:* With loperamide, monitor clients with hepatic impairment for signs of CNS toxicity. Loperamide normally undergoes extensive first-pass metabolism, which may be lessened by liver disease. As a result, a larger portion of the dose reaches the systemic circulation and may cause adverse effects.
9. a. *Rationale:* Diphenoxylate should be used with extreme caution in clients with severe hepatorenal disease because hepatic coma may be precipitated.
10. a. *Rationale:* Diphenoxylate contains atropine, and signs of atropine overdose may occur with usual doses. Diphenoxylate is contraindicated in children younger than 2 years of age.
11. pancreatic enzymes
12. b. *Rationale:* The following oral drugs and dosages are approximately equivalent in antidiarrheal effectiveness:

4 mg morphine, 30 mg codeine, 10 mL paregoric, 5 mg diphenoxylate, and 2 mg loperamide.
13. b. *Rationale:* In antibiotic-associated colitis, stopping the causative drug is the initial treatment.
14. c. *Rationale:* In antibiotic-associated colitis, stopping the causative drug is the initial treatment. If symptoms do not improve within 3 or 4 days, oral metronidazole or vancomycin is given for 7 to 10 days.
15. d. *Rationale:* In ulcerative colitis, sulfonamides, adrenal corticosteroids, and other anti-inflammatory agents such as balsalazide (Colazal), mesalamine (Pentasa), and olsalazine (Dipentum) are the drugs of choice.
16. a and d. *Rationale:* For symptomatic treatment of diarrhea, diphenoxylate with atropine (Lomotil) or loperamide (Imodium) is probably the drug of choice for most people.
17. duration
18. a. *Rationale:* In most cases of acute, nonspecific diarrhea in adults, fluid losses are not severe and clients need only simple replacement of fluids and electrolytes lost in the stool. Acceptable replacement fluids during the first 24 hours include 2 to 3 liters of clear liquids (e.g., flat ginger ale, decaffeinated cola drinks or tea, broth, gelatin).
19. a, b, and d. *Rationale:* Contraindications to the use of antidiarrheal drugs include diarrhea caused by toxic materials, microorganisms that penetrate intestinal mucosa (e.g., pathogenic *E. coli, Salmonella, Shigella*), and antibiotic-associated colitis.
20. Nitazoxanide (Alinia)

Chapter 62: Antiemetics

SECTION II: ASSESSING YOUR UNDERSTANDING

ACTIVITY A
FILL IN THE BLANKS
1. Antiemetic
2. Nausea
3. Vomiting
4. adverse effects
5. vomiting center

ACTIVITY B
MATCHING
1. B   2. D   3. C   4. A   5. E

ACTIVITY C
SHORT ANSWERS
1. Nausea and vomiting are the most common adverse effects of drug therapy. Although the symptoms may occur with most drugs, they are especially associated with alcohol, aspirin, digoxin, anticancer drugs, antimicrobials, estrogen preparations, and opioid analgesics.
2. Nausea and vomiting may be caused by pain and other noxious stimuli, such as unpleasant sights and odors; emotional disturbances; physical or mental stress; radiation therapy; motion sickness; postoperative status, which may include pain; impaired GI motility; and pregnancy.
3. The vomiting center, CTZ, and GI tract contain benzodiazepine, cholinergic, dopamine, histamine, opiate, substance P/neurokinin, and serotonin receptors, which are stimulated by emetogenic drugs and toxins.
4. When stimulated, the vomiting center initiates efferent impulses that stimulate the salivary center, causing closure of the glottis; contraction of abdominal muscles and the diaphragm; relaxation of the gastroesophageal sphincter; and reverse peristalsis, which moves stomach contents toward the mouth for ejection.

5. Anticipatory nausea is triggered by memories, and fear of nausea and vomiting is mediated by afferent signals from the higher centers of the cerebral cortex to the vomiting center.

SECTION III: APPLYING YOUR KNOWLEDGE

ACTIVITY D
CASE STUDIES

1. Metoclopramide (Reglan) is a prokinetic agent that increases GI motility and the rate of gastric emptying by increasing the release of acetylcholine from nerve endings in the GI tract (peripheral cholinergic effects). Historically, metoclopramide has been used intravenously during chemotherapy with cisplatin (Platinol) and other antineoplastic drugs to treat acute nausea and vomiting; however, 5-HT3 receptor antagonists are now the preferred antiemetic for this indication.

2. With oral administration of metoclopramide, action begins in 30 to 60 minutes and peaks in 60 to 90 minutes. With intramuscular (IM) use, action onset occurs in 10 to 15 minutes and peaks in 60 to 90 minutes. With IV use, action onset occurs in 1 to 3 minutes and peaks in 60 to 90 minutes.

3. The sedation that the drug causes may affect her ability to return to work. Other adverse effects include restlessness and extrapyramidal reactions (e.g., akathisia, dystonia, symptoms of Parkinson's disease). Metoclopramide may increase the effects of alcohol and cyclosporine (by increasing their absorption) and decrease the effects of cimetidine and digoxin (by accelerating passage through the GI tract and decreasing time for absorption).

4. The physician will likely discontinue the metoclopramide. Metoclopramide is relatively contraindicated in Parkinson's disease, because it further depletes dopamine and reduces the effectiveness of levodopa, a major antiparkinson drug.

SECTION IV: PRACTICING FOR NCLEX

1. a. *Rationale:* Scopolamine is an anticholinergic drug that is effective in relieving nausea and vomiting associated with motion sickness and radiation therapy for cancer.

2. d. *Rationale:* Dronabinol is a cannabinoid used in the management of nausea and vomiting associated with chemotherapy unrelieved by other antiemetic drugs. It is a Schedule III drug under federal narcotic laws.

3. b. *Rationale:* Substance P, a peptide neurotransmitter in the neurokinin family, plays a role in acute and delayed chemotherapy-induced nausea and vomiting. A precipitant antagonizes the neurokinin 1 receptor, preventing activation by emetogenic chemotherapeutic drugs.

4. c. *Rationale:* 5-HT3 serotonin receptor antagonists such as ondansetron, granisetron, dolasetron, and Palonosetron antagonize serotonin receptors, preventing their activation by emetogenic drugs and toxins. They are used to prevent and treat moderate to severe nausea associated with cancer chemotherapy, radiation therapy, and postoperative status.

5. a. *Rationale:* Prokinetic agents such as metoclopramide increase the release of acetylcholine from nerve endings in the GI tract, thereby increasing GI motility and gastric emptying. Metoclopramide also antagonizes dopamine in the brain. It is prescribed to treat nausea and vomiting associated with gastroparesis and other nonobstructive disorders characterized by gastric retention of food and fluids, and in the treatment of esophageal reflux. It is also useful in prevention of delayed nausea and vomiting associated with chemotherapy.

6. a, b, and d. *Rationale:* Benzodiazepines such as lorazepam produce relaxation, relieve anxiety, and inhibit cerebral cortex input to the vomiting center. They are prescribed for anticipatory nausea associated with cancer chemotherapy.

7. b. *Rationale:* The antiemetic mechanism of action of corticosteroids such as dexamethasone and methylprednisolone is unknown. These drugs are commonly used alone or in combination with 5-HT3 serotonin receptor antagonists and/or substance P/neurokinin 1 receptor antagonists in the management of chemotherapy-induced emesis and postoperative nausea and vomiting.

8. before

9. a, b, and c. *Rationale:* Antiemetics are usually given orally or by rectal suppository in the home setting. The home care nurse may need to assess patients for possible causes of nausea and vomiting and assist patients and caregivers with appropriate use of the drugs and other interventions to prevent fluid and electrolyte depletion. Teaching safety precautions with sedating drugs may also be needed.

10. a. *Rationale:* Phenothiazines are metabolized in the liver and eliminated in urine. In the presence of liver disease (e.g., cirrhosis, hepatitis), metabolism may be slowed and drug elimination half-lives prolonged, with resultant accumulation and increased risk of adverse effects. Therefore, the drugs should be used cautiously in patients with hepatic impairment. Cholestatic jaundice has been reported with promethazine.

11. a. *Rationale:* Most antiemetic drugs are metabolized in the liver and should be used cautiously in patients with impaired hepatic function. With oral ondansetron, do not exceed an 8-mg dose; with IV use, a single, maximal daily dose of 8 mg is recommended.

12. b. *Rationale:* Metoclopramide dosage should be reduced in patients with severe renal impairment to decrease drowsiness and extrapyramidal effects.

13. b. *Rationale:* Most antiemetic drugs cause drowsiness, especially in older adults, and therefore should be used cautiously. Efforts should be made to prevent nausea and vomiting when possible. Older adults are at risk of fluid volume depletion and electrolyte imbalances with vomiting.

14. d. *Rationale:* The American Society of Clinical Oncology recommends the use of a 5-HT3 receptor antagonist plus a corticosteroid before administration of high-dose chemotherapy or chemotherapy with high to moderate emetic risk to pediatric oncology patients.

15. c. *Rationale:* A black box warning alerts nurses that promethazine is contraindicated in children younger than 2 years of age because of the risk of potentially fatal respiratory depression. When using promethazine, the lowest effective dosage should be used, and other drugs with respiratory depressant effects should not be given concurrently. Excessive doses may cause hallucinations, convulsions, and sudden death.

16. 5-HT3 receptor antagonists

17. a, b, and c. *Rationale:* If nausea and vomiting are likely to occur because of travel, administration of emetogenic anticancer drugs, diagnostic tests, or therapeutic procedures, an antiemetic drug should be given before the emetogenic event. Pretreatment usually increases patient comfort and allows use of lower drug doses. It also may prevent aspiration and other potentially serious complications of vomiting.

18. c. *Rationale:* Metoclopramide (Reglan) may be preferred when nausea and vomiting are associated with nonobstructive gastric retention.
19. d. *Rationale:* Antihistamines such as meclizine and dimenhydrinate are useful for vomiting caused by labyrinthitis, uremia, or postoperative status.
20. antihistaminic

Chapter 63: Drugs Used in Ophthalmic Conditions

SECTION II: ASSESSING YOUR UNDERSTANDING

ACTIVITY A
FILL IN THE BLANKS
1. myopia
2. hyperopia
3. presbyopia
4. retina
5. diagnosis

ACTIVITY B
MATCHING
1. A   2. C   3. E   4. B   5. D

ACTIVITY C
SHORT ANSWERS
1. The eyelids and lacrimal system function to protect the eye. The eyelid is a barrier to the entry of foreign bodies, strong light, dust, and other potential irritants. The conjunctiva is the mucous membrane lining of the eyelids. The canthi (singular, *canthus*) are the angles where the upper and lower eyelids meet. The lacrimal system produces a fluid that constantly moistens and cleanses the anterior surface of the eyeball. The fluid drains through two small openings in the inner canthus and flows through the nasolacrimal duct into the nasal cavity. When the conjunctiva is irritated or certain emotions are experienced (e.g., sadness), the lacrimal gland produces more fluid than the drainage system can accommodate. The excess fluid overflows the eyelids and becomes tears.
2. Pupil constriction is called miosis; dilation is called mydriasis.
3. The eyeball is a spherical structure composed of the sclera, cornea, choroid, and retina, plus special refractive tissues. The sclera is a white, opaque, fibrous tissue that covers the posterior five sixths of the eyeball. The cornea is a transparent, special connective tissue that covers the anterior sixth of the eyeball. The cornea contains no blood vessels. The choroid, composed of blood vessels and connective tissue, continues forward to form the iris. The iris is composed of pigmented cells, the opening called the pupil, and muscles that control the size of the pupil by contracting or dilating in response to stimuli.
4. For vision to occur, light rays must enter the eye through the cornea; travel through the pupil, lens, and vitreous body; and be focused on the retina.
5. Light rays do not travel directly to the retina. Instead, they are deflected in various directions according to the density of the ocular structures through which they pass. This process, called *refraction*, is controlled by the aqueous humor, lens, and vitreous body.

SECTION III: APPLYING YOUR KNOWLEDGE

ACTIVITY D
CASE STUDIES
1. Diagnosis of glaucoma is based on the results of a number of tests. Tests for glaucoma include ophthalmoscopic examination of the optic disk, measurement of intraocular pressure (IOP; tonometry), and testing of visual fields. Glaucoma is often characterized by increased IOP (>22 mm Hg) but may also occur with normal IOP (<21 mm Hg); the average IOP is 15 to 16 mm Hg.
2. Mrs. Lincoln has most common type of glaucoma, primary open-angle glaucoma. Its cause is unknown, but contributing factors include advanced age, a family history of glaucoma and elevated IOP, diabetes mellitus, hypertension, myopia, long-term use of corticosteroid drugs, and previous eye injury, inflammation, or infection. Her hypertension put her at risk for this condition. In addition, the incidence of glaucoma in African Americans is about three times higher than in non–African Americans. Glaucoma is one of the leading causes of blindness in the United States and the most common cause of blindness in African Americans.
3. Glaucoma is a group of diseases characterized by optic nerve damage and changes in visual fields.
4. These are signs of closed-angle glaucoma, which is usually an acute situation requiring emergency surgery. It may occur when pupils are dilated and the outflow of aqueous humor is blocked. Darkness and drugs with anticholinergic effects (e.g., atropine, antihistamines, tricyclic antidepressants) may dilate the pupil, reduce outflow of aqueous humor, and precipitate acute glaucoma.

SECTION IV: PRACTICING FOR NCLEX
1. b. *Rationale:* Local eye medications may cause systemic effects; systemic drugs may affect eye function.
2. b. *Rationale:* Eye medications should be kept sterile, to avoid infection.
3. d. *Rationale:* Therapeutic effects of eye drops depend on accurate administration.
4. a, b, and c. *Rationale:* Drug therapy of eye disorders is unique because of the location, structure, and function of the eye.
5. a, b, and c. *Rationale:* The home care nurse may be involved in the care of patients with acute or chronic eye disorders. As with other drug therapies, the nurse may need to teach patients and caregivers reasons for use, accurate administration, and assessment of therapeutic and adverse responses to eye medications.
6. c. *Rationale:* Accurate dosage and occlusion of the nasolacrimal duct in the inner canthus of the eye are needed to prevent adverse drug effects such as hypertension, tachycardia, or dysrhythmias with adrenergic drugs and bradycardia, heart block, or bronchoconstriction with beta blockers.
7. paralyze
8. b. *Rationale:* When treating children, the short-acting mydriatics and cycloplegics (e.g., cyclopentolate, tropicamide) are preferred because they cause fewer systemic adverse effects than atropine or scopolamine.
9. b. *Rationale:* For chronic glaucoma, the goal of drug therapy is to slow disease progression by reducing IOP. Topical beta blockers are first-line drugs and are commonly used.
10. c. *Rationale:* Patients who wear contact lenses are at higher risk of developing abrasions that become infected and ulcerate. For these patients, an antipseudomonal antibiotic (such as gentamicin or a fluoroquinolone) should be used. In addition, the patient should avoid wearing contact lenses until the abrasion is healed and antibiotic therapy is completed.
11. 24 to 72
12. b. *Rationale:* Natamycin (Natacyn) is the drug of choice in fungal eye infections. It has a broad spectrum of antifungal activity and is nonirritating and nontoxic.

13. b. *Rationale:* In severe infections, antibacterial drugs may be given both topically and systemically. Because systemic antibiotics penetrate the eye poorly, large doses are required to attain therapeutic drug concentrations in ocular structures. Drugs that reach therapeutic levels in the eye when given in proper dosage include ampicillin and dicloxacillin.

14. a. *Rationale:* Gentamicin and other antibiotics penetrate the eye when inflammation is present.

15. d. *Rationale:* Drug therapy is usually initiated as soon as culture material (eye secretions) has been obtained and often includes a broad-spectrum antibacterial agent or a combination of two or more antibiotics.

16. a. *Rationale:* Some eye drops contain benzalkonium hydrochloride, a preservative, which is absorbed by soft contact lenses. The medications should not be applied while wearing soft contacts; they should be instilled 15 minutes or longer before soft contacts are inserted.

17. color coded

18. a, b, and c. *Rationale:* Topical ophthalmic medications should not be used after the expiration date; cloudy, discolored solutions should be discarded.

19. a. *Rationale:* Ointments are administered less frequently than drops and often produce higher concentrations of drug in target tissues.

20. hyperemia

Chapter 64: Drugs Used in Dermatologic Conditions

SECTION II: ASSESSING YOUR UNDERSTANDING

ACTIVITY A
FILL IN THE BLANKS
1. environments
2. basal
3. stratum corneum
4. Keratin
5. Melanocytes

ACTIVITY B
MATCHING
1. C   2. A   3. E   4. B   5. D

ACTIVITY C
SHORT ANSWERS
1. Melanocytes are pigment-producing cells located at the junction of the epidermis and the dermis. These cells produce yellow, brown, or black skin coloring in response to genetic influences, melanocyte-stimulating hormone released from the anterior pituitary gland, and exposure to ultraviolet (UV) light (e.g., sunlight).
2. The dermis is composed of elastic and fibrous connective tissue. Dermal structures include blood vessels, lymphatic channels, nerves and nerve endings, sweat glands, sebaceous glands, and hair follicles. The dermis is supported underneath by subcutaneous tissue, which is composed primarily of fat cells.
3. Mucous membranes are composed of a surface layer of epithelial cells, a basement membrane, and a layer of connective tissue. They line body cavities that communicate with the external environment (e.g., mouth, vagina, anus). Mucous membranes receive an abundant blood supply because capillaries lie just beneath the epithelial cells.
4. Dermatologic disorders may be primary (i.e., originating in the skin or mucous membranes) or secondary (i.e., resulting from a systemic condition, such as measles or adverse drug reactions).

5. The skin assists in regulating body temperature through production and elimination of sweat.

SECTION III: APPLYING YOUR KNOWLEDGE

ACTIVITY D
CASE STUDIES
1. "No, the treatment is for a secondary infection on your forearm." Scratching damages the skin and increases the risk of secondary infection, which may be treated by the use of an oral antibiotic.
2. Dermatitis, also called eczema, is not a contagious disease. It is caused by an inflammatory response of the skin to injuries from irritants, allergens, or trauma.
3. Atopic dermatitis is a common disorder characterized by dry skin, pruritus, and lesions that vary according to the extent of inflammation, stages of healing, and scratching. Acute lesions are reddened skin areas containing papules and vesicles; chronic lesions are often thick, fibrotic, and nodular. The cause of atopic dermatitis is uncertain but may involve allergic, hereditary, or psychological elements. Approximately 50% to 80% of patients have asthma or allergic rhinitis; some have a family history of these disorders.
4. Significant stress associated with her profession could be an exacerbating factor in Mrs. Benjamin's condition. Other exacerbating factors are allergens, irritating chemicals, and certain foods, and these should be avoided if possible.
5. Mrs. Benjamin should bring her child to the pediatrician for an assessment. The development of atopic dermatitis may have a hereditary component, so, if she has it, it may be that her child has it too. Furthermore, although atopic dermatitis may occur in all age groups, it is more common in children.

SECTION IV: PRACTICING FOR NCLEX

1. c. *Rationale:* Systemic adverse effects may occur with topical drug therapy; skin disorders may occur with systemic drugs.
2. d. *Rationale:* Special precautions are needed for safe use of oral retinoids in female patients of childbearing potential.
3. c. *Rationale:* Special precautions are needed for safe use of topical corticosteroids, especially in children.
4. a. *Rationale:* Topical drugs are used to treat most skin disorders; accurate application is essential to maximize therapeutic effects.
5. a and c. *Rationale:* Careful assessment of types and locations of lesions can aid diagnosis and treatment of many skin disorders.
6. a and d. *Rationale:* Staphylococci and streptococci are the most common bacterial causes of skin infection, and methicillin-resistant *S. aureus* (MRSA) infections are increasing.
7. a, b, and d. *Rationale:* Skin disorders are commonly treated at home by patients or caregivers. When a home care nurse is involved, responsibilities may include assessing patients, other members of the household, and the home environment for risks of skin disorders; teaching preventive or treatment measures; assisting with treatment; and assessing response to treatment.
8. b. *Rationale:* Older adults often have thin, dry skin and are at risk of pressure ulcers if mobility, nutrition, or elimination is impaired. Principles of topical drug therapy are generally the same as for younger adults. In addition, topical corticosteroids should be used with caution on thinned or atrophic skin.

9. b. *Rationale:* With topical agents, cautious use is recommended. Infants, and perhaps older children, have more permeable skin and are more likely than adults to absorb topical drugs.

10. b and c. *Rationale:* With topical corticosteroids, which are often used to treat atopic dermatitis, suppression of the HPA axis, Cushing's disease, and intracranial hypertension have been reported in children.

11. d. *Rationale:* Because children are at high risk for development of systemic adverse effects with topical corticosteroids, these drugs should be used only if clearly indicated, in the smallest effective dose, for the shortest effective time, and usually without occlusive dressings.

12. c. *Rationale:* With chronic urticaria, the goal of treatment is symptom relief. Antihistamines are most effective when given before histamine-induced urticaria occurs and should be given around the clock, not just when lesions appear.

13. Acitretin

14. d. *Rationale:* Methotrexate is an antineoplastic drug that has long been used to treat psoriasis because it suppresses inflammation and proliferation of T lymphocytes.

15. a. *Rationale:* Sedating, systemic antihistamines such as diphenhydramine or hydroxyzine are often used to relieve itching related to dermatitis and promote rest and sleep.

16. b. *Rationale:* Oral antiandrogens may be given to female patients with high blood levels of androgens (e.g., testosterone). Combination oral contraceptive pills decrease the amount of free testosterone circulating in the bloodstream and therefore may improve acne. Norgestimate/ethinyl estradiol (Ortho Tri-Cyclen) and norethindrone acetate/ethinyl estradiol (Estrostep) are FDA-approved for treatment of acne.

17. d. *Rationale:* Retinoids, in both systemic and topical forms, may be used for moderate to severe acne. All topical retinoids (tretinoin, adapalene, tazarotene) reduce acne lesions, usually within 12 weeks.

18. Oral antimicrobials

19. d. *Rationale:* Combination products of topical clindamycin or erythromycin and benzoyl peroxide are more effective than antibiotics alone.

20. b, c, and d. *Rationale:* When treating skin conditions, dosage depends on the drug concentration, the area of application, and the method of application.

Chapter 65: Drug Use During Pregnancy and Lactation

SECTION II: ASSESSING YOUR UNDERSTANDING

ACTIVITY A
FILL IN THE BLANKS
1. fetotoxic
2. Organogenesis
3. arterial blood pressure
4. tocolytics
5. third week

ACTIVITY B
MATCHING
1. B   2. D   3. A   4. E   5. C

ACTIVITY C
SHORT ANSWERS
1. During pregnancy, mother and fetus undergo physiologic changes that influence drug effects. In pregnant women, physiologic changes alter drug pharmacokinetics In general, drug effects are less predictable because plasma volume expansion decreases plasma drug concentrations, and increased metabolism by the liver and increased elimination by the kidneys shorten the duration of drug actions and effects.

2. After drugs enter the fetal circulation, relatively large amounts are pharmacologically active, because the fetus has low levels of serum albumin and therefore low levels of drug binding. Most drug molecules are transported to the liver, where they are metabolized. Metabolism occurs slowly, because the fetal liver is immature in quantity and quality of drug-metabolizing enzymes. Drugs metabolized by the fetal liver are excreted by fetal kidneys into amniotic fluid. Excretion also is slow and inefficient due to immature development of fetal kidneys.

3. Drugs enter the brain easily because the blood–brain barrier is poorly developed in the fetus.

4. Approximately half of the drug-containing blood is transported through the umbilical arteries to the placenta, where it re-enters the maternal circulation. Thus, the mother can metabolize and excrete some drug molecules for the fetus.

5. The fetus is sensitive to drug effects because it is small, has few plasma proteins that can bind drug molecules, and has a weak capacity for metabolizing and excreting drugs. In addition, the fetus is exposed to any drugs circulating in maternal blood. When drugs are taken on a regular schedule, fetal blood usually contains 50% to 100% of the amount in maternal blood. This means that any drug that stimulates or depresses the central nervous, cardiovascular, respiratory, or other body system in the mother has the potential to stimulate or depress those systems in the fetus. In some cases, fetotoxicity occurs.

SECTION III: APPLYING YOUR KNOWLEDGE

ACTIVITY D
CASE STUDIES
1. The physician will likely prescribe a folic acid supplement. Folic acid deficiency anemia is a type of anemia associated with pregnancy. The recommended daily intake of folic acid doubles during pregnancy, from 400 to 800 mcg, and a folic acid supplement is often prescribed.

2. For many years, it was considered "best practice" to routinely prescribe daily iron supplements for pregnant women, to prevent or treat iron deficiency anemia. More recently, studies indicate that use of the supplements in women who are not anemic may lead to excessive levels of hemoglobin, iron overload, and hypertension in the mother and premature birth or low birth weight (for gestational age) in the infant.

3. Antacids may be used, if necessary, for the treatment of GERD during pregnancy, because little systemic absorption occurs; the drugs are unlikely to harm the fetus if used in recommended doses. A histamine$_2$ (H$_2$) receptor antagonist such as ranitidine (Zantac) may also be used. Proton pump inhibitors such as esomeprazole (Nexium) are thought to be safe, but some clinicians reserve them for patients for whom H$_2$ blockers are ineffective. Nonpharmacologic interventions include eating small meals; not eating for 2 to 3 hours before bedtime; avoiding caffeine, gas-producing foods, and constipation; and sitting in an upright position. For patients who do not obtain adequate relief with these measures, drug therapy may be needed.

4. The patient should use a bulk-producing agent instead of mineral oil. Mineral oil should be avoided, because it interferes with absorption of fat-soluble vitamins. Reduced absorption of vitamin K can lead to bleeding in newborns.

SECTION IV: PRACTICING FOR NCLEX

1. b. *Rationale:* Some drugs should be avoided during lactation; all drugs should be used cautiously.

2. d. *Rationale:* Drugs should be avoided during pregnancy when possible and used cautiously when required.

3. a. *Rationale:* A folic acid supplement is recommended for women who may become pregnant and during pregnancy, to prevent neural tube defects.

4. a. *Rationale:* Fetal organs are formed during the first trimester of pregnancy, possibly before a woman knows she is pregnant. The fetus' brain continues to develop throughout pregnancy and after birth.

5. teratogenicity

6. b. *Rationale:* Many obstetric patients with conditions such as preterm labor, hyperemesis, and elevated blood pressure are managed in the home. The home care nurse who assists in managing these patients should be an obstetric specialist who is knowledgeable about normal pregnancy and potential complications.

7. a. *Rationale:* The American Academy of Pediatrics (AAP) supports breastfeeding as optimal nutrition for infants during the first year of life and does not recommend stopping maternal drug therapy unless necessary. In some instances, mothers may pump and discard breast milk while receiving therapeutic drugs, to maintain lactation.

8. c. *Rationale:* Women with HIV infection should not breastfeed. The virus can be transmitted to the nursing infant.

9. a. *Rationale:* Counsel pregnant women about the use of immunizations during pregnancy. Live-virus vaccines (e.g., measles, mumps, and rubella) should be avoided because of possible harmful effects to the fetus.

10. d. *Rationale:* Regardless of the designated pregnancy risk category or presumed safety, no drug should be used during pregnancy unless it is clearly needed and the potential benefit to the mother outweighs the risk of potential harm to the fetus. The physician should be consulted.

11. c. *Rationale:* When a health care provider is assessing the neonate, drugs received by the mother during pregnancy, labor and delivery, and lactation must be considered.

12. d. *Rationale:* Hemorrhagic disease of the newborn occurs because the intestinal tract lacks the bacteria that normally synthesize vitamin K and there is little if any dietary intake of vitamin K. Vitamin K is required for liver production of several clotting factors, including prothrombin. Therefore, the neonate is at increased risk of bleeding during the first week of life. One dose of phytonadione 0.5 to 1 mg is injected at delivery or on admission to the nursery.

13. proteins

14. b. *Rationale:* Ophthalmia neonatorum is a form of bacterial conjunctivitis that can cause ulceration and blindness. It may be caused by several bacteria, most commonly *Chlamydia trachomatis*, a sexually transmitted organism.

15. a. *Rationale:* With regional anesthesia, the mother is usually conscious and comfortable, and the neonate is rarely depressed.

16. b. *Rationale:* After a cesarean section, a long-acting form of morphine (e.g., Duramorph) may be injected into the epidural catheter to provide analgesia for up to 24 hours. Possible adverse effects include maternal urinary retention, but no significant effects on the fetus have been noted.

17. d. *Rationale:* Parenteral opioid analgesics (e.g., IV or IM meperidine, morphine, or fentanyl) are commonly used to control pain during labor and delivery. They may prolong labor and cause sedation and respiratory depression in the mother and neonate. Meperidine may cause less neonatal depression than other opioid analgesics. Butorphanol is also widely used. If neonatal respiratory depression occurs, it can be reversed by naloxone (Narcan).

18. b. *Rationale:* After delivery, pitocin is the drug of choice for prevention or control of postpartum uterine bleeding. The drug reduces uterine bleeding by contracting uterine muscle. It also plays a role in letdown of breast milk to the nipples during lactation.

19. actin–myosin

20. a. *Rationale:* Magnesium sulfate has long been given IV as a first-line agent. However, studies indicate that the drug is ineffective as a tocolytic, and some clinicians recommend stopping usage for this purpose. In addition, the drug if used, it requires special precautions for administration and monitoring due to potentially severe adverse effects. Safety measures include a unit protocol that standardizes drug concentration, flow rate, type of infusion pump, and frequency and type of assessment data to be documented (e.g., serum magnesium levels, respiratory status, reflexes, uterine activity, urine output). The antidote, calcium gluconate, should be readily available for use if hypermagnesemia occurs.